Cervical Trauma

Surgical Management

Robert F. Heary, MD
Director
Spine Center of New Jersey
Professor of Neurological Surgery
Rutgers, The State University of New Jersey
Newark, New Jersey

102 illustrations

Thieme
New York • Stuttgart • Delhi • Rio de Janeiro

Executive Editor: Timothy Y. Hiscock
Managing Editor: Sarah Landis
Director, Editorial Services: Mary Jo Casey
Production Editor: Sean Woznicki
International Production Director: Andreas Schabert
Editorial Director: Sue Hodgson
International Marketing Director: Fiona Henderson
International Sales Director: Louisa Turrell
Director of Institutional Sales: Adam Bernacki
Senior Vice President and Chief Operating Officer: Sarah Vanderbilt
President: Brian D. Scanlan

Library of Congress Cataloging-in-Publication Data

Names: Heary, Robert F., editor.
Title: Cervical trauma : surgical management / [edited by]
    Robert F. Heary.
Description: New York : Thieme, [2019] | Includes bibliographical
    references.
Identifiers: LCCN 2019010291| ISBN 9781626238534 (hardback) |
    ISBN 9781626238541 (eISBN)
Subjects: | MESH: Cervical Vertebrae–surgery | Spinal Injuries–
    surgery
Classification: LCC RD594.3 | NLM WE 725 | DDC 617.4/82044—dc23
    LC record available at https://lccn.loc.gov/2019010291.

© 2019 Thieme Medical Publishers, Inc.

Thieme Publishers New York
333 Seventh Avenue, New York, NY 10001 USA
+1 800 782 3488, customerservice@thieme.com

Thieme Publishers Stuttgart
Rüdigerstrasse 14, 70469 Stuttgart, Germany
+49 [0]711 8931 421, customerservice@thieme.de

Thieme Publishers Delhi
A-12, Second Floor, Sector-2, Noida-201301
Uttar Pradesh, India
+91 120 45 566 00, customerservice@thieme.in

Thieme Publishers Rio de Janeiro, Thieme Publicações Ltda.
Edifício Rodolpho de Paoli, 25º andar
Av. Nilo Peçanha, 50 – Sala 2508,
Rio de Janeiro 20020-906 Brasil
+55 21 3172-2297 | +55 21 3172-1896
www.thiemerevinter.com.br

Cover design: Thieme Publishing Group
Typesetting by DiTech Process Solutions

Printed in the United States of America   5 4 3 2 1
by King Printing Co., Inc.

ISBN 978-1-62623-853-4

Also available as an e-book:
eISBN 978-1-62623-854-1

Important note: Medicine is an ever-changing science undergoing continual development. Research and clinical experience are continually expanding our knowledge, in particular our knowledge of proper treatment and drug therapy. Insofar as this book mentions any dosage or application, readers may rest assured that the authors, editors, and publishers have made every effort to ensure that such references are in accordance with **the state of knowledge at the time of production of the book.**

Nevertheless, this does not involve, imply, or express any guarantee or responsibility on the part of the publishers in respect to any dosage instructions and forms of applications stated in the book. **Every user is requested to examine carefully** the manufacturers' leaflets accompanying each drug and to check, if necessary in consultation with a physician or specialist, whether the dosage schedules mentioned therein or the contraindications stated by the manufacturers differ from the statements made in the present book. Such examination is particularly important with drugs that are either rarely used or have been newly released on the market. Every dosage schedule or every form of application used is entirely at the user's own risk and responsibility. The authors and publishers request every user to report to the publishers any discrepancies or inaccuracies noticed. If errors in this work are found after publication, errata will be posted at www.thieme.com on the product description page.

Some of the product names, patents, and registered designs referred to in this book are in fact registered trademarks or proprietary names even though specific reference to this fact is not always made in the text. Therefore, the appearance of a name without designation as proprietary is not to be construed as a representation by the publisher that it is in the public domain.

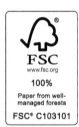

FSC
www.fsc.org
100%
Paper from well-managed forests
FSC® C103101

Contents

Foreword

Robert Heary, in teaming with Thieme, has amassed an amazing collection of treatises on the subject of cervical spine trauma and its surgical management. The book is beautifully constructed and illustrated; the information transmitted is valuable, voluminous, and impeccably portrayed. Content flows seamlessly from one chapter to the next, and the text reads like a single-authored book even though chapters are written by a number of distinguished contributors. The topics comprehensively cover the field of cervical spine trauma, and there seems to be no stone left unturned.

Most books of this type simply fill bookshelves and become out of date within several years of publication. This will not be so for Heary's *Cervical Trauma: Surgical Management.* I seriously doubt that any competition for this book will be forthcoming for at least a decade. This is a testament to its meticulous preparation and attention to detail.

I would be doing the book an injustice by summarizing each chapter. Such would keep you, the reader, from delving into its content. As an aside, such delving is facilitated by the orderly structure of the book and the manner in which it is presented.

I have nothing but accolades for Dr. Heary and his very accomplished authors. Please read and enjoy. Place back on the shelf and use as a reference. Repeat often. This book is a true gem.

Edward C. Benzel, MD
Emeritus Chairman of Neurosurgery
Neurological Institute
Cleveland Clinic
Cleveland, Ohio

Preface

It is a great pleasure to present *Cervical Trauma: Surgical Management* to the spine surgical community. There is a plentiful variety of conditions which require intervention related to trauma involving the cervical spine. This book covers a variety of traumatic injuries and details their management in a comprehensive fashion. While the principle focus of this work is on the surgical management of these injuries, non-operative care is also covered as there are situations where this is the ideal treatment.

An exceptional collection of experts from both the neurosurgical and the orthopaedic spine surgical communities have offered their wealth of experience to provide the depth of knowledge which is required to improve the understanding of cervical spine trauma. Basic understanding of cervical trauma requires thorough knowledge of the anatomy and physiology of the cervical spine. In addition, cervical trauma includes spinal cord injuries, nerve root dysfunction, and painful disorders related to spinal instability which occur with regularity.

The management of spinal cord injuries in the cervical region has been well studied over the past forty years. Developing classification systems and management protocols has enabled spine surgeons to work together with our colleagues in the trauma surgery and critical care communities to provide optimal management to improve long-term outcomes.

Outstanding descriptions of upper cervical spine injuries and their treatments, particularly when the occipitocervical region is involved, include understanding of when surgical treatment is preferable versus the use of non-operative interventions. When surgery is utilized, those various techniques have been covered throughout the earlier chapters of this book. In situations where non-operative management is preferred, the spine surgeon needs to have a complete understanding of the risks and benefits of each of the methods employed. These considerations are examined in great detail in this book as well.

Subaxial injuries involving the third through seventh cervical vertebrae are common and can have devastating effects on long-term outcomes for the victims of these injuries. The various management schema for adults and pediatric patients are covered exhaustively. Beyond just the routine surgical treatments, the specific surgical methods are provided by each of our expert authors with attention to different issues that may arise.

While blunt injuries are far more common, penetrating injuries have specific issues which require expertise to optimize results. Both blunt and penetrating injuries can impact vascular structures, and the care for these types of specific injuries, such as to the vertebral arteries, has been detailed in this book.

Patients with traumatic cervical spine injuries may have had pre-existing conditions which impact their optimal care. Separate chapters are dedicated to providing pearls to assist the spine surgeon in handling situations where the cervical spine was already impaired prior to the traumatic event.

When surgical treatment is indicated, the various methods including minimally invasive surgeries, neurointerventional treatments, and reconstructive therapies utilizing bone grafts or alternative stabilization methods are detailed. Following treatment, cervical trauma patients require rehabilitation to optimize long-term outcomes; this process is discussed as well.

Medications play a role in the treatment of patients with spinal cord injuries. In this book, we present data from various clinical trials studying these medications to assist the spine surgeon in attaining the best possible clinical outcomes.

I am deeply grateful to the outstanding efforts of the leaders in the field of cervical spine surgery who have provided their thoughts and expertise to assist the readers in identifying abnormalities, treating them appropriately, and achieving the best possible results for our patients. I am confident that the readers of this book, whether they be individuals in training or in practice, will benefit from the knowledge conveyed by this elite group of spine surgical experts. I encourage the readers to consider either reading this reference cover-to-cover or using it as a resource to aid in the treatment for specific conditions, as it is designed in such a way to be helpful in each of these situations.

With gratitude to the expert authors, sincerely,

Robert F. Heary, MD
Director, the Spine Center of New Jersey
Professor of Neurological Surgery
Rutgers, the State University of New Jersey
Newark, New Jersey

Acknowledgments

The completion of *Cervical Trauma: Surgical Management* would not have been possible without the continuing support of my amazing children (Declan, Maren, and Conor), and I would like to thank them for understanding all the hours spent putting this book together. In addition, I greatly appreciate the support, energy, and efforts of my administrative support team of Yesenia Sanchez and Roxanne Nagurka. Lastly, Raghav Gupta is a third-year medical student who will be applying to, and matching with, a neurosurgical residency training program next year; his work in assisting with all aspects of this book's preparation are appreciated and will never be forgotten.

Contributors

A. Karim Ahmed, BS
MD Candidate
Department of Neurosurgery
Johns Hopkins School of Medicine
Baltimore, Maryland

Todd J. Albert, MD
Surgeon-in-Chief and Medical Director
Korein-Wilson Professor of Orthopaedic Surgery
Hospital for Special Surgery
Chairman Department of Orthopaedic Surgery
Weill Cornell Medical College
New York, New York

Fawaz Al-Mufti, MD
Associate Professor of Neurology, Neurosurgery and
    Radiology
Division of Neuroendovascular Surgery and Neurocritical
    Care
Westchester Medical Center at New York Medical College
Valhalla, New York

Ilyas Aleem, MD, MS, FRCSC
Assistant Professor
Department of Orthopaedic Surgery
Department of Neurosurgery
University of Michigan
Ann Arbor, Michigan

Paul A. Anderson, MD
Professor
Department of Orthopedics & Rehabilitation
University of Wisconsin
Madison, Wisconsin

Paul M. Arnold, MD
Professor of Neurosurgery
Carle Illinois College of Medicine
Carle Foundation Hospital
Urbana, Illinois

Tyler Atkins, MD
Resident
Department of Neurosurgery
Carolinas Medical Center
Charlotte, North Carolina

Jetan H. Badhiwala, MD
Resident
Department of Surgery
University of Toronto
Toronto, Ontario, Canada

Kelley E. Banagan, MD
Assistant Professor
Assistant Residency Director
Department of Orthopaedics
University of Maryland School of Medicine
Baltimore, Maryland

Edward C. Benzel, MD
Emeritus Chairman of Neurosurgery
Neurological Institute
Cleveland Clinic
Cleveland, Ohio

Amandeep Bhalla, MD
Director of Spine Trauma
Department of Orthopaedic Surgery
Harbor-UCLA Medical Center
Carson, California

Christopher M. Bono, MD
Professor, Executive Vice Chair
Department of Orthopaedic Surgery
Harvard Medical School
Massachusetts General Hospital
Boston, Massachusetts

Domagoj Coric, MD
Chief, Department of Neurosurgery
Carolinas Medical Center
Carolina Neurosurgery and Spine Associates
Charlotte, North Carolina

Bradford L. Currier, MD
Professor
Departments of Orthopedics and Neurosurgery
Director, Spine Fellowship Program
Mayo Clinic
Rochester, Minnesota

Colin T. Dunn, BA
Medical Student
Case Western Reserve University
Cleveland, Ohio

Frank J. Eismont, MD
Leonard M Miller Professor and Chairman
Department of Orthopaedic Surgery
University of Miami Miller School of Medicine
Miami, Florida

Sanford E. Emery, MD, MBA
Professor and Chair
Department of Orthopaedics
West Virginia University
Morgantown, West Virginia

Michael G. Fehlings, MD, PhD, FRCSC, FACS
Professor & Vice Chair Research
Department of Surgery
University of Toronto
Head
Spinal Program
Toronto Western Hospital, University Health Network
Toronto, Ontario, Canada

Domenico A. Gattozzi, MD
Resident
Department of Neurosurgery
University of Kansas Medical Center
Kansas City, Kansas

Alexander D. Ghasem, MD
Department of Orthopedic Surgery
University of Miami/Jackson Memorial Hospital
Miami, Florida

George M. Ghobrial, MD
Staff Neurosurgeon
Novant Health Forsyth Medical Center
Winston Salem, North Carolina

Joseph P. Gjolaj, MD, FACS
Assistant Professor
Department of Orthopaedics
University of Miami Miller School of Medicine
Miami, Florida

Rahul Goel, MD
Resident
Department of Orthopaedic Surgery
Emory University
Atlanta, Georgia

Gaurav Gupta, MD, FAANS
Assistant Professor
Department of Neurosurgery
Rutgers – Robert Wood Johnson Medical School
New Brunswick, New Jersey

Raghav Gupta, BS
Medical Student
New Jersey Medical School
Rutgers University
Newark, New Jersey

Christine Hammer, MD
Resident
Department of Neurosurgery
Thomas Jefferson University
Philadelphia, Pennsylvania

James S. Harrop, MD, FACS
Professor, Departments of Neurological and Orthopedic Surgery
Director, Division of Spine and Peripheral Nerve Surgery
Neurosurgery Director of Delaware Valley SCI Center
Thomas Jefferson University
Philadelphia, Pennsylvania

Robert F. Heary, MD
Director
Spine Center of New Jersey
Professor of Neurological Surgery
Rutgers, The State University of New Jersey
Newark, New Jersey

Fady Y. Hijji, MD
Resident
Department of Orthopaedic Surgery
Wright State University
Dayton, Ohio

Alan S. Hilibrand, MD, MBA
Joseph and Marie Field Professor of Spinal Surgery
Department of Orthopaedic Surgery
Jefferson Medical College / The Rothman Institute
Philadelphia, Pennsylvania

Randall J. Hlubek, MD
Resident
Department of Neurosurgery
Barrow Neurological Institute
St. Joseph's Hospital and Medical Center
Phoenix, Arizona

Jacob Hoffmann, MD
Resident
Department of Orthopaedic Surgery
McGovern Medical School, The University of Texas at Houston
Houston, Texas

Justin Iorio, MD
Department of Orthopedic Surgery
Hospital for Special Surgery
New York, New York

Megan M. Jack, MD, PhD
Resident
Department of Neurosurgery
The University of Kansas Medical Center
Kansas City, Kansas

Darnell T. Josiah, MD, MS
Assistant Professor
Department of Neurosurgery
University of Wisconsin–Madison
Madison, Wisconsin

I. David Kaye, MD
Assistant Professor
Department of Orthopedic Surgery
Thomas Jefferson University Hospital
The Rothman Institute
Philadelphia, Pennsylvania

Steven Kirshblum, MD
Senior Medical Officer and Director of Spinal Cord Injury
  Services
Kessler Institute for Rehabilitation
West Orange, New Jersey
Professor and Chair
Department of Physical Medicine and Rehabilitation
Rutgers – New Jersey Medical School
Newark, New Jersey

Krishna T. Kudaravalli, BS
Department of Orthopaedic Surgery
Rush University Medical Center
Chicago, Illinois

Michaela Lee, MD
Resident
Department of Neurosurgery
George Washington University Medical Center
Washington, DC

Mayan Lendner, BS
Research Fellow
Spine
Rothman Orthopaedics
Philadelphia, Pennsylvania

Allan D. Levi, MD, PhD
Professor and Chairman
Department of Neurosurgery
University of Miami Miller School of Medicine
Miami, Florida

Steven C. Ludwig, MD
Professor and Chief of Spine Surgery
Director of Spine Fellowship
Department of Orthopaedic Surgery
University of Maryland School of Medicine
Baltimore, Maryland

Neil Majmundar, MD
Resident
Department of Neurological Surgery
Rutgers – New Jersey Medical School
Newark, New Jersey

Catherine A. Mazzola, MD
Department of Neurological Surgery
Division of Pediatric Neurological Surgery
Clinical Assistant Professor
Rutgers – New Jersey Medical School
Newark, New Jersey

Hamadi Murphy, MD, MS
Resident
Department of Orthopaedic Surgery
Southern Illinois University School of Medicine
Springfield, Illinois

Anil Nanda, MD, MPH, FACS
Professor and Chairman
Department of Neurosurgery
Rutgers – New Jersey Medical School & Robert Wood
  Johnson Medical School
Peter W. Carmel M.D. Endowed Chair of Neurological Surgery
Senior Vice President of Neurosurgical Services,
  RWJBarnabas Health
New Brunswick, New Jersey

Ankur S. Narain, MD
Orthopaedic Surgery Resident
Department of Orthopaedic Surgery
University of Massachusetts Medical Center
Worcester, Massachusetts

Michael Nosko, MD, PhD
Associate Professor
Department of Neurosurgery
Rutgers University – Robert Wood Johnson Medical School
New Brunswick, New Jersey

Mark L. Prasarn, MD
Chief of Spine Surgery
Department of Orthopaedic Surgery
University of Texas
Houston, Texas

Daniel K. Resnick, MD, MS
Professor and Vice Chairman
Department of Neurosurgery
University of Wisconsin School of Medicine and Public
    Health
Madison, Wisconsin

Samuel Rosenbaum, MD
Department of Orthopaedic Surgery
University of Michigan
Ann Arbor, Michigan

Michael K. Rosner, MD
Professor
Department of Neurosurgery
George Washington University School of Medicine and
    Health Sciences
Washington, DC

Sudipta Roychowdhury, MD
Clinical Associate Professor of Radiology
Department of Radiology
Rutgers – Robert Wood Johnson Medical School
New Brunswick, New Jersey

Hanna Sandhu, BS
Medical Student
Sidney Kimmel Medical College at Thomas Jefferson
    University
Philadelphia, Pennsylvania

Rick C. Sasso, MD
Professor
Chief of Spine Surgery
Department of Orthopaedic Surgery
Indiana University School of Medicine
Indiana Spine Group
Indianapolis, Indiana

Arash J. Sayari, MD
Resident Physician
Department of Orthopaedic Surgery
Rush University Medical Center
Chicago, Illinois

Nicole Silva, BS
Medical Student
Department of Neurosurgery
Rutgers – New Jersey Medical School
Newark, New Jersey

Kern Singh, MD
Professor, Department of Orthopaedic Surgery
Co-Director, Minimally Invasive Spine Institute at Rush
Founder and President, Minimally Invasive Spine Study
    Group
Rush University Medical Center
Chicago, Illinois

Joseph D. Smucker, MD
Orthopaedic Spine Surgeon
Indiana Spine Group
Carmel, Indiana

Ryan Solinsky, MD
Spinal Cord Injury Medicine Physician-Scientist
Spaulding Rehabilitation Hospital
Instructor
Department of Physical Medicine & Rehabilitation
Harvard Medical School
Boston, Massachusetts

Michael P. Steinmetz, MD
Professor and Chairman Department of Neurosurgery
Cleveland Clinic Lerner College of Medicine
Cents for Spine Health
Neurologic Institute
Cleveland Clinic
Cleveland, Ohio

Assem A. Sultan, MD
Clinical Fellow of Spine Surgery
Center for Spine Health
McGovern Medical School
Cleveland, Ohio

Derrick Sun, MD
Assistant Professor
Department of Neurosurgery
UT Health San Antonio
San Antonio, Texas

Swetha J. Sundar, MD
Resident
Department of Orthopaedic Surgery
Cleveland Clinic
Cleveland, Ohio

Fadi B. Sweiss, MD
Resident
Department of Neurosurgery
George Washington University
Washington, DC

Nicholas Theodore, MD
Donlin M. Long Professor of Neurosurgery
Professor of Neurosurgery, Orthopaedics & Biomedical
  Engineering
Director, Neurosurgical Spine Program
Johns Hopkins University School of Medicine
Baltimore, Maryland

Evan J. Trapana, MD
Resident
Department of Orthopaedic Surgery
Jackson Memorial Hospital and University of Miami Miller
  School of Medicine
Miami, Florida

Alexander R. Vaccaro, MD, PhD, MBA
Richard H. Rothman Professor and Chairman, Department
  of Orthopaedic Surgery
Professor of Neurosurgery
Co-Director, Delaware Valley Spinal Cord Injury Center
Co-Chief of Spine Surgery
Sidney Kimmel Medical Center of Thomas Jefferson University
President, Rothman Institute
Philadelphia, Pennsylvania

Scott C. Wagner, MD
Assistant Professor of Orthopaedics
Uniformed Services University of the Health Sciences
Department of Orthopaedics
Walter Reed National Military Medical Center
Bethesda, Maryland

Kelly H. Yom, BA
Clinical Research Assistant
Department of Orthopedic Surgery
Rush University Medical Center
Chicago, Illinois

1 Anatomy of the Cervical Spine

Ilyas Aleem, Samuel Rosenbaum, and Bradford L. Currier

Abstract

A thorough understanding of cervical spine anatomy is essential for those involved in the care of cervical trauma patients. Every effort must be made to gain a clear understanding of the three-dimensional relationship between vital structures prior to surgical exposure and treatment. This chapter explores the anatomy of the craniovertebral junction and subaxial spine with respect to osteology, ligamentous structures, intervertebral discs, musculature, and neurovascular structures.

Keywords: cervical anatomy, cervicothoracic junction, foramen magnum, atlas, axis, subaxial spine

1.1 Craniovertebral Junction

The craniovertebral junction (CVJ) is highly complex and is composed of the foramen magnum, occiput, atlas, axis, and their associated ligamentous, muscular, and neurovascular structures. This together represents the transition between the brain and cervical spine, and provides an extremely complex unit of stability and flexibility not found in any other region of the spine.[1]

1.1.1 Osteology of the Craniovertebral Junction

Foramen Magnum and Occipital Condyle

The foramen magnum is an oval shaped opening in the occipital bone that allows for the transition between the cranium and the spinal column (▶ Fig. 1.1). The opisthion and basion are the midpoints on the posterior and anterior margins of the foramen magnum, respectively. The average sagittal diameter of the foramen magnum measures 34.7 ± 2.5 mm.[2] The foramen magnum is flanked anterolaterally by the occipital condyles, which form bilateral inferior convexities allowing articulation with the atlas.[3] The lateral-faced occipital condyles articulate with the superomedially facing concave articular surfaces on the superior aspect of the atlas lateral masses, permitting flexion and extension of the cranium on the anterior half of the foramen magnum.[3,4] In articulating with the trapezoidal lateral mass of the atlas below, the condylar external surface is convex downward, facing outward and sloping cephalocaudal in both sagittal and coronal views.[5] Mean intercondylar distance is 29.4 mm (range: 26.2–37.0 mm).[5]

The Atlas (C1)

The atlas (C1) is an atypical vertebra without a body or spinous process, resulting in a ring-like appearance (▶ Fig. 1.2).[6] It comprises a short anterior arch and longer posterior arch connected by two dense, cortical lateral masses on either side. Instead of a body, it has an anterior tubercle that serves as an attachment for the longus colli muscle. The posterior tubercle serves as an attachment point for the rectus capitis posterior minor muscle and the suboccipital membrane. The obliquus capitis superior and inferior muscles originate from the transverse process of C1 and insert into the base of the occipital bone and into the spinous process of C2, respectively. The transverse process contains the foramen transversarium, through which the vertebral

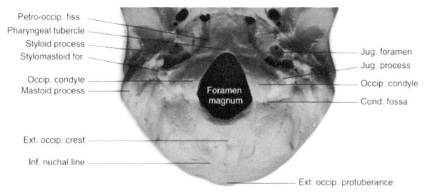

Fig. 1.1 Foramen magnum flanked by the occipital condyles. (Reproduced with permission from Kim et al.[6])

Petro-occip. fiss.
Pharyngeal tubercle
Styloid process
Stylomastoid for.
Occip. condyle
Mastoid process
Foramen magnum
Jug. foramen
Jug. process
Occip. condyle
Cond. fossa
Ext. occip. crest
Inf. nuchal line
Ext. occip. protuberance

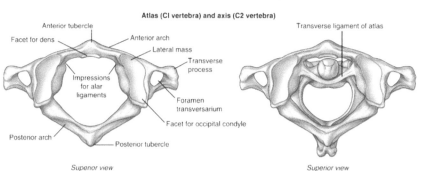

Fig. 1.2 Axial illustrations of the atlas and axis. (Reproduced with permission from Drake RL, Vogl W, Mitchell AWM. Gray's Anatomy for Students. 2nd Ed. Elsevier; 2010.)

Atlas (CI vertebra) and axis (C2 vertebra)

Anterior tubercle
Facet for dens
Anterior arch
Lateral mass
Transverse process
Impressions for alar ligaments
Foramen transversarium
Posterior arch
Facet for occipital condyle
Posterior tubercle
Superior view

Transverse ligament of atlas
Superior view

artery passes. The lateral masses are located at the junction of the anterior and posterior arch providing a secure anchor for placement of lateral mass screws. The concave superior facet of the lateral mass articulates above with the occipital condyle, and the flatter inferior facet of the lateral mass articulates below with C2. Just posterior to the lateral mass is the groove for the vertebral artery. When exposing the posterior arch of C1, it is recommended that exposure not go beyond 1 to 1.5 cm from midline to avoid injury to the vertebral artery. The atlanto-occipital articulation primarily permits extension and flexion, as well as lateral flexion.[7]

C1 lateral mass screw insertion places the vertebral and carotid arteries, hypoglossal nerve, and C2 nerve roots at risk.[8] The depth of bicortical screw insertion is approximately 19.3 mm in the axial plane and 20.9 mm in the sagittal plane.[8,9,10] The ideal start point for a C1 lateral mass screw is at the junction of the medial edge of the posterior arch attaching to the lateral mass with 10 to 15 degree angulation upward and 5 to 10 degrees medially.[11,12] The height for lateral mass screw placement, measured as the cephalad–caudad distance from the bottom of the inferior facet to the top of the posterior arch at the vertebral artery groove, measures 9.0 mm with a minimum height of 4.7 mm. In a computed tomography (CT) study of 50 head and neck scans, Currier et al found the mean distance from the internal carotid artery (ICA) to the anterior aspect of the C1 lateral mass to be 2.9 mm (range: 0–7.2 mm) (▶ Fig. 1.3).[13] Furthermore, the proximity of the ICA to C1 posed a high risk of arterial injury from a drill bit or screw in 12% of cases. An alternative entrance point that avoids the troublesome bleeding often encountered when dissecting in the region of the lateral mass is on the inferior third of the posterior arch through the pedicle analog. However, prior to the use of this entry point, the preoperative imaging must be carefully evaluated to ensure that the bone caudal to the groove of the vertebral artery is sufficient to allow screw placement.[14]

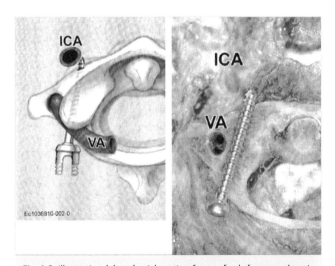

Fig. 1.3 Illustration **(a)** and axial section from a fresh frozen cadaveric specimen **(b)** showing proximity of C1 screw placement relative to the location of the internal carotid artery (ICA). VA, vertebral artery. (Reproduced with permission from Currier et al.[13])

The Axis (C2)

The axis (C2) was so named because it functions as a pivot for the atlas, allowing the head to rotate. Like the atlas, the axis is also unique due to the odontoid process or dens, which is a bony process that protrudes upward from the body of C2 (▶ Fig. 1.2). It is generally 1.0 to 1.5 cm long and 1 cm wide, inclining posteriorly up to 30 degrees relative to the body of C2.[15] The ventral surface of the odontoid articulates with the posterior aspect of the anterior arch of C1. The transverse ligament traverses from one side of the C1 ring to the other side in the transverse groove on the dorsal surface of the dens, providing stability to the dens. Fifty percent of cervical spine rotation occurs at the atlantoaxial joint.

The C2 pedicle averages approximately 8.7 mm high with a mean width of 5.8 mm and an overall transverse angle of 43.2 degrees which makes it a robust option for C2 pedicle screw placement.[16,17] The anatomic median angle of the pedicle is 10.4 degrees and the angle of declination is 28.4 degrees. The safe site of screw entry is the superior and medial third of the posterior surface of the C2 pedicle. The safe trajectory for a C2 pedicle screw is 40 degrees medial and 20 degrees superior.[18] In a radiographic analysis of C2 pedicle screws, Chin et al found the mean distance along the laminar surface between the isthmus and starting point to be 8.1 mm, and the mean distance from the superior border of the lamina to the starting point to be 5.7 mm.[19] The transverse processes of the axis are small lateral projections demarcating the lateral margin of the foramen transversarium, in which the vertebral artery courses upward before deviating medially over the C1 superior sulcus (▶ Fig. 1.4).

Translaminar axis screws are a robust option when fixation through the C2 pedicle or pars is problematic from either an anatomic or technical perspective.[20,21,22] Saetia and Phankhongsab described transverse diameters of the C2 lamina, C2 laminar length, and spinolaminar angles in 200 adult C2 CT scans.[23] They found the mean inner and outer transverse diameter of the C2 lamina to be 4.2 and 6.6 mm, respectively. The mean C2 laminar length was 37.3 mm and the mean spinolaminar angle was 56.4 degrees.[23] In another study of 420 adult C2 specimens, Cassinelli et al found 71% of specimens had a laminar thickness of ≥ 5 mm, and 93% of specimens had a laminar thickness of ≥ 4 mm.[24]

1.1.2 Ligamentous Anatomy of the Craniovertebral Junction

The ligamentous components of the CVJ can be classified as either extrinsic or intrinsic.[6,25] The extrinsic ligaments include the fibroelastic membranes, the ligamentum flavum, and the ligamentum nuchae. The ligamentum nuchae extends from the occipital protuberance to the posterior aspects of the atlas and upper cervical spinous processes. The intrinsic ligaments are composed of the tectorial membrane, accessory atlantoaxial, cruciate, and odontoid ligaments, and the anterior atlantooccipital membranes (▶ Fig. 1.5). All of the ligaments that make up the intrinsic layer are located anterior to the dura.[25]

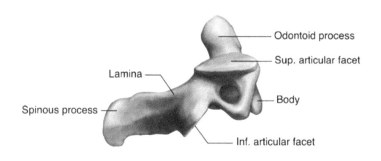

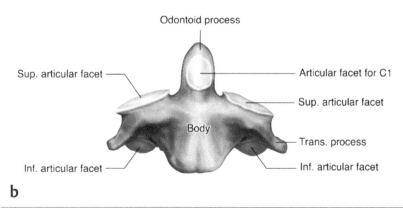

Fig. 1.4 (a) Lateral and (b) anterior illustrations of the axis. (Reproduced with permission from Kim et al.[6])

Cruciform Ligaments

The cruciform ligaments, as their name suggests, are composed of transverse and vertical components crossing behind the dens. The transverse atlantal ligament attaches to a small bony tubercle on the medial side of the lateral masses of the atlas on either side, arching across the ring of the atlas behind the dens. As it crosses behind the dens in the transverse groove, small bands are directed upward and downward, toward the clivus and C2 body, respectively.[6] The transverse atlantal ligament is the strongest ligament of the CVJ and is the predominant stabilizer of the atlas.[26] The transverse ligament serves as an anteroposterior stabilizer holding the odontoid in its vertical position, thus allowing stable rotation of the head.[3,25,26] Laxity or injury to the transverse ligament can lead to atlantoaxial instability.[27]

Alar Ligaments

Paired alar ligaments originate on the upper portion of the posterior surface of the dens and travel laterally to insert on the C1 lateral masses (atlantoalar band) and occiput (occipitoalar band).[15] The alar ligaments play an important role in the stabilization of the head during movement and are the primary restraint to axial rotation.[25] If the transverse ligament ruptures, the alar ligaments become responsible for preventing atlantoaxial subluxation. Damage to the alar ligaments results in further instability with axial rotation.

Tectorial Membrane

The tectorial membrane is a cephalad extension of the posterior longitudinal ligament (PLL), attaching to the body of C2 caudally

and basilar groove of the occiput cranially. The tectorial membrane is firmly adherent at its cranial and caudal regions. It serves as a significant secondary stabilizer in the prevention of ventral compression of the thecal sac by the odontoid.[6,25] The tectorial membrane is composed of a lateral part (also referred to as the accessory atlantoaxial ligament) joining the atlanto-occipital capsular ligaments (Arnold ligaments) and a central part that merges with the dura mater.[25] Superior and inferior crura arise from the transverse ligament as it crosses the dens, attaching to the anterior foramen magnum and body of the dens, respectively.[3]

Capsular Ligaments and Atlanto-occipital Membranes

Capsular joint ligaments connect the occiput to the C2 complex. Capsular ligaments extend across the convex-concave articulations, ensuring stable movement through a wide range of motion. The atlanto-occipital articulation is reinforced by the cephalic extension of the anterior longitudinal ligament (ALL) and ligamentum flavum, respectively termed the anterior and posterior atlanto-occipital membranes at this level. The anterior and posterior atlanto-occipital membranes extend from the foramen magnum to the anterior and posterior arch of the atlas, respectively. They contribute very little to CVJ stability.[3,25]

Accessory Atlantoaxial Ligament and Apical Ligament

The accessory atlantoaxial ligament and apical ligament offer little to no contribution to CVJ stabilization.[25] The accessory

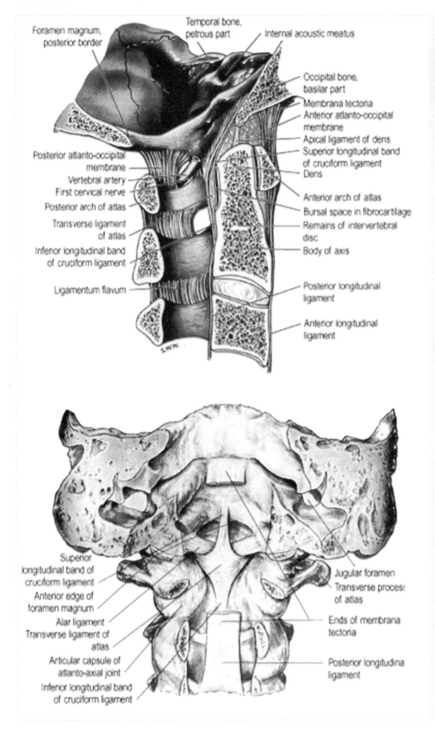

Fig. 1.5 Illustrations of the osseoligamentous structures of the craniocervical junction: (*above*) right lateral view of sagittally sectioned craniocervical junction in a median plane; (*below*) posterior view of the coronally sectioned craniocervical junction; the tectorial membrane has been partly removed to expose deeper ligaments. (Reproduced with permission from Standring S, ed. Gray's Anatomy: The Anatomical Basis of Clinical Practice. 39 ed. The Back, Elsevier; 2005.)

atlantoaxial ligament connects the lateral mass of the atlas to the body of the axis and extends to the occipital bone. The apical ligament, also known as the suspensory ligament or odontoid ligament, extends from the tip of the dens to the anterior border of the foramen magnum. It lies between the anterior atlanto-occipital membrane and the cruciform ligament, in the triangular space created by the paired alar ligaments inside of which is connective tissue, fat, and a small venous plexus.[6,25]

1.2 Subaxial Cervical Spine Anatomy

1.2.1 Osteology

The C3 to C6 vertebrae are considered typical vertebrae while C7 (along with C1 and C2) is considered atypical as it has several unique characteristics leading to the spine's transition at the cervicothoracic junction. Each vertebra in the subaxial spine consists of a body anteriorly which connects to two lateral masses through posterolateral bony projections, the pedicles and transverse processes which form the anterolateral and posteromedial walls of the transverse foramen. The lateral masses contain the superior and inferior articular facets and connect to the spinous process posteromedially through the lamina. Together, the lamina and the pedicles form the vertebral arch (▶ Fig. 1.6).

Vertebral Body

The vertebral body consists of a thin cortical shell filled with softer cancellous bone. The superior and inferior endplates of the vertebral body are typically saddle shaped with the superior endplate convex in the sagittal plane and concave in the coronal plane while the inferior endplate is concave in the sagittal plane and convex in the coronal plane. The anterior lip inferiorly will occasionally overlap the superior endplate at the next level.[28] The endplates are elliptical with their widths greater than depths. The widths and depths of both the superior and inferior endplates increase from C3 to C7. The depth ranges from 15 mm at C3 to 18.1 mm at C7 and the width ranges from 15.8 to 23.4 mm. Posterior vertebral body heights range from 10.9 to 15.14 mm and remain relatively constant from C3 to C7, whereas anterior vertebral body height increases from 14.37 mm at C3 to 14.97 mm at C7.[29,30]

Uncinate Process

The uncinate process (also termed uncal process or uncus) is an articular projection at the posterolateral aspect of the superior endplate unique to the cervical spine. It forms the uncovertebral joint or joint of Luschka with the inferior beveled aspect of the vertebra above. It generally is positioned more posteriorly and increases in height and width from C3 to C7. It functions as a "guide rail" for anterior–posterior motion during flexion and extension, assists with coupling of rotation and lateral bending, contributes to stability to the spinal column in the medial–lateral plane, and protects the neural foramen from herniated disc material.[31] The uncinate process helps define the outer limits of anterior decompression and serves as a key guide to avoid injury to the vertebral artery that lies in the foramen transversarium just lateral to it. The width of the uncinate process (and therefore distance to the foramen) ranges from 3.5 to 6 mm.[31,32,33,34,35]

Transverse Process

The transverse processes in the subaxial spine are unique when compared to the thoracic and lumbar spine. They project poster-

olaterally off the vertebral body and contain the foramen transversarium or transverse foramen, which transmits the vertebral artery (usually entering at C6) and the venous plexus at C7. The transverse process begins at the anterior root that extends medially from the vertebral body to the anterior tubercle, from which the anterior scalene, longus capitis, longus colli, and ventral intertransverse muscles originate. The anterior tubercle of C6 is larger and termed the carotid tubercle or Chassaignac tubercle. The costotransverse bar connects the anterior tubercle to the posterior tubercle and has a concave groove superiorly for the exiting nerve root. The posterior tubercle serves as the origin of the splenius cervicis, longissimus, levator scapulae, middle scalene, posterior scalene, and iliocostalis muscles.[36,37]

Pedicles

The pedicles are cylindrical bony corridors that connect the vertebral body posterolaterally to the lateral masses. They are formed by a cortical shell with a soft cancellous interior. A vertebral notch is located on the superior and inferior aspects of each pedicle to contribute to the neural foramen. Morphometric and cadaveric measurements of pedicles are numerous.[38,39,40,41,42,43,44,45,46] Mean pedicle lengths range from 5.2 mm at C3 to 5.7 mm at C7 while mean pedicle axis length from the posterior pedicle cortex to the anterior body cortex is relatively similar and ranges from 32.3 mm at C7 to 34.2 mm at C6 (C3–C5 lying somewhere in between). Mean pedicle width increases from 5.2 mm at C3 to 6.6 mm at C7 and mean pedicle height is quite similar from C3 to C7 ranging from 6.7 mm at C6 to 7.0 mm at C4. The mean medial pedicle transverse angles range between 47 and 49 degrees at C3 to C5, 44.2 degrees at C6, and 38.7 degrees at C7. The mean pedicle sagittal angle in reference to the horizontal decreases considerably from 14.2 degrees at C3 to –3.27 degrees at C6 and –1.9 degrees at C7.[42]

From an anterior cervical approach, the pedicle, which is the anatomic landmark defining the boundaries of the foramen, is hidden from view intraoperatively. This can potentially lead to incomplete surgical decompression of the foramen. In a radiographic CT analysis of 100 patients, we recently showed that the posterior endplate valley (PEV), defined as the posterior margin of the caudal vertebral body of the segment to be decompressed, is an accurate surgical landmark that is consistently at most 1 mm from the superior aspect of the cervical pedicle in the subaxial spine (▶ Fig. 1.7).[47]

Lateral Mass

The lateral mass is a flat elliptical pillar of bone that connects the pedicle to the transverse process to complete the vertebral

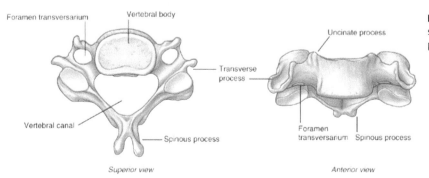

Foramen transversarium

Vertebral body

Uncinate process

Transverse process

Vertebral canal

Spinous process

Foramen transversarium   Spinous process

Superior view

Anterior view

Fig. 1.6 Illustrations of typical subaxial vertebra, superior and anterior views. (Reproduced with permission from Kim et al.[6])

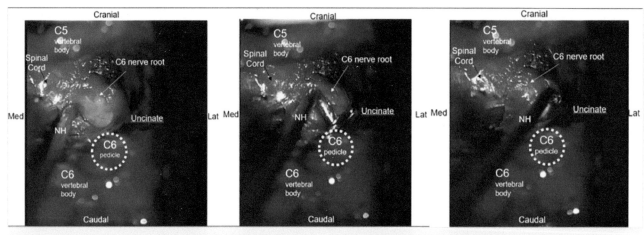

Fig. 1.7 Intraoperative images showing the location of the C6 pedicle, C6 nerve root with respect to the uncinate.

arch. It also serves as the pars interarticularis of the cervical vertebrae with the horizontally oriented superior and inferior articular facets projecting off of it, and provides the posterior border of the transverse foramen. The dimensions of the lateral masses are critical in lateral mass screw fixation given its intimate relationship with the vertebral artery and exiting nerve roots.[48,49] Measurements of the lateral mass using the Roy-Camille trajectory and Magerl trajectory have been repeated in the literature with variable results.[50,51,52,53,54,55] Average depth of the lateral mass ranges from 8.6 to 15.7 mm and generally decreases from C3 to C7 with a large drop from C6 to C7.

Lamina and Spinous Process

The laminae project posteromedially from the lateral masses to join at the spinous processes. Translaminar length generally increases from C3 to C7 ranging from 21 mm at C3 to 25.5 mm at C7. Laminar thickness decreases from C3 to C5, where it is the thinnest in the entire spine, and then increases to C7 ranging from 1.9 mm at C5 to 6.3 mm at C7.[56,57] The spinous process projects posteroinferiorly from the confluence of the laminae and is bifid from C3 to C6. It is largest and most prominent on the skin at C7.[58]

1.2.2 Joints, Ligaments, and Intervertebral discs

The complex discoligamentous anatomy of the subaxial cervical spine serves principally for stability and flexibility. The posterior discoligamentous complex is well known as a key component to spinal stability in cervical and thoracolumbar trauma classification systems.

Anterior Longitudinal Ligament

The ALL runs superior to inferior along the anterior vertebral bodies from the skull base to the sacrum. It acts as a tension band along the anterior spine. It is attached firmly to the vertebral bodies and loosely to the disc space.[59] Despite most illustrations depicting it with lateral margins anteriorly, it sweeps around laterally under the longus colli muscles and connects to the PLL forming a continuous layer surrounding the vertebral body.[60] Defining the fibers at the lateral border, it becomes narrower at C1–C2 and C2–C3.[61]

Posterior Longitudinal Ligament

The PLL runs superior to inferior along the posterior vertebral body in the vertebral foramen. Superiorly it is an inferior extension of the tectorial membrane. It is adherent to the annulus fibrosus and loosely attached to the vertebral body (reverse of ALL). It is 3 to 5 times thicker in the cervical spine than the thoracolumbar spine and attenuates in width as well as in thickness as it descends, perhaps contributing to disc herniations being much more common in the lumbar spine.[59,60]

Intervertebral Disc

The intervertebral disc lies between the cartilaginous endplates forming a fibrocartilaginous joint between the endplates. It functions to provide shock absorption with axial loads as well as flexibility to the spinal column.[62,63] It consists of a thick, layered fibrous outer ring termed the annulus fibrosus and an inner gelatinous nucleus pulposus. The annulus consists of concentric layered rings, or lamellae, with parallel collagen fibers in each layer oriented about 60 degrees to the vertical axis. The nucleus pulposus is a gelatinous structure composed of randomly organized collagen fibers with radially oriented elastin fibers surrounded by an extracellular matrix consisting largely of aggrecans and water. Chondrocyte-like cells are dispersed thinly throughout the matrix. The endplate consists of a thin (< 1 mm) layer of hyaline cartilage.[63] In general, the disc space is wider in the mediolateral direction than the anteroposterior direction. Disc space height is lowest at C4–C5 (3.3 mm average) and highest at C5–C6 (4.3 mm average).[62]

Ligamentum Flavum

The ligamentum flavum connects the lamina from C2 to the sacrum. It forms an inverted V shape in the cervical spine as a result of the shape of the lamina themselves. Its width stays relatively constant from about 9 to 11 mm. It increases in length from an average of 10.3 mm at C2–C3 to 17.5 mm at C7–T1.[61]

Facet Joints and Capsule

The facet joint is a synovial joint formed by the articulation between the inferior articular facet of the superior vertebra and superior articular facet of the inferior vertebra. In contrast to the more sagittally oriented facet joints of the lumbar spine, cervical facet joints are generally coronally oriented, transitioning from being posteromedially oriented at C3–C4 to posterolaterally oriented at C6–C7. This limits extension but allows for increased motion in other planes.[64,65] Cartilage thickness increases centrally and decreases peripherally along the articular surface and is consistently thicker in the upper cervical spine compared to the subaxial cervical spine.[66] Within the joint is a meniscus analog. Alternatively called a meniscoid, synovial fold, or intra-articular inclusion, this structure is an extension of the synovium that lies between the joint and is thought to provide increased congruence and improved joint lubrication, and likely plays a role in chronic neck pain after injury.[67,68,69,70]

Interspinous Ligament

The interspinous ligament connects the spinous processes. It is not well developed in the cervical spine. This thin, membranous structure originates predictably along the entire superior aspect of the inferior spinous process and inserts variably on the inferior edge of the superior spinous process, often with gaps or tears superiorly. It is angled anteriorly and gradually increases in length from C2–C3 to C6–C7.[61]

Supraspinous Ligament and Ligamentum Nuchae

The supraspinous ligament connects the tips of the spinous processes. This ligament is often absent in the cervical spine. When present, it is thin and not well developed. Similar to the interspinous ligament, it tends to increase in length from C2–C3 to C6–C7.[61] The ligamentum nuchae consists of a dorsal fibrous band, or dorsal raphe, that attaches C7 to the external occipital protuberance and less firmly to C6, and a ventral midline septum which connects the dorsal raphe to the tips of the cervical spinous processes and superiorly to external occipital protuberance and external occipital crest. It is not a true ligament but a confluence of tendinous fibers of the surrounding trapezius, splenius capitis, and rhomboid minor posteriorly and a fascial band or intermuscular septum anteriorly.[71]

1.3 Cervical Musculature

1.3.1 Anterolateral Musculature[72,73,74,75]

Superficial Muscles

The superficial layer anteriorly includes the platysma and sternocleidomastoid muscles (SCM). The platysma is a broad thin subcutaneous muscle that extends from the superior pectoralis and deltoid fascia to the mandible and lower lip. It is innervated by the cervical branch of the facial nerve. It acts to depress the lower lip and corners of the mouth, as well as the mandible, and creates tense ridges in the neck. The SCM originates from two heads at the sternum and clavicle and runs obliquely to insert on the mastoid process and superior nuchal line. It is innervated by the spinal accessory nerve (cranial nerve, CN XI) and acts to tilt the head toward the ipsilateral shoulder and rotate the head toward the contralateral shoulder.

Deep Muscles

The deep anterolateral musculature can be broadly grouped into the anterior, lateral, suprahyoid, and infrahyoid muscles (▶ Fig. 1.8). The suprahyoid group consists of the digastric, stylohyoid, mylohyoid, and geniohyoid muscles. In general, these muscles act to elevate the hyoid during swallowing. The infrahyoid group (strap muscles) includes the sternohyoid, sternothyroid, omohyoid, and thyrohyoid muscles. All are innervated

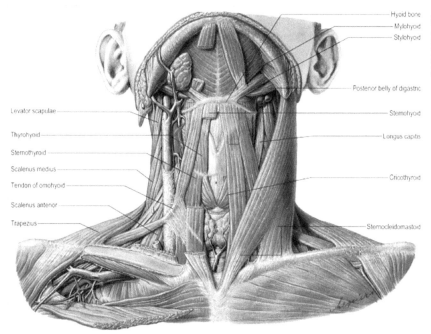

Fig. 1.8 Musculature of the anterior neck. (Reproduced with permission from Standring S, ed. Gray's Anatomy: The Anatomical Basis of Clinical Practice. 41 ed. New York: Elsevier Limited; 2016.)

by the ansa cervicalis (C1–C3) except the thyrohyoid which is innervated by C1 via the hypoglossal nerve. In general, they act to depress the hyoid and larynx during swallowing and speech.

The anterior vertebral muscles include the longus colli, longus capitis, rectus capitis anterior, and rectus capitis lateralis. The rectus capitis anterior originates from the anterior aspect of the lateral mass of C1 and root of the transverse process and inserts on the occipital bone anterior to the occipital condyle. It is innervated by the ventral rami of C1–C2 and acts to flex the head at the atlanto-occipital joints. The rectus capitis lateralis originates on the superior surface of the lateral mass of C1 and inserts on the jugular process of the occipital bone. It is similarly supplied by the ventral rami of C1–C2 and acts to laterally flex the head. The longus capitis originates from the anterior tubercles of C3–C6 and inserts on the inferior surface of the basilar part of the occipital bone. It is innervated by the ventral rami of C1–C3 and acts to flex the head. The longus colli lies on the anterior aspect of the vertebral bodies from C1 to T3. It is innervated by the ventral rami of C2–C6 and acts to flex the neck.

1.3.2 Posterior Musculature[72,73,74,75]

Superficial Layer

The superficial layer of the cervical posterior musculature includes the trapezius and levator scapulae muscles. The trapezius originates from the ligamentum nuchae, superior nuchal ridge, external occipital protuberance, and spinous processes and supraspinous ligaments of C7–T1. It inserts on the scapular spine, acromion, and lateral third of the clavicle. It is innervated by the spinal accessory nerve (CN XI). It acts to stabilize and move the scapula during shoulder movement, and assists with extension and lateral bending of the head and neck when the scapula is stabilized. The levator scapulae originates on the transverse processes of C1 and C2 as well as the posterior tubercles of C3 and C4. It inserts on the medial border of the scapula and is innervated directly by C3 and C4 as well as C5 via the dorsal scapular nerve. The levator scapulae acts to elevate the superior angle of the scapula.

Intermediate Layer

The intermediate layer includes the splenius and the erector spinae groups. The splenius capitis originates from the mastoid process and the occipital bone below the lateral third of the superior nuchal line and inserts on the spinous processes (and their supraspinous ligaments) of C7 through T3 or T4. Its tendinous fibers interlace in the midline at the dorsal raphe of the ligamentum nuchae. It is innervated by the second and third dorsal rami and acts to rotate the head to the same side and to extend the head. The splenius cervicis arises from the transverse processes of C1 and C2 and the posterior tubercle of C3; it inserts on the spinous processes of T3–T6. The muscle is innervated by the lower cervical dorsal rami and acts unilaterally to rotate upper cervical vertebra and bilaterally to extend the upper cervical spine (similar to the action of the splenius capitis muscle on the head). The erector spinae group consists of the spinalis, longissimus, and iliocostalis muscles. These are innervated by the cervical dorsal rami. The spinalis is the most medial portion of the erector spinae and is poorly developed in

the cervical spine but when present it consists of the spinalis cervicis, which extends from the spinous processes of C2–C4 to the ligamentum nuchae and spinous processes of C7 (and occasionally T1 and T2), and the spinalis capitis (which extends from the occipital bone between the superior and inferior nuchal lines to the spinous processes of C7 and T1). The longissimus is the middle portion of the erector spinae. The longissimus capitis originates from the mastoid process and typically inserts on the transverse processes of C5–T4. The longissimus cervicis originates from the posterior tubercles of the transverse processes of C2–C6 and inserts on the transverse processes of T1–T4 or T5. The iliocostalis is the most lateral muscle of the erector spinae group. The iliocostalis cervicis originates from the posterior tubercles of C4–C6 and inserts at the angles of the third through sixth ribs. The exact function of the erector spinae in the cervical spine is unknown given their small sizes and low force generation abilities. However, the other erector muscles of the thoracic and lumbar region act concentrically to extend the spine and eccentrically to control flexion against gravity.

Deep Layer

The deep posterior muscles extend between the spinous and transverse processes at various levels. The rotatores, multifidus, and semispinalis muscles are collectively termed as the spinotransverse group. These are innervated by cervical dorsal rami except for the semispinalis capitis which is innervated by C2 via the greater occipital nerve and by C3. They act as extensors of the head and spine depending on their origin. The multifidus extends from the lateral edge of the spinous process at one level to the superior articular facet of the levels below (can be anywhere from 2–5 levels below). The semispinalis is the longest muscle of the spinotransverse group. The semispinalis cervicis originates from the spinous processes of C2–C5 and runs over the multifidus to insert on the transverse processes of T1–T5 or T6. The semispinalis capitis lies over the semispinalis cervicis. It originates on the occipital bone between the superior and inferior nuchal lines and inserts on the superior articular facets of C4–C7 and the tips of the transverse processes of T1–6 or T7.

1.4 Neurovascular Anatomy of the Cervical Spine

1.4.1 Cervical Spinal Cord and Meninges

The spinal cord extends from the foramen magnum into the vertebral (or spinal) canal, a bony corridor defined anteriorly by the posterior vertebral bodies and discs, laterally by the pedicles and lateral masses, and posteriorly by the lamina and ligamentum flavum. The vertebral canal is roughly triangular. It is wider in the medial-lateral direction than the anteroposterior direction at all levels in the cervical spine. The width is relatively constant from C2 to C7 at around 23 to 26 mm.[30] Spinal cord morphometry has been studied extensively.[76,77,78,79,80,81,82,83] A review of published studies showed the spinal cord is widest at the C4 level (mean 13.3 mm), tapering off to 11.5 mm at C1 and 11 mm at C7.[78]

The spinal cord is surrounded by three layers of connective tissue termed the meninges.[82,83] The pia mater lies closest to the cord and forms the denticulate ligaments which attach to the arachnoid and dura mater, helping to stabilize it in space. The second layer, the arachnoid mater, overlies the pia mater and is continuous with the cerebral arachnoid. A fenestrated intermediate layer between the pia and arachnoid mater forms a meshwork of ligaments attaching the spinal cord to the arachnoid mater. The cerebrospinal fluid (CSF) runs in the subarachnoid space. The dura mater is the outermost layer surrounding the spinal cord. It is attached superiorly to the foramen magnum and posterior aspect of the C2 and C3 vertebral bodies as well as to the PLL.

1.4.2 Spinal Cord Blood Supply and Venous Drainage

The primary blood supply to the spinal cord comes from the segmental arteries and the longitudinal arteries (namely the anterior spinal artery and the paired posterior spinal arteries). The anterior spinal artery supplies the anterior two-thirds of the spinal cord and runs longitudinally along the anterior median fissure. It begins cranially from joined branches of the vertebral arteries. The anterior spinal artery gives off central branches which penetrate posteriorly into the cord and branches to the pial plexus on the surface of the cord. The paired longitudinal posterior spinal arteries originate from the vertebral arteries or the posterior inferior cerebellar branches of the vertebral arteries. They are smaller than their anterior counterparts and supply the posterior third of the cord.[84,85] Segmental arteries supplying the cervical spinal cord come from the vertebral arteries, ascending cervical arteries, and deep cervical arteries.[84,85]

The venous drainage of the spinal cord is divided into intrinsic, extrinsic, and extradural systems.[84,85] The intrinsic system forms a complex network of anastomoses and drains into the extrinsic system. The extradural system consists of the vertebral venous plexus that lies outside the dura in the vertebral canal, and the extraspinal efferents consisting of the vertebral, deep cervical, and jugular veins connected to the previous systems via intervertebral veins. This system also plays a role in CSF reabsorption via the arachnoid granulations in the spinal nerve roots.[86]

1.4.3 Spinal Nerves and Nerve Roots

The nerve roots exit the spinal cord at the anterolateral sulcus (motor or ventral rootlets) and the posterolateral sulcus (sensory or dorsal rootlets). These rootlets unite into the dorsal and ventral nerve roots. The dorsal rootlets are shortest in length at C5 and the longest in length at T1.[87] The ventral and dorsal roots are surrounded by their own pia mater and run in a sleeve of dura and arachnoid mater which then fuses with the epineurium as it exits the neural foramen and forms a spinal nerve. The dorsal root ganglion is a thickening in the dorsal root, usually in the neural foramen, that contains numerous sensory (efferent) nerve cell bodies. The roots take up about one-third of the neural foramen, with the rest being occupied by fat and vascular structures. The roots fuse shortly after, forming the spinal nerve proper within the neural foramen, and then split into dorsal and ventral rami. The early sinuvertebral (recurrent

meningeal) branches quickly innervate the facet joints, annulus fibrosus, PLL, and periosteum of the vertebral canal. In the cervical spine, the nerves exit above the numbered pedicle (except for C8 which exits between C7 and T1) and tend to exit more obliquely than in the lumbar spine.[87,88,89]

1.4.4 Sympathetic Chain

The cervical sympathetic chain is located posteromedial to the carotid sheath deep to the prevertebral fascia running over the longus colli and capitis muscles. While the longus muscles diverge laterally from superior to inferior, the sympathetic trunk runs obliquely in the opposite direction converging medially at C6. The average distance from the medial border of the longus colli to the sympathetic trunk at C6 is about 10.6 to 11.6 mm. The trunk itself is 2.7 to 3.3 mm and expands up to 5.3 to 7.2 mm.[90,91,92]

1.4.5 Vertebral Artery

The vertebral artery branches from the subclavian artery and has four segments (▶ Fig. 1.9).[93] V1 most commonly courses superiorly from the subclavian artery anterior to the transverse

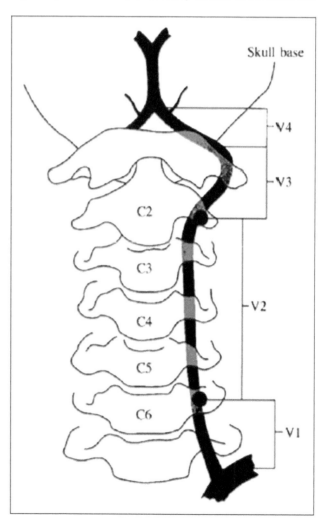

Fig. 1.9 Four segments of the vertebral artery. (Reproduced with permission from Schroeder and Hsu.[93])

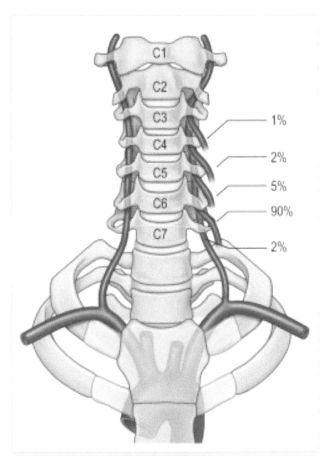

Fig. 1.10 Incidence of variations in vertebral artery anatomy. (Reproduced with permission from Standring S, ed. Gray's Anatomy: The Anatomical Basis of Clinical Practice. 41 ed. New York: Elsevier Limited; 2016.)

process of C7 into the foramen transversarium of C6. V2 is the portion most susceptible to injury in the subaxial spine and includes the artery from its entry into the C6 foramen through the C1 foramen. V3 curves laterally over the arch of C1 and extends superiorly to the foramen magnum, and V4 is the final segment from the foramen magnum, where it joins with the contralateral vertebral artery to become the basilar artery.[94] The left vertebral artery is larger in diameter than the right one in 42.9% of cases, and is equal in size in 21.4% of cases.[95] The vertebral artery is not in the C6 foramen 8% of the cases, is hypoplastic in 10% of patients, and has migrated medially in 7.6% of patients (▶ Fig. 1.10).[94]

References

[1] White AA, III, Panjabi MM. The clinical biomechanics of the occipitoatlantoaxial complex. Orthop Clin North Am. 1978; 9(4):867–878

[2] Naderi S, Korman E, Citak G, et al. Morphometric analysis of human occipital condyle. Clin Neurol Neurosurg. 2005; 107(3):191–199

[3] Lopez AJ, Scheer JK, Leibl KE, Smith ZA, Dlouhy BJ, Dahdaleh NS. Anatomy and biomechanics of the craniovertebral junction. Neurosurg Focus. 2015; 38(4):E2

[4] Avci E, Dagtekin A, Ozturk AH, et al. Anatomical variations of the foramen magnum, occipital condyle and jugular tubercle. Turk Neurosurg. 2011; 21(2):181–190

[5] de Oliveira E, Rhoton AL, Jr, Peace D. Microsurgical anatomy of the region of the foramen magnum. Surg Neurol. 1985; 24(3):293–352

[6] Kim DH, Vaccaro AR, Dickman CA, Cho D, Lee S, Kim I. Surgical Anatomy and Techniques to the Spine. 2nd ed. Elsevier; 2013

[7] Panjabi M, Dvorak J, Crisco J, III, Oda T, Hilibrand A, Grob D. Flexion, extension, and lateral bending of the upper cervical spine in response to alar ligament transections. J Spinal Disord. 1991; 4(2):157–167

[8] Ma XY, Yin QS, Wu ZH, Xia H, Liu JF, Zhong SZ. Anatomic considerations for the pedicle screw placement in the first cervical vertebra. Spine. 2005; 30(13):1519–1523

[9] Gupta T. Cadaveric morphometric anatomy of C-1 vertebra in relation to lateral mass screw placement. Surg Radiol Anat. 2008; 30(7):589–593

[10] Wait SD, Ponce FA, Colle KO, Parry PV, Sonntag VK. Importance of the C1 anterior tubercle depth and lateral mass geometry when placing C1 lateral mass screws. Neurosurgery. 2009; 65(5):952–956, discussion 956–957

[11] Blagg SE, Don AS, Robertson PA. Anatomic determination of optimal entry point and direction for C1 lateral mass screw placement. J Spinal Disord Tech. 2009; 22(4):233–239

[12] Christensen DM, Eastlack RK, Lynch JJ, Yaszemski MJ, Currier BL. C1 anatomy and dimensions relative to lateral mass screw placement. Spine. 2007; 32(8):844–848

[13] Currier BL, Maus TP, Eck JC, Larson DR, Yaszemski MJ. Relationship of the internal carotid artery to the anterior aspect of the C1 vertebra: implications for C1-C2 transarticular and C1 lateral mass fixation. Spine. 2008; 33(6): 635–639

[14] Kesman TJ, Currier BL. C1–C2 fusion: transarticular screws versus Harms/Melcher procedure. In: Jandial R, Garfin SR, eds. Best Evidence for Spine Surgery: 20 Cardinal Cases. Philadelphia, PA: Saunders Elsevier; 2012

[15] Tun K, Kaptanoglu E, Cemil B, Karahan ST, Esmer AF, Elhan A. A neurosurgical view of anatomical evaluation of anterior C1-C2 for safer transoral odontoidectomy. Eur Spine J. 2008; 17(6):853–856

[16] Kazan S, Yildirim F, Sindel M, Tuncer R. Anatomical evaluation of the groove for the vertebral artery in the axis vertebrae for atlanto-axial transarticular screw fixation technique. Clin Anat. 2000; 13(4):237–243

[17] Smith ZA, Bistazzoni S, Onibokun A, Chen NF, Sassi M, Khoo LT. Anatomical considerations for subaxial (C2) pedicle screw placement: a radiographic study with computed tomography in 93 patients. J Spinal Disord Tech. 2010; 23(3):176–179

[18] Gupta S, Goel A. Quantitative anatomy of the lateral masses of the atlas and axis vertebrae. Neurol India. 2000; 48(2):120–125

[19] Chin KR, Mills MV, Seale J, Cumming V. Ideal starting point and trajectory for C2 pedicle screw placement: a 3D computed tomography analysis using perioperative measurements. Spine J. 2014; 14(4):615–618

[20] Gorek J, Acaroglu E, Berven S, Yousef A, Puttlitz CM. Constructs incorporating intralaminar C2 screws provide rigid stability for atlantoaxial fixation. Spine. 2005; 30(13):1513–1518

[21] Lehman RA, Jr, Dmitriev AE, Helgeson MD, Sasso RC, Kuklo TR, Riew KD. Salvage of C2 pedicle and pars screws using the intralaminar technique: a biomechanical analysis. Spine. 2008; 33(9):960–965

[22] Matsubara T, Mizutani J, Fukuoka M, Hatoh T, Kojima H, Otsuka T. Safe atlantoaxial fixation using a laminar screw (intralaminar screw) in a patient with unilateral occlusion of vertebral artery: case report. Spine. 2007; 32(1): E30–E33

[23] Saetia K, Phankhongsab A. C2 anatomy for translaminar screw placement based on computerized tomographic measurements. Asian Spine J. 2015; 9(2):205–209

[24] Cassinelli EH, Lee M, Skalak A, Ahn NU, Wright NM. Anatomic considerations for the placement of C2 laminar screws. Spine. 2006; 31(24):2767–2771

[25] Debernardi A, D'Aliberti G, Talamonti G, Villa F, Piparo M, Collice M. The craniovertebral junction area and the role of the ligaments and membranes. Neurosurgery. 2015; 76 Suppl 1:S22–S32

[26] Naderi S, Cakmakçi H, Acar F, Arman C, Mertol T, Arda MN. Anatomical and computed tomographic analysis of C1 vertebra. Clin Neurol Neurosurg. 2003; 105(4):245–248

[27] Spektor S, Anderson GJ, McMenomey SO, Horgan MA, Kellogg JX, Delashaw JB, Jr. Quantitative description of the far-lateral transcondylar transtubercular approach to the foramen magnum and clivus. J Neurosurg. 2000; 92(5): 824–831

[28] Clark CR, Benzel EC, Currier BL. Cervical Spine: The Cervical Spine Research Society Editorial Committee. 3rd ed. Wolters Kluwer Health; 2004

[29] Oh S-HMD, Perin NIMD, Cooper PRMD. Quantitative three-dimensional anatomy of the subaxial cervical spine: implication for anterior spinal surgery. Neurosurgery. 1996; 38(6):1139–1144

[30] Panjabi MM, Duranceau J, Goel V, Oxland T, Takata K. Cervical human vertebrae. Quantitative three-dimensional anatomy of the middle and lower regions. Spine. 1991; 16(8):861–869

[31] Hartman J. Anatomy and clinical significance of the uncinate process and uncovertebral joint: A comprehensive review. Clin Anat. 2014; 27(3):431–440

[32] Ebraheim NA, Lu J, Haman SP, Yeasting RA. Anatomic basis of the anterior surgery on the cervical spine: relationships between uncus-artery-root complex and vertebral artery injury. Surg Radiol Anat. 1998; 20(6):389–392

[33] Lu J, Ebraheim NA, Yang H, Skie M, Yeasting RA. Cervical uncinate process: an anatomic study for anterior decompression of the cervical spine. Surg Radiol Anat. 1998; 20(4):249–252

[34] Park MS, Moon S-H, Kim T-H, et al. Surgical Anatomy of the Uncinate Process and Transverse Foramen Determined by Computed Tomography. Global Spine J. 2015; 5(5):383–390

[35] Yilmazlar S, Kocaeli H, Uz A, Tekdemir I. Clinical importance of ligamentous and osseous structures in the cervical uncovertebral foraminal region. Clin Anat. 2003; 16(5):404–410

[36] Kawashima M, Tanriover N, Rhoton AL, Jr, Matsushima T. The transverse process, intertransverse space, and vertebral artery in anterior approaches to the lower cervical spine. J Neurosurg. 2003; 98(2) Suppl:188–194

[37] Nourbakhsh A, Yang J, Gallagher S, Nanda A, Vannemreddy P, Garges KJ. A safe approach to explore/identify the V(2) segment of the vertebral artery during anterior approaches to cervical spine and/or arterial repairs: anatomical study. J Neurosurg Spine. 2010; 12(1):25–32

[38] Chazono M, Tanaka T, Kumagae Y, Sai T, Marumo K. Ethnic differences in pedicle and bony spinal canal dimensions calculated from computed tomography of the cervical spine: a review of the English-language literature. Eur Spine J. 2012; 21(8):1451–1458

[39] Karaikovic EE, Kunakornsawat S, Daubs MD, Madsen TW, Gaines RW, Jr. Surgical anatomy of the cervical pedicles: landmarks for posterior cervical pedicle entrance localization. J Spinal Disord. 2000; 13(1):63–72

[40] Li Y, Liu J, Liu Y, Wu Y, Zhu Q. Cervical pedicle screw fixation at C6 and C7: A cadaveric study. Indian J Orthop. 2015; 49(4):465–470

[41] Liao W, Guo L, Bao H, Wang L. Morphometric analysis of the seventh cervical vertebra for pedicle screw insertion. Indian J Orthop. 2015; 49(3):272–277

[42] Liu J, Napolitano JTMS, Ebraheim NA. Systematic review of cervical pedicle dimensions and projections. Spine. 2010; 35(24):E1373–E1380

[43] Ludwig SC, Kramer DL, Vaccaro AR, Albert TJ. Transpedicle screw fixation of the cervical spine. Clin Orthop Relat Res. 1999(359):77–88

[44] Onibokun A, Khoo LT, Bistazzoni S, Chen NF, Sassi M. Anatomical considerations for cervical pedicle screw insertion: the use of multiplanar computerized tomography measurements in 122 consecutive clinical cases. Spine J. 2009; 9(9):729–734

[45] Panjabi MM, Shin EK, Chen NCBS, Wang J-L. Internal morphology of human cervical pedicles. [Miscellaneous Article]. Spine. 2000; 25(10):1197–1205

[46] Shin EK, Panjabi MM, Chen NC, Wang JL. The anatomic variability of human cervical pedicles: considerations for transpedicular screw fixation in the middle and lower cervical spine. Eur Spine J. 2000; 9(1):61–66

[47] Alder JA. Ilyas; Popper, Joseph; Freedman, Brett; Nassr, Ahmad; Bydon, Mohamad; Yaszemski, Michael; Currier, Bradford. A Novel Anatomic Landmark to Assess Adequate Decompression in Anterior Cervical Spine Surgery: The Posterior Endplate Valley (PEV) AOSpine Fellows Forum; 2017; Banff

[48] Ebraheim NA, Lu J, Skie M, Heck BE, Yeasting RA. Vulnerability of the recurrent laryngeal nerve in the anterior approach to the lower cervical spine. [Miscellaneous Article]. Spine. 1997; 22(22):2664–2667

[49] Xu R, Ebraheim NA, Nadaud MC, Yeasting RA, Stanescu S. The location of the cervical nerve roots on the posterior aspect of the cervical spine. Spine. 1995; 20(21):2267–2271

[50] Barrey C, Mertens P, Jund J, Cotton F, Perrin G. Quantitative anatomic evaluation of cervical lateral mass fixation with a comparison of the Roy-Camille and the Magerl screw techniques. Spine. 2005; 30(6):E140–E147

[51] Ebraheim NA, Klausner T, Xu R, Yeasting RA. Safe lateral-mass screw lengths in the Roy-Camille and Magerl techniques. An anatomic study. Spine. 1998; 23(16):1739–1742

[52] Merola AA, Castro BA, Alongi PR, et al. Anatomic consideration for standard and modified techniques of cervical lateral mass screw placement. Spine. 2002; 2(6):430–435

[53] Mohamed E, Ihab Z, Moaz A, Ayman N, Haitham AE. Lateral mass fixation in subaxial cervical spine: anatomic review. Global Spine J. 2012; 2(1):39–46

[54] Sangari SK, Heinneman TE, Conti MS, et al. Quantitative Gross and CT measurements of Cadaveric Cervical Vertebrae (C3-C6) as Guidelines for the Lateral mass screw fixation. Int J Spine Surg. 2016; 10:43

[55] Stemper BD, Marawar SV, Yoganandan N, Shender BS, Rao RD. Quantitative anatomy of subaxial cervical lateral mass: an analysis of safe screw lengths for Roy-Camille and magerl techniques. Spine. 2008; 33(8):893–897

[56] Alvin MDBS, Abdullah KGBS, Steinmetz MPMD, et al. Translaminar screw fixation in the subaxial cervical spine: quantitative laminar analysis and feasibility of unilateral and bilateral translaminar virtual screw placement. Spine. 2012; 37(12):E745–E751

[57] Xu R, Burgar A, Ebraheim NA, Yeasting RA. The quantitative anatomy of the laminas of the spine. Spine. 1999; 24(2):107–113

[58] Saluja S, Patil S, Vasudeva N. Morphometric Analysis of Sub-axial Cervical Vertebrae and Its Surgical Implications. J Clin Diagn Res. 2015; 9(11):AC01–AC04

[59] Bland JH, Boushey DR. Anatomy and physiology of the cervical spine. Semin Arthritis Rheum. 1990; 20(1):1–20

[60] Hayashi K, Yabuki T, Kurokawa T, Seki H, Hogaki M, Minoura S. The anterior and the posterior longitudinal ligaments of the lower cervical spine. J Anat. 1977; 124(Pt 3):633–636

[61] Panjabi MM, Oxland TR, Parks EH. Quantitative anatomy of cervical spine ligaments. Part II. Middle and lower cervical spine. J Spinal Disord. 1991; 4(3):277–285

[62] Pait TGMD, Killefer JAMD, Arnautovic KIMD. Surgical anatomy of the anterior cervical spine: the disc space, vertebral artery, and associated bony structures. Neurosurgery. 1996; 39(4):769–776

[63] Raj PP. Intervertebral disc: anatomy-physiology-pathophysiology-treatment. Pain Pract. 2008; 8(1):18–44

[64] Pal GP, Routal RV, Saggu SK. The orientation of the articular facets of the zygapophyseal joints at the cervical and upper thoracic region. J Anat. 2001; 198(Pt 4):431–441

[65] Panjabi MM, Oxland T, Takata K, Goel V, Duranceau J, Krag M. Articular facets of the human spine. Quantitative three-dimensional anatomy. Spine. 1993; 18(10):1298–1310

[66] Yoganandan N, Knowles SAMS, Maiman DJMD, Pintar FA. Anatomic study of the morphology of human cervical facet joint. Spine. 2003; 28(20):2317–2323

[67] Farrell SF, Osmotherly PG, Cornwall J, Rivett DA. The anatomy and morphometry of cervical zygapophyseal joint meniscoids. Surg Radiol Anat. 2015; 37(7):799–807

[68] Farrell SF, Osmotherly PG, Cornwall J, Sterling M, Rivett DA. Cervical spine meniscoids: an update on their morphological characteristics and potential clinical significance. Eur Spine J. 2017; 26(4):939–947

[69] Inami S, Kaneoka K, Hayashi K, Ochiai N. Types of synovial fold in the cervical facet joint. J Orthop Sci. 2000; 5(5):475–480

[70] Yu SW, Sether L, Haughton VM. Facet joint menisci of the cervical spine: correlative MR imaging and cryomicrotomy study. Radiology. 1987; 164(1):79–82

[71] Mercer SR, Bogduk N. Clinical anatomy of ligamentum nuchae. Clin Anat. 2003; 16(6):484–493

[72] Grodinsky M, Holyoke EA. The fasciae and fascial spaces of the head, neck and adjacent regions. Am J Anat. 1938; 63(3):367–408

[73] Guidera AK, Dawes PJD, Stringer MD. Cervical fascia: a terminological pain in the neck. ANZ J Surg. 2012; 82(11):786–791

[74] Som PM, Curtin HD. Fascia and Spaces of the Neck. Head and Neck Imaging. 5 ed. Philadelphia, PA: Mosby; 2011:2203–2234

[75] Watkinson JC, Gleeson M. Neck. In: Standring S, ed. Gray's Anatomy: The Anatomical Basis of Clinical Practice. 41 ed. Philadelphia, PA: Elsevier; 2016:442–474

[76] Elliott HC. Cross-sectional diameters and areas of the human spinal cord. Anat Rec. 1945; 93(3):287–293

[77] Fradet L, Arnoux P-J, Ranjeva J-P, Petit Y, Callot V. Morphometrics of the entire human spinal cord and spinal canal measured from in vivo high-resolution anatomical magnetic resonance imaging. Spine. 2014; 39(4):E262–E269

[78] Frostell A, Hakim R, Thelin EP, Mattsson P, Svensson M. A Review of the Segmental Diameter of the Healthy Human Spinal Cord. Front Neurol. 2016; 7:238

[79] Kameyama T, Hashizume Y, Ando T, Takahashi A. Morphometry of the normal cadaveric cervical spinal cord. Spine. 1994; 19(18):2077–2081

[80] Ko HY, Park JH, Shin YB, Baek SY. Gross quantitative measurements of spinal cord segments in human. Spinal Cord. 2004; 42(1):35–40

[81] Okada Y, Ikata T, Katoh S, Yamada H. Morphologic analysis of the cervical spinal cord, dural tube, and spinal canal by magnetic resonance imaging in normal adults and patients with cervical spondylotic myelopathy. Spine. 1994; 19(20):2331–2335

[82] Sherman JL, Nassaux PY, Citrin CM. Measurements of the normal cervical spinal cord on MR imaging. AJNR Am J Neuroradiol. 1990; 11(2):369–372

[83] Yanase M, Matsuyama Y, Hirose K, et al. Measurement of the cervical spinal cord volume on MRI. J Spinal Disord Tech. 2006; 19(2):125–129

[84] Bosmia AN, Hogan E, Loukas M, Tubbs RS, Cohen-Gadol AA. Blood supply to the human spinal cord: part I. Anatomy and hemodynamics. Clin Anat. 2015; 28(1):52–64

[85] Colman MW, Hornicek FJ, Schwab JH. Spinal Cord Blood Supply and Its Surgical Implications. J Am Acad Orthop Surg. 2015; 23(10):581–591

[86] Griessenauer CJ, Raborn J, Foreman P, Shoja MM, Loukas M, Tubbs RS. Venous drainage of the spine and spinal cord: a comprehensive review of its history, embryology, anatomy, physiology, and pathology. Clin Anat. 2015; 28(1):75–87

[87] Alleyne CH, Jr, Cawley CM, Barrow DL, Bonner GD. Microsurgical anatomy of the dorsal cervical nerve roots and the cervical dorsal root ganglion/ventral root complexes. Surg Neurol. 1998; 50(3):213–218

[88] Bogduk N. The clinical anatomy of the cervical dorsal rami. Spine. 1982; 7(4):319–330

[89] Zhang J, Tsuzuki N, Hirabayashi S, Saiki K, Fujita K. Surgical anatomy of the nerves and muscles in the posterior cervical spine: a guide for avoiding inadvertent nerve injuries during the posterior approach. Spine. 2003; 28(13):1379–1384

[90] Civelek E, Karasu A, Cansever T, et al. Surgical anatomy of the cervical sympathetic trunk during anterolateral approach to cervical spine. Eur Spine J. 2008; 17(8):991–995

[91] Ebraheim NA, Lu J, Yang H, Heck BE, Yeasting RA. Vulnerability of the sympathetic trunk during the anterior approach to the lower cervical spine. Spine. 2000; 25(13):1603–1606

[92] Yin Z, Yin J, Cai J, Sui T, Cao X. Neuroanatomy and clinical analysis of the cervical sympathetic trunk and longus colli. J Biomed Res. 2015; 29(6):501–507

[93] Schroeder GD, Hsu WK. Vertebral artery injuries in cervical spine surgery. Surg Neurol Int. 2013; 4 Suppl 5:S362–S367

[94] Eskander MS, Drew JM, Aubin ME, et al. Vertebral artery anatomy: a review of two hundred fifty magnetic resonance imaging scans. Spine. 2010; 35(23):2035–2040

[95] Abd el-Bary TH, Dujovny M, Ausman JI. Microsurgical anatomy of the atlantal part of the vertebral artery. Surg Neurol. 1995; 44(4):392–400, discussion 400–401

2 Classification of Spinal Cord Injury

Ryan Solinsky and Steven Kirshblum

Abstract

This chapter details the clinical examination and scoring as well as classification with the most broadly accepted tool, the International Standards for Neurological Classification of Spinal Cord Injury (ISNCSCI) exam and the American Spinal Injury Association Impairment Scale. Recommended terminology regarding classification and description of spinal cord injury is discussed. Common incomplete spinal cord syndromes are described in detail, including central cord syndrome, Brown-Sequard syndrome, anterior cord syndrome, posterior cord syndrome, and discomplete injuries. Lastly, assessing remaining autonomic function following spinal cord injury is described.

Keywords: international standards, motor scoring, sensory scoring, classification, SCI syndromes, autonomic standards

2.1 Introduction

Accurate neurological assessment is essential after a patient sustains a spinal cord injury (SCI). The most accurate tool for assessing SCI is to perform the standardized neurological examination as endorsed by the International Standards for Neurological Classification of Spinal Cord Injury (ISNCSCI).[1] These Standards define common terms used by clinicians in the assessment of SCI and describe the neurological examination (Appendix 2.1 (p.22)). The examination and classification of a person with SCI are two different skills, and therefore will be described separately. The examination is recorded on a standardized worksheet (▶ Fig. 2.1) and allows for efficient classification of the sensory, motor, and neurological levels, as well as generation of sensory and motor index scores, determination of the clinical completeness of the injury, and impairment classification.

The ISNCSCI was developed to document selected neurological parameters at the time the exam is conducted in a clinical setting[2] as opposed to incorporating all aspects of a neurological exam. While not the initial intention, these Standards have been used for inclusion/exclusion criteria for research studies, outcome measures, as well as for prognostication of neurological recovery for large groups of persons with SCI.

2.2 Examination

2.2.1 Sensory Examination

The sensory examination is performed on 28 key dermatomal points (▶ Fig. 2.1), each tested for light touch appreciation and sharp/dull discrimination bilaterally. Deep anal pressure (DAP), described below, is also a required portion of the exam. A three-point grading scale (0–2) is used, with the cheek of the face used as the control point. Testing is performed with the patient's eyes closed or vision blocked so the patient cannot identify the site being tested. For light touch, a tapered wisp of cotton from a cotton tip applicator is moved across the skin (not exceeding 1 cm). A score of "2" (intact) corresponds to the same touch sensation as on the face and "1" if felt different from the face (either hypo or hyperesthesia). A score of "0" (absent) is used if there is no appreciation of sensation.

For the sharp/dull discrimination, a clean, disposable safety pin is used. A score of "2" is documented for sensation that is perceived the same as the face with intact ability to differentiate sharp (pin end of the safety pin) from dull (rounded edge of the pin) edge. A score of "1" corresponds to altered sensation (hypo or hyperesthesia) relative to the face while maintaining the ability to differentiate sharp from dull. A score of "0"

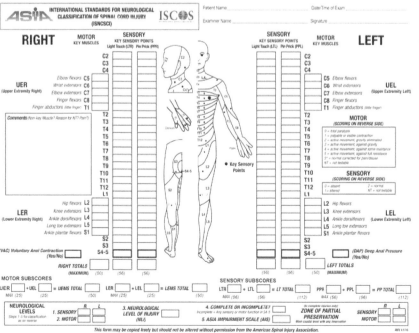

Fig. 2.1 International Standards for Neurological Classification of Spinal Cord Injury (ISNCSCI) flowsheet. (Reproduced with permission.)[1]

represents absent sensation, and is also given for the inability to differentiate the sharp from dull end of the pin. If accurate sensory testing is unable to be performed due to extenuating circumstances (i.e., burns, casts, amputations, etc.), the level is designated as not testable, or "NT," on the worksheet for that dermatome, or an alternate location within the dermatome can be tested with a notation in the comment box on the worksheet. If there is a question whether the patient can definitively discriminate between the sharp and dull edges, 8/10 correct answers is considered accurate, as this reduces the probability of correct guessing to < 5%.

A prominent pitfall in performing sensory testing is variation in the caudal extent of the C4 dermatome, at times referred to as the "C4 cape." Variably, this cervical dermatome can extend in close proximity to the nipple line, making it easy to confuse it with the T3 dermatome. In accordance with the International Standards, if T1 and T2 dermatomes are absent and T3 appears intact, T3 should be scored as absent if there is no sensation at T4 (thereby assuming an extended C4 cape).

It is important to test the S4–S5 dermatome (< 1 cm lateral to the mucocutaneous junction of the anus) for both sharp/dull discrimination and light touch, as this represents function of the most caudal aspect of the sacral spinal cord. In addition, DAP is tested by inserting a lubricated gloved finger into the anus and applying pressure to the anorectal wall using the thumb to gently squeeze the anus against an inserted index finger.[4] The patient is asked if they can appreciate this digital pressure. Consistently perceived pressure is recorded as either present (YES) or absent (NO) on the worksheet. If a patient has intact sensation to sharp/dull discrimination or light touch at S4/S5, DAP is not required for classification in the current ISNCSCI exam (though the motor portion of the anorectal exam, described below, is still required). Optional elements of the sensory examination include joint movement appreciation and position sense, and awareness of deep pressure/pain, each of which can add to better characterization of an injury. Details of this testing are reviewed elsewhere (www.asialearning.com).

2.2.2 Motor Examination

The motor examination encompasses testing 10 key muscles bilaterally, which are featured on the scoring worksheet (▶ Fig. 2.1 and Appendix 2.1 (p. 22)). It is recommended that the muscles should be examined in a rostral to caudal sequence, starting with the elbow flexors (C5 tested muscle) and finishing with the ankle plantar flexors (Sl muscle) with the patient in supine positioning to maximize reproducibility over time post injury. Muscles are graded and recorded on the standard worksheet, on a 6-point scale from 0 to 5[5] without pluses or minuses to maximize interrater reliability.

Although each of the key muscles has one root listed, usually two segments innervate these muscles (i.e., for biceps—C5 and C6). If a particular muscle has a grade of 3/5, it is considered to have full innervation by at least the more rostral nerve root segment and is considered useful for functional activities. A muscle initially graded as 5/5 would be considered fully innervated by both spinal root segments (▶ Fig. 2.2).

Placing the joints in the proper position during manual muscle testing (MMT) and stabilizing above and below the joint tested is important especially if the muscles do not have antigravity

strength.[1] Careful consideration toward muscle substitution masquerading as key muscle movements must be considered. Common substitutions include forearm supination mimicking wrist extension (C6), shoulder external rotation substituting for elbow extension (C7), wrist extension with tenodesis substituting for long finger flexion (C8), and finger extension appearing as small finger abduction (T1). Triggering of co-contracting spasticity (e.g., use of active elbow flexion to trigger elbow extension spasms) may also cause inaccuracies in the motor exam if not appreciated. In the lower extremities, abdominal or adductor contractions may also appear (with or without the addition of spasticity) as hip flexion and ankle dorsiflexion may mimic long toe extension. The InSTeP training videos are recommended to fully appreciate all of these positions (www.asialearning.com).

Patient's clinical condition may prevent the completion of an accurate examination. Limiting factors such as pain and deconditioning may be present such that the patient's MMT only grades a 4/5. If the examiner feels that the patient would otherwise have normal strength, the muscle should be graded as a 5* to indicate that inhibiting factors were present and these should be documented in the comment box on the worksheet. When the patient is not fully testable due to any reason, such as spasticity that prevents accurate stabilization of the joint, uncontrolled clonus, severe pain, a fracture limiting the exam, the cognitive status impacting participation, or a contracture limiting > 50% of full range of motion, the examiner should record "NT" instead of a numerical score for the specific myotome.

In a patient with a potentially unstable spine, care must be taken when performing MMT. When examining a newly injured individual with a lesion below T8, the hip should not be flexed passively or actively beyond 90 degrees, as this may place too great a kyphotic stress on the lumbar spine. In this circumstance, isometric assessment of hip flexion is appropriate.

Voluntary anal contraction (VAC) is tested by inserting a lubricated gloved finger into the anus and asking the patient to "squeeze my finger as if to hold back a bowel movement." This is graded as either present (YES) or absent (NO) in the appropriate box on the worksheet. Care must be taken during this exam

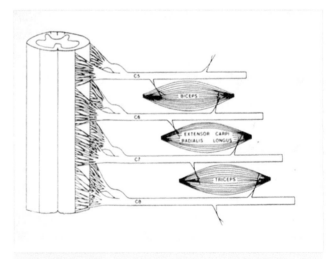

Fig. 2.2 Muscle innervation by level of injury. (Reproduced with permission.)[1]

for patient modesty, as well as to differentiate volitional contraction from anal spasm when the finger is inserted, or anal contraction triggered by Valsalva.

A number of optional muscles (diaphragm, deltoids, abdominal muscles, medial hamstrings, and hip adductors) may also be tested, and these may be helpful in determining motor sparing of certain regions of the spinal cord and motor incompleteness, but are not used to obtain a motor index score. Beevor sign may also be helpful in specific clinical circumstances to supporting variable thoracic denervation, though this test should not be performed during the acute stages of thoracic/lumbar injuries. The hip adductor muscles, while not used as part of the motor score, are important muscles to monitor, as they are often the first muscles to recover in the lower extremity. Outside of the key 10 key muscles, non-key muscles are also tested in limited scenarios (as described below).

Although not a part of the ISNCSCI, deep tendon reflex testing may be useful to regularly assess along with anal wink and bulbocavernosus reflex for identifying phases of spinal shock[6] and identification of upper versus lower motor neuron dysfunction. Spasticity and autonomic assessments can also help providers develop a more comprehensive understanding of an individual's deficits, and are described elsewhere.

2.3 Terminology

Tetraplegia: It is preferred to the term *quadriplegia* and is defined as impairment or loss of motor and/or sensory function in the cervical segments of the spinal cord due to damage of neural elements within the spinal cord. It does not include injury to the peripheral nerves outside the neural canal.[1]

Paraplegia: It refers to an impairment of motor and/or sensory function in the thoracic, lumbar, or sacral (but not cervical) segments of the spinal cord secondary to the damage of neural elements within the spinal canal. The terms quadriparesis (tetraparesis) and paraparesis are discouraged because they describe incomplete lesions imprecisely.

Sensory level: It is the most caudal dermatome to have normal (score of 2) sensation for both sharp/dull discrimination and light touch. This is determined by a grade of 2 (normal/intact) in all dermatomes beginning with C2 and extending caudally to the first segment that has a score of < 2 for either sharp/dull discrimination or light touch. The intact dermatome level located immediately above the first dermatome level with impaired or absent light touch or sharp/dull discrimination is designated as the sensory level (one for each side of the body).

If sensation is abnormal at C2, the sensory level is designated as C1.[1] If sensation is intact through S4–S5, the sensory level should be recorded as intact ("INT") rather than as S4–S5. If the patient is unable to reliably appreciate sensation when tested on the face, then "NT" should be recorded and "ND" (not determinable) should be documented in the appropriate area on the worksheet with no sensory level given.

Sensory index scoring: This provides a means of numerically documenting changes in sensory function and is calculated by adding the scores for all dermatomes. If "NT" has been documented at any level, then a sensory score cannot be calculated.

Motor level: It is defined as the lowest key muscle that has a grade of at least 3, provided all key muscles represented by segments rostral to that level are graded as 5.[1] The motor level

may differ by side of the body; a single motor level would be the more rostral of the two. If "NT" has been documented as part of the exam and this muscle is required for determination of the motor level, the designation of the motor level for that side should be deferred and "ND" is documented on the worksheet.

The myotomes that are not clinically testable by MMT (i.e., above C5, T2–L1, and S2–S5) are assumed to have full innervation if sensory innervation for sharp/dull discrimination and light touch are also intact at the level and rostrally. For example, if the sensory level is C4 and there is no C5 motor function strength (or strength graded as < 3), the motor level is C4. In a case where the C5 motor function is graded ≥ 3 on both sides of the body, with a sensory level on the left at C4 and on the right at C3 (the right C4 dermatome is impaired); the motor level on the left would be C5 and on the right it would be C3. Since the C4 dermatome on the right is impaired, it is presumed that the C4 myotome is also impaired. Therefore, the motor level is designated as C3, since the patient does not meet the criteria of having a key muscle function (in this case the C5 muscle) ≥ 3/5 with the levels above (in this case C4) scoring as normal. On the left side, the C4 dermatome is normal so the C4 myotome is considered normal, and as a result the left motor level is C5.

It is important to recognize and document if neurological injury is unrelated to SCI. For example, in a patient with a thoracic level injury who also has a brachial plexus injury, a note should be made in the comment box on the worksheet to correctly classify the patient's spinal level of injury (thoracic level), rather than assigning a higher (cervical) level due to a non-SCI-related injury.

Motor index scoring: It is calculated by adding the muscle scores of each key muscle group. It is recommended to separate the motor scores into two scores: one for the upper limbs and one for the lower limbs.[1,7] The motor scores provide a means of numerically documenting changes in motor function. If "NT" has been documented, then a motor index score cannot be calculated.

Neurological level of injury: This is used when determining the American Spinal Injury Association [ASIA] Impairment Scale (AIS) classification grade and refers to the most caudal segment of the spinal cord with normal sensory and antigravity muscle function on both sides of the body, provided that there is normal (intact) sensory and motor function rostrally. If the motor level is C7 and the sensory level is C8, the overall single neurological level of injury (NLI) is C7. The motor level and upper extremity motor index score better reflect the degree of function as well as the severity of impairment and disability, relative to the NLI, after motor complete tetraplegia.[8] This is because the sensory level may place the neurological level more rostral, thereby incorrectly implying poorer function.

Zone of partial preservation: It is defined as the dermatomes and myotomes caudal to the sensory and motor levels that remain partially innervated in an individual with a neurologically complete (AIS A) injury (see below).[1] The zone of partial preservation (ZPP) should be recorded on the worksheet by documenting the most caudal segment with some sensory and/or motor function. A single segment for each ZPP rather than the entire range of partially innervated segments should be documented. For example, in an individual with AIS A tetraplegia, if the right sensory level is C5 and some sensation extends to C8, then C8 is recorded as the right sensory ZPP. For ZPP description, motor function does not follow sensory function (i.e., in a case of a T6 level of injury, impaired sensation at T7 does not imply there is intact/impaired motor function at T7). If there is no ZPP (no partially innervated segments below a motor or sensory level), the motor or sensory level should be entered as the ZPP.[1] With an incomplete injury, the ZPP is not applicable and "NA" is recorded.

2.4 Classification of Injury

Utilizing a standard method of neurological assessment is important to help determine the course of recovery and the effect of interventions in the treatment of SCI. There have been many systems developed for the classification of SCI that have been based on bony patterns of injury, mechanism of injury, neurological function, and functional outcome,[9,10,11,12,13,14,15] and a full history is reviewed elsewhere.[16,17] The ISNCSCI is currently the most valid and reliable classification to assess SCI and is used by the Model System Spinal Cord Injury database. A computerized classification program has been developed utilizing this schema[18,19] and algorithms are available at www.ISNCSCIalgorithm.com and http://ais.emsci.org. The ISNCSCI exam is composed of determining the NLI and assigning a grade based on completeness of injury through the AIS.

A number of articles have posed challenging cases as well as some potential improvements to the classification[20,21,22,23,24,25]; however, the current classification has remained unchanged since 2015. Other scales and examination techniques have also been described,[26,27,28,29] some of which utilize additional muscle groups, such as used in the NASCIS trials.[29] El Masry et al, however, found the ASIA and NASCIS motor scoring systems comparable in representing motor deficits and recovery.[30] The ISNCSCI has been found overall to be valid, reliable, and sensitive to change, most especially in patients with neurologically complete injuries.[25,31,32,33,34,35,36,37]

A neurologically *complete* injury is defined as the absence of sensory and motor function in the lowest sacral segments (*no sacral sparing*), whereas an *incomplete* injury is partial preservation of sensory and/or motor function as determined by examination of the most caudal segment (S4–S5) (*sacral sparing*). Sacral sparing is tested by sharp/dull discrimination and light touch at the anal mucocutaneous junction (S4/S5 dermatome) on both sides, as well as testing VAC of the external anal sphincter (the motor aspect) and DAP as part of the rectal examination. If any of these are present (representing sacral sparing), intact or impaired, even on one side, the individual has an incomplete injury. According to this definition, a patient with cervical SCI can have sensory and motor function in the trunk or even in the legs, but unless sacral sparing is present, the injury is classified as "complete" with a large ZPP. When sacral sparing is used to define incompleteness, motor recovery is significantly more likely to occur than when it is not.[9] The *sacral sparing* definition of the completeness of the injury was adopted by the ASIA Standards Committee in 1992.[10] Prior to this, an injury was considered "incomplete" if motor or sensory function extended more than three levels below the injury. The sacral sparing definition has been considered a more stable definition, because fewer patients convert from incomplete to complete status over time post injury.[9]

The AIS has five grades, which are listed in ▶ Table 2.1. The determination of the AIS is described in ▶ Table 2.2.

Table 2.1 ASIA Impairment Scale

AIS A (complete)	No motor or sensory function is preserved in the sacral segments S4–S5
AIS B (sensory incomplete)	Sensory but not motor function is preserved at the most caudal sacral segments S4–S5, **AND** no motor function is preserved more than three levels below the motor level on either side of the body
AIS C (Motor incomplete)	Motor function is preserved at the most caudal sacral segments (S4–S5) on VAC **OR** the patient meets the criteria for sensory incomplete status (sensory function preserved at the most caudal sacral segments (S4–S5) by LT, *sharp/dull discrimination* or DAP), with sparing of motor function more than three levels below the *motor level* on *either* side of the body. This includes key or non-key muscle functions more than 3 levels below the motor level to determine motor incomplete status. For AIS C – less than half of key muscle functions below the single NLI have a muscle grade ≥ 3.
AIS D (Motor incomplete)	Motor incomplete status as defined above, with at least half (half or more) of key muscle functions below the single NLI having a muscle grade ≥ 3.
AIS E (Normal)	If sensation and motor function as tested with the ISNCSCI are graded as normal in all segments, and the patient had prior deficits, then the AIS grade is E. Someone without an SCI does not receive an AIS grade.

Abbreviations: AIS, ASIA Impairment Scale; DAP, deep anal pressure; ISNCSCI, International Standards for Neurological Classification of Spinal Cord Injury; LT, light touch; NLI, neurological level of injury; SCI, spinal cord injury; VAC, voluntary anal contraction.
Source: International Standards for Neurological Classification of Spinal Cord Injury.[1]

AIS A: Motor and sensory complete. No sacral sparing including sharp/dull discrimination or light touch sensation at any of the S4–S5 dermatomes; no VAC and no DAP. In this case, a ZPP is documented on the worksheet. If the injury is complete, the worksheet will read "N-O-O-O-O-N" across the bottom—"no" for VAC, the four 0s for no S4–S5 sensation for light touch or sharp/dull discrimination modalities on either side of the body, and another "no" for DAP.[2]

AIS B: Motor complete and sensory incomplete. Sensory but not motor function is preserved at the most caudal sacral segments S4–S5, and no motor function is preserved more than three levels below the *motor* level on either side of the body.

AIS C: Motor incomplete. Motor function is preserved at the most caudal sacral segments on VAC or the patient meets the criteria for sensory incomplete status (sensory function preserved at the most caudal sacral segments (S4–S5) by light touch, sharp/dull discrimination or DAP), with sparing of motor function more than three levels below the ipsilateral motor level on either side of the body. This spared motor function includes key or non-key muscles (see ▶ Table 2.3) or VAC to determine motor incomplete status. For AIS C, less than half of a key muscle functions below the single NLI have a muscle grade of 3/5.[3]

Non-key muscles more than three levels below the motor level on each side should be tested[1] in case of sensory sacral sparing when there are no key muscle functions present more than three levels below the motor level to differentiate between AIS B and AIS C. The presence of any muscle function in these muscles should be documented in the comments section of the worksheet.

Table 2.2 Steps in classifying the injury according to the AIS

a) Determine *sensory levels* for right and left sides.
- Starting from the top of the worksheet for sensory function, go down the column until you see a "1" or "0."
- Going up one level gives you the sensory level.

b) Determine *motor levels* for right and left sides.
- The motor level is the most caudal key muscle group that is graded ≥ 3/5 with all segments above graded 5/5 strength.
- In regions where there is no myotome to test, the motor level is presumed to be the same as the sensory level, if testable motor function above that level is also normal.

c) Determine the neurological level of injury.
The most rostral of the sensory and motor levels determined in steps 1 and 2.

d) Determine whether the injury is complete or incomplete (sacral sparing).
Sacral sparing = sensory or motor function in the lowest sacral segments, that includes sharp/dull edge discrimination or LT at S4–S5, VAC, or DAP.

e) Determine AIS grade.
1. Is injury complete (i.e., no sacral sparing)?
If yes, AIS = A; and record ZPP, if present.
2. If incomplete, is injury motor incomplete?
- No: AIS = B. (AIS B refers to a case where there is no voluntary anal contraction OR motor function more than 3 levels below the *motor level* on a given side, if the patient has sensory incomplete classification).
- Yes: presence of VAC OR motor function > three levels below the *motor level* on a given side if the patient has sensory incomplete classification.
3. If motor incomplete, are ≥ 50% of the key muscles below the *neurological level* graded 3 or better? If no, AIS = C. If yes, AIS – D.
4. If sensation and motor function is normal in all segments, AIS = E.
- Note: AIS E is used in follow-up testing when an individual with a documented SCI has recovered normal function. If no deficits are found at initial testing, the individual is considered neurologically intact, and the AIS does not apply.

Abbreviations: AIS, ASIA Impairment Scale; DAP, deep anal pressure; LT, light touch; SCI, spinal cord injury; VAC, voluntary anal contraction; ZPP, zone of partial preservation.

AIS D: Motor incomplete status as described above, with at least half (half or more) of the key muscles below the single NLI having a muscle grade of ≥ 3.

It is important to note that to distinguish AIS C versus AIS D, the motor scores below the single NLI are used, whereas to distinguish between an AIS B and AIS C, the motor level on each side of the body is utilized. The reason for using the motor level to distinguish an AIS B versus AIS C is to avoid the possible situation when a patient may regain sensation in a single additional caudal level, changing the AIS from "C" to a "B." For example: a patient initially had a motor level of C5 and a sensory level of C4 with sensory sparing at S4/S5 and some motor sparing only in C6–C8. Using the neurological level, this patient would qualify for AIS C, since C8 motor is more than three levels below the neurological level (C4). If the patient regains normal sensation over time in the C5 dermatome (with no other changes), the neurological level becomes C5 and the patient would revert from an AIS C to B because C8 is no longer more than three levels below the neurological level, indicating "worsening" despite neurological improvement. This is avoided by using the motor level, since the designation is independent of the sensory level.

Table 2.3 Non-key muscles for ISNCSCI classification of individuals as AIS B versus AIS C

Primary movement	Root level
Shoulder: flexion, extension, adduction, internal and external rotation *Elbow:* supination	C5
Elbow: pronation *Wrist:* flexion	C6
Finger: flexion at proximal joint, extension *Thumb:* flexion, extension, and abduction in plane of thumb	C7
Finger: flexion at MCP joint *Thumb:* opposition, adduction, and abduction perpendicular to palm	C8
Finger: abduction of the index finger	T1
Hip: adduction	L2
Hip: external rotation	L3
Hip: extension, abduction, internal rotation *Knee:* flexion *Ankle:* inversion and eversion *Toe:* MP and IP extension	L4
Hallux and toe: DIP and PIP flexion and abduction	L5
Hallux: adduction	S1

Source: International Standards for Neurological Classification of Spinal Cord Injury.[1]
Abbreviations: DIP, distal interphalangeal; IP, interphalangeal; MCP, metacarpophalangeal; MP, metatarsophalangeal; PIP, proximal interphalangeal.

AIS E: All components of the standardized neurological examination are normal. The grade E is used in follow-up when testing an individual with a previously documented SCI that has recovered normal function. If at initial testing no neurological deficits are found, then the AIS does not apply.

For pediatric patients, training for the examination is well described in the WeeSTeP (www.http://asia-spinalinjury.org/learning/). The comprehensive examination of the ISNCSCI is thought to be too complex for the cognitive abilities and tolerance of children younger than 6 years[38,39,40,41] and some patients as old as 8 years may have difficulty with the exam.[38,40] As periodic updates to the ISNCSCI classification occur, the reader is encouraged to visit the ASIA learning website for the most up to date classification rules.

2.5 Incomplete SCI Syndromes

A variety of clinical SCI syndromes have been previously described and include central cord, Brown-Sequard, anterior cord, posterior cord, and discomplete syndromes. Majority of these syndromes have remained largely unchanged since they were originally noted in literature, with the exception of central cord syndrome. Cauda equina and conus medullaris syndromes are also important to understand with respect to SCI, though are outside of the scope of this text.

Central cord syndrome (CCS) is the most common of the incomplete injury syndromes, accounting for 9% of all traumatic SCI and approximately 50% of incomplete injuries. CCS is characterized by motor weakness, which is greater in the upper extremities than the lower extremities, in association with sacral sparing.[42,43] At the level of injury there is lower motor neuron (LMN) weakness as well as sensory loss, with upper motor neuron (UMN) paralysis below the lesion level. In addition to the motor weakness, other features include bladder dysfunction and varying sensory loss below the level of the lesion. CCS most commonly occurs in older persons with existing cervical spondylosis who suffer a hyperextension injury, typically from a fall, followed by motor vehicle crashes. However, CCS may occur in persons of any age and is associated with other etiologies, predisposing factors, and injury mechanisms also. The postulated mechanism of injury involves compression of the cord both anteriorly and posteriorly by degenerative changes of the bony structures, with inward bulging of the ligamentum flavum during hyperextension in an already narrowed spinal canal.[42,43,44,45,46,47] Occurring with or without fracture or dislocation, CCS was initially described to be caused by hemorrhage to the central cord. Subsequent research, however, has not supported this and instead identifies that the deficits are predominately due to white matter lesions, with potential further gray matter involvement (when accompanied with LMN findings in upper extremities).[44,45] The finding that the upper extremities are relatively more involved than the lower extremities was initially postulated due to more central location of fibers of the upper limb within spinal cord motor tracts (with the lower limbs more peripherally located).[42,46] This has been challenged, with more recent studies being supportive of a disproportionate distribution of the corticospinal tract contributing to hand and upper extremity function, thereby any injury to the tract leading to more accentuated symptoms in these areas.[48] Definitive diagnostic criteria for traumatic CCS remain unclear with a lack of consensus on the degree of upper extremity weakness or lower extremity sparing required for classification.[49,50]

Research has demonstrated the degree of motor discrepancy between upper and lower extremities does not prognosticate recovery, instead, the AIS remains most predictive of recovery.[51] CCS usually has a favorable prognosis.[47,52,53,54] The typical pattern of recovery occurs first and to the greatest extent in the lower extremities, followed by bowel and bladder function, upper extremity (proximal), and finally intrinsic (distal) hand function. The prognosis for functional recovery of ambulation, activities of daily living (ADL), and bowel and bladder function are dependent upon the patient's age, with a less optimistic prognosis in older patients relative to younger patients.[53,54] Patients < 50 years of age are more successful in achieving independent ambulation than older patients (87–97 vs. 31–41%). Similar differences were seen between the younger and older patients in independent bladder function (83 vs. 29%), independent bowel function (63 vs. 24%), and dressing (77 vs. 12%). However, for patients with initial neurological examinations (within 72 hours) classification of AIS D tetraplegia, prognosis for recovery of independent ambulation is excellent, even for those whose age is > 50 years.[55]

A syndrome with similar clinical features of upper extremity paresis or paralysis, with minimal to no lower extremity involvement is *cruciate paralysis*.[56,57,58,59,60,61] This may occur with fractures of C1 and C2, and subsequent neurological compromise of the brainstem at the cervicomedullary junction.[57] This contrasts CCS that is usually localized in the mid to lower segments of the cervical spinal cord (i.e., C4–C5). Respiratory insufficiency occurs in roughly 25% of patients with cruciate paralysis and cranial nerves can also demonstrate deficits.

Overall, the prognosis for cruciate paralysis is excellent, with studies noting more than 50% of patients with complete recovery.[57] Wallenberg proposed an anatomical explanation for this clinical syndrome,[62] suggesting that the decussation of the fibers to the upper limb lay in a more rostral, medial, and ventral location in the cervicomedullary junction compared to a more lateral and caudal location of the lower limb decussating fibers. Therefore, injury to the canal, where the upper extremity fibers travel alone after decussation, causes preferential injury to the upper limbs. Neuroanatomical evidence to support this hypothesis, however, has not been found.[63]

Brown-Sequard syndrome (BSS) is characterized by asymmetric paresis with hypoalgesia more marked on the less paretic side and accounts for 2 to 4% of all traumatic SCI.[62,63,64,65,66,67,68] In the classic presentation of BSS, there is: (a) ipsilateral loss of all sensory modalities *at* the level of the lesion; (b) ipsilateral flaccid paralysis *at* the level of the lesion; (c) ipsilateral loss of position sense and vibration *below* the lesion; (d) contralateral loss of pain and temperature *below* the lesion; and (e) ipsilateral motor loss (UMN) *below* the level of the lesion.

Understanding the underlying neuroanatomy allows for insight into this constellation of signs. Spinothalamic tract decussation within the spinal cord leads to contralateral loss of pain and temperature when injured. Corticospinal and dorsal column tracts decussate within the brainstem, explaining for clinical findings of loss of motor, proprioception, and vibration sense ipsilateral to the lesion.

Although BSS has traditionally been associated with knife injuries, a variety of etiologies, including those that result in closed spinal injuries with or without vertebral fractures may be the cause.[67,68,69] In addition, neoplastic causes and intramedullary inflammatory lesions, such as in multiple sclerosis, can result in partial or complete BSS. In clinical practice, the presentation of pure BSS is relatively rare. More often, patients present clinically with a combination of features of BSS and CCS, with varying degrees of ipsilateral hemiplegia and contralateral hemianalgesia. This has been termed as ***Brown-Sequard-plus syndrome***.[67]

Despite the variation in presentation, considerable consistency is found in the prognosis of BSS. Recovery usually takes place in the ipsilateral proximal extensors and then in the distal flexors.[70,71] Motor recovery of any extremity having pain/temperature sensory deficit occurs before the opposite extremity and these patients may expect functional gait recovery by 6 months.

Of the patients with BSS, 75 to 90% ambulate independently at discharge from rehabilitation and nearly 70% perform functional skills and ADL independently.[51,69,73] The most important predictor of function is whether the upper or lower limb is the predominant site of weakness. When the upper limb is weaker than the lower limb, patients are more likely to ambulate at discharge.[67] Recovery of bowel and bladder function is also favorable, with continence achieved in 82 and 89% patients, respectively.[67]

The ***anterior cord syndrome (ACS)*** accounts for 2.7% of traumatic SCI and classically involves a lesion affecting the anterior two-thirds of the spinal cord while preserving the posterior columns. ACS may occur from retropulsed disc or bone fragments,[72] direct injury to the anterior spinal cord, or most commonly with vascular injury or occlusion of the anterior spinal artery that provides the blood supply to the anterior spinal cord.[73] This vascular etiology can occur during surgery to the aorta (especially with clamping above the renal artery) or other processes that could decrease blood flow to the spinal cord (i.e., vertebral burst fracture). In ACS, there is a variable loss of motor as well as pinprick sensation with a relative preservation of light touch, proprioception, and deep-pressure sensation. Usually patients with ACS have only 10 to 20% chances of muscle recovery and even in those with some recovery, there is poor muscle power and coordination.[74]

The *posterior cord syndrome* is the least frequent of incomplete SCI syndromes and has been omitted from recent versions of the International Standards. It is characterized by preservation of pain, temperature, and touch appreciation with varying degrees of motor preservation, and an absence of all dorsal column function. Prognosis for ambulation is poor, secondary to the proprioceptive deficits.

Neurological pathways within the spinal cord may be spared even after a neurologically complete injury on clinical exam. The term *discomplete injury* was introduced by Dimitrevic and colleagues[75,76] to describe a clinically complete SCI with neurophysiological evidence of residual function and connectivity above and below the injury. Subsequent studies have demonstrated degrees of intact localization with quantitative sensory testing below the neurological level of injury in complete injuries (AIS A) without sparing of clinical motor, light touch or sharp/dull edge discrimination.[44,77,78,79,80]

Finnerup et al performed quantitative sensory testing (including thermal stimulation, pressure, pinch, and pain sensitivity) in 24 subjects with AIS A (with no sparing of voluntary motor function or preserved sharp/dull edge discrimination or light touch sensation below the injury), they found that 50% had vague localized sensation to the stimuli.[80] All patients had no cortical response to lower extremity (posterior tibial nerve) somatosensory evoked potentials. There was no relationship between the presence of this sensory perception and the level of injury or etiology. There was also no correlation between the presence of sensory perception and the presence or severity of spasticity or chronic neuropathic pain.[80]

Neuropathological studies found a similar percentage (50%) of anatomically discomplete injuries in persons with clinical evidence of complete injuries.[44,75] Furthermore, recent research on epidural stimulation in clinically complete injuries suggests the presence of such latent tracts.[81] However, it is still unclear where the spared information travels and what the preservation of these pathways represents. Knowledge of retained neural communication across a spinal cord injury may have consequences for treatment strategies and enhancing functional recovery. Further study is required in this area.

2.6 Autonomic Assessment

In addition to paralysis and sensory deficits following SCI, autonomic dysfunction may also play a prominent role and it includes difficulty with regulation of cardiovascular, bronchopulmonary, sexual, sudomotor, and other autonomic functions.[82,83] Assessment of autonomic function is inherently complicated by the complexity of the autonomic nervous system. However, a systemic evaluation tool, the International Standards to determine remaining Autonomic Function after Spinal Cord Injury (ISAFSCI),

has been developed by ASIA and the International Spinal Cord Society.[84] (▶ Fig. 2.3). The Autonomic Standards allow for documentation of general autonomic, urinary bladder, bowel, and sexual function. Recent evaluations have shown moderate to good interrater reliability of the ISAFSCI (Kappa 0.41–0.88 for its various subscales),[85] though planned revisions are ongoing.[86] Previous versions of these standards[87] also contained guidelines for documenting urodynamic evaluations, though this is not currently included in the required forms.

Urodynamic evaluation is a urologic procedure which involves filling the bladder with sterile water and monitoring pressure within the bladder, urethral sphincters, and rectum. In addition to noting the presence of sensation of filling and ability to volitionally void, live observation of developing pressure gradients allows for characterization of neurogenic lower urinary tract abnormalities which are common after SCI including bladder spasticity and detrusor sphincter dyssynergia. Furthermore, electromyography of the urethral sphincter may also be done. Urodynamics may induce autonomic dysreflexia in individuals with SCI at or above T6. This condition, marked by progressive, sympathetically mediated rise in systolic blood pressure > 20 mm Hg over baseline,[84] is caused by a typically noxious stimulus below the level of injury and is only symptomatic in approximately 40% of patients.[88,89,90] As overdistension of the bladder is the primary cause of autonomic dysreflexia,[91] documentation is appropriate.

Further formal assessments of autonomic function are possible through specialized electrophysiologic laboratory tests,[92] though are not routinely performed as part of standard assessment. The most widespread of these tests is the sympathetic skin responses.[93,94] This test assesses the autonomic nervous system's ability to generate a sweat response similar to the galvanic skin response used in "lie detector tests." The absence of this response in patients anatomically at risk for autonomic dysreflexia has been shown to be 93% predictive of autonomic dysreflexia occurrence on urodynamic testing.[95] Twenty-four-

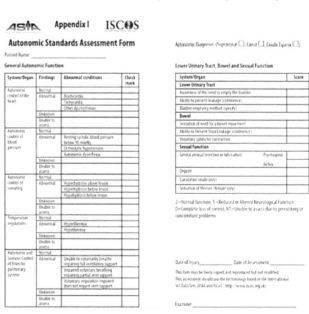

Fig. 2.3 International Standards to document remaining autonomic function after spinal cord injury (ISAFSCI) flowsheet. (Reproduced with permission.)[86]

hour ambulatory blood pressure monitoring has also been shown to be effective and quantifying the frequency and degree of autonomic dysreflexia throughout a patient's normal day[95,96] can be useful to more fully characterize the impact of autonomic dysfunction. Consideration and quantification of autonomic function remains important in fully characterizing function and is recommended for all patients following SCI.

References

[1] Kirshblum SC, Burns SP, Biering-Sorensen F, et al. International Standards for Neurological Classification of Spinal Cord Injury (revised 2011). J Spinal Cord Med. 2011; 34(6):535–546

[2] Kirshblum SC, Waring W, Biering-Sorensen F, et al. Reference for the 2011 revision of the International Standards for Neurological Classification of Spinal Cord Injury. J Spinal Cord Med. 2011; 34(6):547–554

[3] Waring WP, III, Biering-Sorensen F, Burns S, et al. 2009 review and revisions of the international standards for the neurological classification of spinal cord injury. J Spinal Cord Med. 2010; 33(4):346–352

[4] Vogel L, Samdani A, Chafetz R, Gaughan J, Betz R, Mulcahey MJ. Intra-rater agreement of the anorectal exam and classification of injury severity in children with spinal cord injury. Spinal Cord. 2009; 47(9):687–691

[5] Daniels L, Worthingham C. Muscle Testing Techniques of Manual Examination, 5th ed. Philadelphia, PA: WB Sanders; 1986

[6] Ditunno JF, Little JW, Tessler A, Burns AS. Spinal shock revisited: a four-phase model. Spinal Cord. 2004; 42(7):383–395

[7] Marino RJ, Graves DE. Metric properties of the ASIA motor score: subscales improve correlation with functional activities. Arch Phys Med Rehabil. 2004; 85(11):1804–1810

[8] Marino RJ, Rider-Foster D, Maissel G, Ditunno JF. Superiority of motor level over single neurological level in categorizing tetraplegia. Paraplegia. 1995; 33(9):510–513

[9] Waters RL, Adkins RH, Yakura JS. Definition of complete spinal cord injury. Paraplegia. 1991; 29(9):573–581

[10] American Spinal Injury Association/International Medical Society of Paraplegia (ASIA/IMSOP). International Standards for Neurological and Functional Classification of Spinal Cord Injury Patients (Revised). Chicago, IL: American Spinal Injury Association; 1992

[11] Bracken MB, Webb SB, Jr, Wagner FC. Classification of the severity of acute spinal cord injury: implications for management. Paraplegia. 1978-78; 15(4):319–326

[12] Roaf R. International classification of spinal injuries. Paraplegia. 1972; 10(1):78–84

[13] Chehrazi B, Wagner FC, Jr, Collins WF, Jr, Freeman DH, Jr. A scale for evaluation of spinal cord injury. J Neurosurg. 1981; 54(3):310–315

[14] Jochheim KA. Problems of classification in traumatic paraplegia and tetraplegia. Paraplegia. 1970; 8(2):80–82

[15] Mabray MC, Talbott JF, Whetstone WD, et al. Multidimensional analysis of magnetic resonance imaging predicts early impairment in thoracic and thoracolumbar spinal cord injury. J Neurotrauma. 2016; 33(10):954–962

[16] Kirshblum SC, Donovan W. Neurological assessment and classification of traumatic spinal cord injury. In: Kirshblum SC, Campagnolo D, DeLisa JE, eds. Spinal Cord Medicine. Philadelphia. Lippincott/Williams and Wilkins. 2002:82–95

[17] Kirshblum S, Waring W, III. Updates for the International Standards for Neurological Classification of Spinal Cord Injury. Phys Med Rehabil Clin N Am. 2014; 25(3):505–517, vii

[18] Chafetz RS, Prak S, Mulcahey MJ. Computerized classification of neurologic injury based on the International Standards for Classification of Spinal Cord Injury. J Spinal Cord Med. 2009; 32(5):532–537

[19] Walden K, Bélanger LM, Biering-Sørensen F, et al. Development and validation of a computerized algorithm for International Standards for Neurological Classification of Spinal Cord Injury (ISNCSCI). Spinal Cord. 2016; 54(3): 197–203

[20] Kirshblum SC, Biering-Sørensen F, Betz R, et al. International Standards for Neurological Classification of Spinal Cord Injury: cases with classification challenges. J Spinal Cord Med. 2014; 37(2):120–127

[21] Schuld C, Franz S, van Hedel HJ, et al. EMSCI study group. International Standards for Neurological Classification of Spinal Cord Injury: classification skills of clinicians versus computational algorithms. Spinal Cord. 2015; 53(4):324–331

[22] Franz S, Kirshblum SC, Weidner N, Rupp R, Schuld C, EMSCI study group. Motor levels in high cervical spinal cord injuries: implications for the International Standards for Neurological Classification of Spinal Cord Injury. J Spinal Cord Med. 2016; 39(5):513–517

[23] Hales M, Biros E, Reznik JE. Reliability and validity of the sensory component of the International Standards for Neurological Classification of Spinal Cord Injury (ISNCSCI): a systematic review. Top Spinal Cord Inj Rehabil. 2015; 21(3):241–249

[24] Gündoğdu İ, Akyüz M, Öztürk EA, Çakci FA. Can spinal cord injury patients show a worsening in ASIA Impairment Scale Classification despite actually having neurological improvement? The limitation of ASIA Impairment Scale Classification. Spinal Cord. 2014; 52(9):667–670

[25] Spiess MR, Müller RM, Rupp R, Schuld C, van Hedel HJ, EM-SCI Study Group. Conversion in ASIA Impairment Scale during the first year after traumatic spinal cord injury. J Neurotrauma. 2009; 26(11):2027–2036

[26] Lucas JT, Ducker TB. Motor classification of spinal cord injuries with mobility, morbidity and recovery indices. Am Surg. 1979; 45(3):151–158

[27] Bracken MB, Hildreth N, Freeman DH, Jr, Webb SB. Relationship between neurological and functional status after acute spinal cord injury: an epidemiological study. J Chronic Dis. 1980; 33(2):115–125

[28] Bracken MB, Collins WF, Freeman DF, et al. Efficacy of methylprednisolone in acute spinal cord injury. JAMA. 1984; 251(1):45–52

[29] Bracken MB, Shepard MJ, Collins WF, et al. A randomized, controlled trial of methylprednisolone or naloxone in the treatment of acute spinal-cord injury. Results of the Second National Acute Spinal Cord Injury Study. N Engl J Med. 1990; 322(20):1405–1411

[30] El Masry WS, Tsubo M, Katoh S, El Miligui YHS, Khan A. Validation of the American Spinal Injury Association (ASIA) motor score and the National Acute Spinal Cord Injury Study (NASCIS) motor score. Spine. 1996; 21(5):614–619

[31] Cohen ME, Bartko JJ. Reliability of the ISCSCI-92. In: Ditunno JF, Donovan WH, Maynard FM, eds. Reference Manual for the International Standards for Neurological and functional Classification of Spinal Cord Injury. ASIA, Chicago; 1994: 59–66

[32] Marino RJ, Jones L, Kirshblum S, Tal J, Dasgupta A. Reliability and repeatability of the motor and sensory examination of the international standards for neurological classification of spinal cord injury. J Spinal Cord Med. 2008; 31(2):166–170

[33] Jonsso, n M, Tollbäck A, Gonzales H, Borg J. Inter-rater reliability of the 1992 international standards for neurological and functional classification of incomplete spinal cord injury. Spinal Cord. 2000; 38(11):675–679

[34] Savic G, Bergström EM, Frankel HL, Jamous MA, Jones PW. Inter-rater reliability of motor and sensory examinations performed according to American Spinal Injury Association standards. Spinal Cord. 2007; 45(6):444–451

[35] Marino RJ. Neurological and functional outcomes in spinal cord injury: review and recommendations. Top Spinal Cord Inj Rehabil. 2005; 10:51–64

[36] Schuld C, Wiese J, Franz S, et al. EMSCI Study Group. Effect of formal training in scaling, scoring and classification of the International Standards for Neurological Classification of Spinal Cord Injury. Spinal Cord. 2013; 51(4):282–288

[37] Liu N, Zhou MW, Krassioukov AV, Biering-Sørensen F. Training effectiveness when teaching the International Standards for Neurological Classification of Spinal Cord Injury (ISNCSCI) to medical students. Spinal Cord. 2013; 51(10):768–771

[38] Mulcahey MJ, Gaughan JP, Chafetz RS, Vogel LC, Samdani AF, Betz RR. Interrater reliability of the international standards for neurological classification of spinal cord injury in youths with chronic spinal cord injury. Arch Phys Med Rehabil. 2011; 92(8):1264–1269

[39] Chafetz RS, Gaughan JP, Vogel LC, Betz R, Mulcahey MJ. The international standards for neurological classification of spinal cord injury: intra-rater agreement of total motor and sensory scores in the pediatric population. J Spinal Cord Med. 2009; 32(2):157–161

[40] Mulcahey MJ, Gaughan J, Betz RR, Johansen KJ. The International Standards for Neurological Classification of Spinal Cord Injury: reliability of data when applied to children and youths. Spinal Cord. 2007; 45(6):452–459

[41] Krisa L, Mulcahey MJ, Gaughan JP, Smith B, Vogel LC. Using a limited number of dermatomes as a predictor of the 56-dermatome test of the international standards for neurological classification of spinal cord injury in the pediatric population. Top Spinal Cord Inj Rehabil. 2013; 19(2):114–120

[42] Schneider RC, Cherry G, Pantek H. The syndrome of acute central cervical spinal cord injury; with special reference to the mechanisms involved in hyperextension injuries of cervical spine. J Neurosurg. 1954; 11(6):546–577

[43] Quencer RM, Bunge RP, Egnor M, et al. Acute traumatic central cord syndrome: MRI-pathological correlations. Neuroradiology. 1992; 34(2):85–94

[44] Bunge RP, Puckett WR, Becerra JL, Marcillo A, Quencer RM. Observations on the pathology of human spinal cord injury. A review and classification of 22 new cases with details from a case of chronic cord compression with extensive focal demyelination. Adv Neurol. 1993; 59:75–89

[45] Kakulas BA, Bedbrook GM. Pathology of injuries of the vertebral column. In: Vinken PJ and Bruyn GW, eds. Handbook of Clinical Neurology, Vol 25. Amsterdam; N. Holland Pub Co. 1976:27–42

[46] Taylor AR. The mechanism of injury to the spinal cord in the neck without damage to vertebral column. J Bone Joint Surg Br. 1951; 33-B(4):543–547

[47] McKinley W, Santos K, Meade M, Brooke K. Incidence and outcomes of spinal cord injury clinical syndromes. J Spinal Cord Med. 2007; 30(3):215–224

[48] Levi AD, Tator CH, Bunge RP. Clinical syndromes associated with disproportionate weakness of the upper versus the lower extremities after cervical spinal cord injury. Neurosurgery. 1996; 38(1):179–183, discussion 183–185

[49] Pouw MH, van Middendorp JJ, van Kampen A, et al. EM-SCI study group. Diagnostic criteria of traumatic central cord syndrome. Part 1: a systematic review of clinical descriptors and scores. Spinal Cord. 2010; 48(9):652–656

[50] van Middendorp JJ, Pouw MH, Hayes KC, et al. EM-SCI Study Group Collaborators. Diagnostic criteria of traumatic central cord syndrome. Part 2: a questionnaire survey among spine specialists. Spinal Cord. 2010; 48(9):657–663

[51] Pouw MH, van Middendorp JJ, van Kampen A, Curt A, van de Meent H, Hosman AJ. Diagnostic criteria of traumatic central cord syndrome. Part 3: descriptive analyses of neurological and functional outcomes in a prospective cohort of traumatic motor incomplete tetraplegics. Spinal Cord. 2011; 49(5):614–622

[52] Merriam WF, Taylor TKF, Ruff SJ, McPhail MJ. A reappraisal of acute traumatic central cord syndrome. J Bone Joint Surg Br. 1986; 68(5):708–713

[53] Penrod LE, Hegde SK, Ditunno JF, Jr. Age effect on prognosis for functional recovery in acute, traumatic central cord syndrome. Arch Phys Med Rehabil. 1990; 71(12):963–968

[54] Roth EJ, Lawler MH, Yarkony GM. Traumatic central cord syndrome: clinical features and functional outcomes. Arch Phys Med Rehabil. 1990; 71(1):18–23

[55] Burns SP, Golding DG, Rolle WA, Jr. Graziani V, Ditunno JF, Jr. Recovery of ambulation in motor-incomplete tetraplegia. Arch Phys Med Rehabil. 1997; 78(11):1169–1172

[56] Bell HS. Paralysis of both arms from injury of the upper portion of the pyramidal decussation: "cruciate paralysis". J Neurosurg. 1970; 33(4):376–380

[57] Dickman CA, Hadley MN, Pappas CTE, Sonntag VKH, Geisler FH. Cruciate paralysis: a clinical and radiographic analysis of injuries to the cervicomedullary junction. J Neurosurg. 1990; 73(6):850–858

[58] Erlich V, Snow R, Heier L. Confirmation by magnetic resonance imaging of Bell's cruciate paralysis in a young child with Chiari type I malformation and minor head trauma. Neurosurgery. 1989; 25(1):102–105

[59] Marano SR, Calica AB, Sonntag VKH. Bilateral upper extremity paralysis (Bell's cruciate paralysis) from a gunshot wound to the cervicomedullary junction. Neurosurgery. 1986; 18(5):642–644

[60] Schneider RC, Crosby EC, Russo RH, Gosch HH. Chapter 32. Traumatic spinal cord syndromes and their management. Clin Neurosurg. 1973; 20:424–492

[61] Hatzakis MJ, Jr, Bryce N, Marino R. Cruciate paralysis, hypothesis for injury and recovery. Spinal Cord. 2000; 38(2):120–125

[62] Wallenberg A. Anatomischer Befund in einem als "acute bulbaraffection (embolie der cerebellar post inf sinista?)" beschreiben falle. Arch Phychiatr. 1901; 34:923–959

[63] Pappas CTE, Gibson AR, Sonntag VKH. Decussation of hind-limb and fore-limb fibers in the monkey corticospinal tract: relevance to cruciate paralysis. J Neurosurg. 1991; 75(6):935–940

[64] Bohlman HH. Acute fractures and dislocations of the cervical spine. An analysis of three hundred hospitalized patients and review of the literature. J Bone Joint Surg Am. 1979; 61(8):1119–1142

[65] Bosch A, Stauffer ES, Nickel VL. Incomplete traumatic quadriplegia. A ten-year review. JAMA. 1971; 216(3):473–478

[66] Brown-Sequard CE. Lectures on the physiology and pathology of the central nervous system and the treatment of organic nervous affections. Lancet. 1868; 2:593–595, 659–662, 755–757, 821–823

[67] Roth EJ, Park T, Pang T, Yarkony GM, Lee MY. Traumatic cervical Brown-Sequard and Brown-Sequard-plus syndromes: the spectrum of presentations and outcomes. Paraplegia. 1991; 29(9):582–589

[68] Tattersall R, Turner B. Brown-Séquard and his syndrome. Lancet. 2000; 356(9223):61–63

[69] Koehler PJ, Endtz LJ. The Brown-Séquard syndrome. True or false? Arch Neurol. 1986; 43(9):921–924

[70] Graziani V, Tessler A, Ditunno JF. Incomplete tetraplegia: sequence of lower extremity motor recovery. J Neurotrauma. 1995; 12:121

[71] Little JW, Halar E. Temporal course of motor recovery after Brown-Sequard spinal cord injuries. Paraplegia. 1985; 23(1):39–46

[72] Bauer RD, Errico TJ. Cervical spine injuries. In: Errico TJ, Bauer RD, Waugh T, eds. Spinal Trauma. Philadelphia, PA: JB Lippincott; 1991:71–121

[73] Cheshire WP, Santos CC, Massey EW, Howard JF, Jr. Spinal cord infarction: etiology and outcome. Neurology. 1996; 47(2):321–330

[74] Bohlman HH, Ducker TB. Spine and spinal cord injuries. In: Rothman RH, ed. The Spine. 3rd ed. Philadelphia, PA: WB Saunders; 1992:973–1011

[75] Dimitrijevic MR. Neurophysiology in spinal cord injury. Paraplegia. 1987; 25(3):205–208

[76] Sherwood AM, Dimitrijevic MR, McKay WB. Evidence of subclinical brain influence in clinically complete spinal cord injury: discomplete SCI. J Neurol Sci. 1992; 110(1–2):90–98

[77] Dimitrijevic MR, Dimitrijevic MM, Faganel J, Sherwood AM. Suprasegmentally induced motor unit activity in paralyzed muscles of patients with established spinal cord injury. Ann Neurol. 1984; 16(2):216–221

[78] Kakulas BA. The applied neuropathology of human spinal cord injury. Spinal Cord. 1999; 37(2):79–88

[79] Sabbah P, Lévêque C, Pfefer F, et al. Functional MR imaging and traumatic paraplegia: preliminary report. J Neuroradiol. 2000; 27(4):233–237

[80] Finnerup NB, Gyldensted C, Fuglsang-Frederiksen A, Bach FW, Jensen TS. Sensory perception in complete spinal cord injury. Acta Neurol Scand. 2004; 109(3):194–199

[81] Angeli CA, Edgerton VR, Gerasimenko YP, Harkema SJ. Altering spinal cord excitability enables voluntary movements after chronic complete paralysis in humans. Brain. 2014; 137(Pt 5):1394–1409

[82] Krassioukov A, Claydon VE. The clinical problems in cardiovascular control following spinal cord injury: an overview. Prog Brain Res. 2006; 152:223–229

[83] Mathias CJ, Frankel HL. Autonomic disturbances in spinal cord lesions. In: Bannister R, Mathias CJ, eds. Autonomic Failure: A Textbook of Clinical Disorders of the Autonomic Nervous System. Oxford Medical Publications; 2002:839–881

[84] Krassioukov A, Biering-Sørensen F, Donovan W, et al. Autonomic Standards Committee of the American Spinal Injury Association/International Spinal Cord Society. International standards to document remaining autonomic function after spinal cord injury. J Spinal Cord Med. 2012; 35(4):201–210

[85] Davidson RA, Carlson M, Fallah N, et al. Inter-rater reliability of the International Standards to document remaining autonomic function after spinal cord injury. J Neurotrauma. 2017; 34(3):552–558

[86] Round AM, Park SE, Walden K, Noonan VK, Townson AF, Krassioukov AV. An evaluation of the International Standards to document remaining autonomic function after spinal cord injury: input from the international community. Spinal Cord. 2017; 55(2):198–203

[87] Krassioukov AV, Karlsson AK, Wecht JM, Wuermser LA, Mathias CJ, Marino RJ, Joint Committee of American Spinal Injury Association and International Spinal Cord Society. Assessment of autonomic dysfunction following spinal cord injury: rationale for additions to International Standards for Neurological Assessment. J Rehabil Res Dev. 2007; 44(1):103–112

[88] Kirshblum SC, House JG, O'connor KC. Silent autonomic dysreflexia during a routine bowel program in persons with traumatic spinal cord injury: a preliminary study. Arch Phys Med Rehabil. 2002; 83(12):1774–1776

[89] Linsenmeyer TA, Campagnolo DI, Chou IH. Silent autonomic dysreflexia during voiding in men with spinal cord injuries. J Urol. 1996; 155(2):519–522

[90] Ekland MB, Krassioukov AV, McBride KE, Elliott SL. Incidence of autonomic dysreflexia and silent autonomic dysreflexia in men with spinal cord injury undergoing sperm retrieval: implications for clinical practice. J Spinal Cord Med. 2008; 31(1):33–39

[91] Liu N, Fougere R, Zhou MW, Nigro MK, Krassioukov AV. Autonomic dysreflexia severity during urodynamics and cystoscopy in individuals with spinal cord injury. Spinal Cord. 2013; 51(11):863–867

[92] Low PA. Laboratory evaluation of autonomic function. Suppl Clin Neurophysiol. 2004; 57:358–368

[93] Cariga P, Catley M, Mathias CJ, Savic G, Frankel HL, Ellaway PH. Organisation of the sympathetic skin response in spinal cord injury. J Neurol Neurosurg Psychiatry. 2002; 72(3):356–360

[94] Hubli M, Krassioukov AV. How reliable are sympathetic skin responses in subjects with spinal cord injury? Clin Auton Res. 2015; 25(2):117–124

[95] Curt A, Nitsche B, Rodic B, Schurch B, Dietz V. Assessment of autonomic dysreflexia in patients with spinal cord injury. J Neurol Neurosurg Psychiatry. 1997; 62(5):473–477

[96] Hubli M, Krassioukov AV. Ambulatory blood pressure monitoring in spinal cord injury: clinical practicability. J Neurotrauma. 2014; 31(9):789–797

Appendix 2.1 Glossary of Key Terms

Dermatome: The area of the skin innervated by the sensory axons within each segmental nerve root.

Myotome: The collection of muscle fibers innervated by the motor axons within each segmental nerve root.

Key muscle groups: Ten muscle groups that are tested as part of the standardized spinal cord examination.

Root level	Muscle group	Root level	Muscle group
C5	Elbow flexors	L2	Hip flexors
C6	Wrist extensors	L3	Knee extensors
C7	Elbow extensors	L4	Ankle dorsiflexors
C8	Long Finger flexors	L5	Long toe extensor
T1	Small finger abductors	S1	Ankle plantarflexors

Non-key muscle function: Muscle functions that are not part of the key muscle functions that are routinely tested. In a patient with an apparent AIS B classification, non-key muscle functions > three levels below the motor level on each side should be tested to most accurately classify the injury and differentiate between AIS B vs. C.

Motor level: The most caudal key muscle group that is graded 3/5 or greater with the segments cephalad graded normal (5/5) strength.

Motor index score: Calculated by adding the muscle scores of each key muscle group; a total score of 100 is possible. It is now recommended to separate the motor scores into 2 scores; one for the upper limb and one for the lower limb.

Sensory level: The most caudal dermatome to have normal sensation for both pin prick/dull and light touch on both sides.

Nondeterminable (ND): This term is used on the worksheet when any component of the scoring cannot be determined based upon the examination results.

Neurological level of injury (NLI): The most caudal level at which both motor and sensory modalities are intact.

Sacral sparing: The presence of residual preserved neurological function at the most caudal aspect of the cord determined by examination of sensory and motor functions. This includes the preservation of light touch or pin (intact or impaired) on either side at the S4–S5 dermatome, presence of DAP or VAC.

Complete injury: The absence of sensory and motor function in the lowest sacral segments (i.e. no sacral sparing).

Incomplete injury: Preservation of motor and/or sensory function below the neurologic level that includes the lowest sacral segments (i.e., presence of sacral sparing).

Zone of partial preservation (ZPP): Used only with complete injuries, refers to the dermatomes and myotomes caudal to the motor and sensory levels that remain partially innervated. The most caudal segment with some sensory and/or motor function defines the extent of the ZPP.

Abbreviations: DAP, deep anal pressure; VAC, voluntary anal contraction.

Source: International Standards for Neurological Classification of Spinal Cord Injury.[1]

3 Pathophysiology of Spinal Cord Injury

Assem A. Sultan and Edward C. Benzel

Abstract

Spinal cord injury may result from traumatic or nontraumatic events. Treatment options for traumatic spinal cord injury depend on the pathophysiology of the spinal cord injury. In this chapter, we discuss the two pathophysiologic phases of injury to help determine appropriate treatment interventions. The secondary phase is further divided into four stages: the acute stage, the subacute stage, the intermediate stage, and the chronic stage. We briefly discuss the neuroprotective and neuroregenerative effects at the cellular and biochemical levels.

Keywords: spinal cord injury, pathophysiologic mechanism, phases of injury, neuroprotective effect, neuroregenerative effect

3.1 Introduction

Acute traumatic spinal cord injury (SCI) is a devastating sequela of physical trauma to the spinal cord. Depending on the severity of trauma, partial to complete loss of neurological functions will result at or below the level of the injury. It is estimated that of the 12,000 new patients diagnosed with SCI each year in the United States, 4,000 die before they reach hospital while 1,000 die during hospitalization.[1,2,3,4] Therefore, the sequelae of SCI extend beyond affecting patients and their families and carries a substantial socioeconomic impact globally.[5,6,7] Despite the demonstrated value of supportive care, particularly in reducing mortality due to SCI,[8] the natural history of irreversible paralysis due to SCI continues to burden both patients and health care systems.[5,9] Therefore, ongoing research efforts have attempted to investigate potential neuroprotective and neuroregenerative interventions through a better understanding of the pathophysiological events involved in SCI on both the macroscopic and the molecular scales. The purpose of this chapter is to elucidate the pathophysiologic mechanisms implicated in SCI. Detailed discussion of the clinical presentation as well as management options for SCI has not been provided as that is the focus of the other chapters in this text.

3.2 Epidemiology

The annual incidence of SCI is estimated to be 12 to 53 cases per million population individuals in developed countries and 15 to 40 cases per million individuals worldwide.[8,10,11,12] In the United States, 12,000 new cases of SCI are recorded each year.[7,13] Cervical spine injury is the most common anatomical location for injury and associated with the greatest morbidity and cost. Of all SCI cases, 54 to 75% occur in the cervical spine, while 15% are estimated to occur in the thoracic spine, and 10% in the lumbar spine.[5,7,8,14]

Analysis of National Spinal Cord Injury Database (NSCID) records revealed important trends on the incidence and prevalence of SCI. Increasing mean age at injury has been observed from a mean of 28.7 years between 1973 and 1979 to 38.0 years between 2000 and 2003.[12] In addition, the prevalence has markedly risen in the elderly population from 4.7% between 1973 and 1979 to almost 11% between 2000 and 2003.[12] Conversely, the prevalence has fallen for children between 0 and 15 years from 6.4 to 2% during the same period.[12] The increasing incidence of SCI among the elderly population can have clinical implications on the management of this subset of patients with specific needs and age-related co-morbidities. However, young male patients continue to be the most often impacted by SCI, the majority of whom are healthy and at their physical peak.[7,14]

Etiologically, motor vehicle accidents are the dominant cause of SCI accounting for 50% of all causes of injury in all age groups. Alcohol consumption is linked to 25% of cases.[8,9] In addition, falls are the second most common cause of SCI in all age groups and the most common cause for patients who are aged 60 years and more.[9] Furthermore, the overall incidence for SCI from falls and work-related injuries has consistently increased over the past 30 years and accounts for 30% of all SCIs.[12] Other causes for SCI include violence which accounts for 11% of injuries and sports-related injuries which accounts for 9% of all SCIs.[8,9]

SCI is associated with significant mortality and morbidity with a mortality rate ranging between 4 to 17% during the initial admission.[2] In addition, morbidity is largely affected by the high incidence of cervical spine injuries among patients with acute SCI with the most common injury pattern being incomplete tetraplegia (34.5%), followed by complete paraplegia (23.1%), complete tetraplegia (18.4%), and incomplete paraplegia (17.5%). For these patients, quality of life is determined by pain, extent of loss of visceral functions, and hand functions.[15]

3.3 Pathological Phases of Injury

The pathogenesis of acute traumatic SCI is a biphasic process.[16,17,18] In the primary phase, immediate damage is caused by the initial physical trauma leading to local deformation of the neural elements and disruption of the local circulation. This is followed by a secondary phase of progressive injury caused by an interplay of complex biochemical, cellular, and systemic reactions to the primary insult.[16,19,20] Although the changes in the secondary phase aim to provide a neuroprotective effect, the true end result is progressive neural destruction that can continue for several weeks or months following the initial trauma. Understanding the order and timing of pathophysiologic changes in the secondary phase may help guide different treatment regimen instituted in the context of acute SCI. Historically, the model of primary and secondary phases of injury was first demonstrated in animal studies.[21] Since then, multiple mechanisms have been uncovered, some of which have been implicated in the secondary phase of acute SCI.[18,22,23,24,25,26,27,28,29]

3.3.1 Primary Spinal Cord Injury

In this phase, primary injury forces can result from acute compression, shearing, laceration, distraction, or acceleration-deceleration, all of which can subject the spinal cord to contusion and persistent compression.[30,31] Common clinical scenarios include burst fractures, flexion–distraction injuries, and penetrating missile injuries. Anatomical disruption can lead to complete spinal cord transection, but more commonly partial disruption is encountered.[7] In this situation, spared neural axons may traverse the damaged area. However, these axons are frequently demyelinated and are subsequently dysfunctional.[32,33,34,35,36] Biochemically, this phase is marked by local elevation of proinflammatory mediators including tumor necrosis factor-α (TNF-α), interleukin 1-beta (IL-1β), and cytotoxic levels of glutamate due to cellular disruption.[37] The injury process involved in this phase can last for up to two hours following the initial trauma.[37]

3.3.2 Secondary Spinal Cord Injury

A growing body of evidence has demonstrated that a cascade of complex cellular and biochemical reactions follows the primary phase of injury and leads to progressive and delayed local neural elements destruction.[18,20,22,23,24,25,26,33,38,39,40] Multiple studies have attempted to identify key processes that may be targeted by neuroprotective interventions to improve clinical outcomes. Chronologically, the secondary phase can be divided into the early acute stage (first 48 hours), the subacute stage (2 weeks), the intermediate stage (6 months), and the chronic stage (beyond 6 months).[41] Each stage is mediated by specific pathological mechanisms. Ionic dysregulation, apoptosis, vascular mechanisms, and free radical generation are among the most widely accepted pathways implicated in the pathogenesis of this phase.[8,18,25,26]

In the early acute secondary phase, ionic dysregulation (particularly intracellular hypercalcemia) initiates a multitude of damaging processes including mitochondrial dysfunction and cell death.[42] This is triggered via a rapid increase in extracellular excitatory amino acids, namely glutamate and aspartate, following the primary injury phase. This leads to an influx of intracellular calcium.[25] Mitochondrial dysfunction and depletion of intracellular energy stores further impair ionic regulation through a disruption in the adenosine triphosphate (ATP)-dependent cell membrane Na$^+$/K$^+$ transporters. Furthermore, the Na$^+$/K$^+$/glutamate pump is disrupted leading to elevated levels of excitatory glutamate which in turn act on the N-methyl-D-aspartate, alpha-amino-3-hydroxy-5-methyl-4-isoxazolepropionic acid, and kainate receptors.[25] Consequently, this leads to a further influx of Ca^{2+} and Na$^+$ and a vicious cycle ensues. Moreover, with intracellular hypercalcemia, enzymes involved in cell degradation and death pathways are activated including phospholipases, calpain, caspase, and nitric oxide synthase (NOS).[43]

Free radicals also play an important role in mediating cell damage in the early phase.[44,45] Peaking during the first 12 hours, rising levels of intracellular free radicals progressively disrupt cell membranes by lipid peroxidation resulting in further ionic dysregulation, membrane transport, and eventually cell lysis. In addition, a rise in intracellular calcium inactivates cellular antioxidants that normally bind free radicals.[46] Free radicals also activate apoptotic pathways, with recent animal studies demonstrating that this role is largely mediated by the peroxynitrite radical molecule.[46] Calcium-induced mitochondrial dysfunction is believed to initiate free radical generation. Antioxidants therapy has thus gained interest as a potential treatment option during this phase.[46] High-dose methylprednisolone administration in the first 8 hours following neurological insult had previously gained popularity in clinical practice and was believed to provide a neuroprotective effect via counteracting lipid peroxidation in the early acute phase.[47,48,49,50,51,52] Modest clinical effect and demonstrated flaws in the methodology of supporting studies have prompted discontinuation of this in clinical practice.

Vascular impairment and spinal cord ischemia result from a myriad of systemic and local factors and are thought to significantly contribute to injury during the secondary phase.[38] Systemic factors are commonly seen in polytrauma patients who suffer from hemorrhagic shock with subsequent tissue hypoperfusion. Moreover, neurogenic shock can result from acute SCI with profound hypotension and bradycardia in complete cord injury. Decreased cardiac function and loss of the vascular sympathetic activity can lead to a prolonged systemic cardiovascular depression for several weeks or months following the onset of the injury. In addition, thoracic injuries and respiratory failure caused by respiratory muscle paralysis or fatigue may also contribute to local spinal cord hypoxemia. Locally there are also several mechanisms that lead to impaired microcirculation and tissue oxygenation.[38] Vasoactive amine release causes local vasospasm.[38] In addition, endothelial cell damage is one of the early acute phase events that can lead to increased local vascular permeability and interstitial edema which can also worsen the local ischemia. Furthermore, the central cord gray matter is more susceptible to ischemic insult than the peripheral white matter.[53,54] Normally, the central gray matter to peripheral white matter blood flow ratio is maintained at 3:1, which helps to explain ischemic susceptibility.[53,54,55] In addition, multiple animal studies have demonstrated loss of local spinal blood flow autoregulatory mechanisms in SCI and it is believed to contribute to local ischemic injury.[18,56] Moreover, impaired venous drainage and thrombosis has also been reported to play a pathogenic role.[57]

Necrosis and apoptosis are two important mechanisms involved in cell death in SCI.[58,59] Apoptosis has gained substantial attention in the literature, although it was mainly demonstrated in animal models.[39] Apoptosis or programmed cell death has been demonstrated to primarily affect oligodendrocytes resulting in axonal demyelination.[60] This process becomes evident between the first day to the end of the first week following initial injury.[59] However, this mechanism was not clearly demonstrated in human models of SCI.[61,62] Several extrinsic and intrinsic signals can activate apoptosis with activation of the intracellular caspases and proapoptotic proteins. The result is deoxyribonucleic acid (DNA) cleavage and proteolysis of cellular proteins followed by phagocytosis of shrunken cells, without an associated inflammatory response. Blocking the caspase pathway and suppressing apoptosis may provide a therapeutic benefit during the secondary phase of acute SCI.[25] As demonstrated, apoptosis is an active process that requires cellular energy expenditure, gene expression, and de novo enzyme synthesis. On the other hand, necrosis is a passive process of cellular damage that involves mitochondrial and cell membrane disruption and an intense local inflammatory response. Necroptosis is another newly described mechanism involving programmed necrosis and is believed to play a role in early neural cell damage following SCI.[63] Understanding this pathway paved the way for a new class of potentially cytoprotective agents that target key molecules involved in necroptosis.[64]

Although current evidence on necroptosis inhibition is largely driven from animal studies, the results hold promise for future human application.[65,66]

Cellular inflammatory response in the secondary phase is regulated by numerous proinflammatory cells. Neutrophils and microglial cells predominate the cellular response during the first few days.[67,68] Over the next 5 to 10 days activated microglial cells and macrophages become the predominant mediators. In addition, proinflammatory mediators are released by these cells including TNF-α, interferons, and ILs. Overall, multiple studies have demonstrated that this neuroinflammatory response can have both deleterious and protective effects.[37] Therefore, it is still unclear whether this response can be a target for therapeutic intervention.

Following the acute phase, a subacute phase begins which is characterized by astrocytic cell proliferation and phagocytosis of cellular and myelin debris, paving the way for axonal regeneration.[41] However, astroglial scar tissue also starts to form and studies have suggested that this may interfere with neural regeneration.[41] This occurs between 2 days and 2 weeks following the initial injury. Next, the intermediate phase follows and continues for 6 months. This phase is characterized by scar maturation and continued axonal regeneration. Finally, a chronic phase starts at 6 months and may continue for years; this is characterized by the formation of a stable glial scar, formation of a syrinx, and Wallerian degeneration.[41] A target for future research efforts may include attempt to improve the regenerative capacity and neural plasticity of spared axons.

3.4 Discussion

Traumatic SCI remains a challenge in clinical practice and more effective treatment options are yet to be discovered. Understanding the pathophysiologic phases of injury will help guide treatment interventions to alter the inevitable loss of neurological function. In the primary SCI phase, preventive measures which are aimed at enhancing safety on the road, in the house, or at work, are essential. In the secondary phase of SCI, complex cellular and biochemical reactions may add damage to the insult and render the healing environment hostile to neuronal regeneration. Despite the exponential expansion of our knowledge of secondary phase interactions, further studies are needed to help us better understand the unique reactions in human subjects and possibly guide future interventions.

References

[1] Sances A, Jr, Myklebust JB, Maiman DJ, Larson SJ, Cusick JF, Jodat RW. The biomechanics of spinal injuries. Crit Rev Biomed Eng. 1984; 11(1):1–76

[2] Kraus JF. Epidemiologic features of head and spinal cord injury. Adv Neurol. 1978; 19:261–279

[3] Carter RE, Jr. Etiology of traumatic spinal cord injury: statistics of more than 1,100 cases. Tex Med. 1977; 73(6):61–65

[4] Albin MS, White RJ. Epidemiology, physiopathology, and experimental therapeutics of acute spinal cord injury. Crit Care Clin. 1987; 3(3):441–452

[5] Harvey C, Wilson SE, Greene CG, Berkowitz M, Stripling TE. New estimates of the direct costs of traumatic spinal cord injuries: results of a nationwide survey. Paraplegia. 1992; 30(12):834–850

[6] Cripps RA, Lee BB, Wing P, Weerts E, Mackay J, Brown D. A global map for traumatic spinal cord injury epidemiology: towards a living data repository for injury prevention. Spinal Cord. 2011; 49(4):493–501

[7] Ackery A, Tator C, Krassioukov A. A global perspective on spinal cord injury epidemiology. J Neurotrauma. 2004; 21(10):1355–1370

[8] Sekhon LH, Fehlings MG. Epidemiology, demographics, and pathophysiology of acute spinal cord injury. Spine. 2001; 26(24) Suppl:S2–S12

[9] National Spinal Cord Injury Statistical Center. Spinal cord injury. Facts and figures at a glance. J Spinal Cord Med. 2014; 37(3):355–356

[10] Singh A, Tetreault L, Kalsi-Ryan S, Nouri A, Fehlings MG. Global prevalence and incidence of traumatic spinal cord injury. Clin Epidemiol. 2014; 6: 309–331

[11] Botterell EH, Jousse AT, Kraus AS, Thompson MG, WynneJones M, Geisler WO. A model for the future care of acute spinal cord injuries. Can J Neurol Sci. 1975; 2(4):361–380

[12] Jackson AB, Dijkers M, Devivo MJ, Poczatek RB. A demographic profile of new traumatic spinal cord injuries: change and stability over 30 years. Arch Phys Med Rehabil. 2004; 85(11):1740–1748

[13] van den Berg MEL, Castellote JM, de Pedro-Cuesta J, Mahillo-Fernandez I. Survival after spinal cord injury: a systematic review. J Neurotrauma. 2010; 27(8):1517–1528

[14] Pirouzmand F. Epidemiological trends of spine and spinal cord injuries in the largest Canadian adult trauma center from 1986 to 2006. J Neurosurg Spine. 2010; 12(2):131–140

[15] National Spinal Cord Injury Statistical Center. Spinal cord injury. Facts and figures at a glance. J Spinal Cord Med. 2005; 28(4):379–380

[16] Hagg T, Oudega M. Degenerative and spontaneous regenerative processes after spinal cord injury. J Neurotrauma. 2006; 23(3–4):264–280

[17] Amar AP, Levy ML. Pathogenesis and pharmacological strategies for mitigating secondary damage in acute spinal cord injury. Neurosurgery. 1999; 44(5):1027–1039, discussion 1039–1040

[18] Tator CH, Fehlings MG. Review of the secondary injury theory of acute spinal cord trauma with emphasis on vascular mechanisms. J Neurosurg. 1991; 75(1):15–26

[19] Sandler AN, Tator CH. Effect of acute spinal cord compression injury on regional spinal cord blood flow in primates. J Neurosurg. 1976; 45(6):660–676

[20] Collins WF. A review and update of experiment and clinical studies of spinal cord injury. Paraplegia. 1983; 21(4):204–219

[21] Allen AR. Aurgery of experimental lesion of spinal cord equivalent to crush injury of fracture dislocation of spinal column. J Am Med Assoc. 1911 (11):878

[22] Pehar M, Vargas MR, Robinson KM, et al. Peroxynitrite transforms nerve growth factor into an apoptotic factor for motor neurons. Free Radic Biol Med. 2006; 41(11):1632–1644

[23] McCord JM, Edeas MA. SOD, oxidative stress and human pathologies: a brief history and a future vision. Biomed Pharmacother. 2005; 59(4):139–142

[24] Popovich PG. Immunological regulation of neuronal degeneration and regeneration in the injured spinal cord. Prog Brain Res. 2000; 128:43–58

[25] Park E, Velumian AA, Fehlings MG. The role of excitotoxicity in secondary mechanisms of spinal cord injury: a review with an emphasis on the implications for white matter degeneration. J Neurotrauma. 2004; 21(6):754–774

[26] Mautes AE, Weinzierl MR, Donovan F, Noble LJ. Vascular events after spinal cord injury: contribution to secondary pathogenesis. Phys Ther. 2000; 80(7):673–687

[27] Ackery A, Robins S, Fehlings MG. Inhibition of Fas-mediated apoptosis through administration of soluble Fas receptor improves functional outcome and reduces posttraumatic axonal degeneration after acute spinal cord injury. J Neurotrauma. 2006; 23(5):604–616

[28] Buss A, Pech K, Merkler D, et al. Sequential loss of myelin proteins during Wallerian degeneration in the human spinal cord. Brain. 2005; 128(Pt 2):356–364

[29] Casha S, Yu WR, Fehlings MG. Oligodendroglial apoptosis occurs along degenerating axons and is associated with FAS and p75 expression following spinal cord injury in the rat. Neuroscience. 2001; 103(1):203–218

[30] Tator CH. Update on the pathophysiology and pathology of acute spinal cord injury. Brain Pathol. 1995; 5(4):407–413

[31] Baptiste DC, Fehlings MG. Pharmacological approaches to repair the injured spinal cord. J Neurotrauma. 2006; 23(3–4):318–334

[32] McDonald JW, Belegu V. Demyelination and remyelination after spinal cord injury. J Neurotrauma. 2006; 23(3–4):345–359

[33] Totoiu MO, Keirstead HS. Spinal cord injury is accompanied by chronic progressive demyelination. J Comp Neurol. 2005; 486(4):373–383

[34] Radojicic M, Reier PJ, Steward O, Keirstead HS. Septations in chronic spinal cord injury cavities contain axons. Exp Neurol. 2005; 196(2):339–341

[35] Nashmi R, Fehlings MG. Changes in axonal physiology and morphology after chronic compressive injury of the rat thoracic spinal cord. Neuroscience. 2001; 104(1):235–251

[36] Bunge RP, Puckett WR, Becerra JL, Marcillo A, Quencer RM. Observations on the pathology of human spinal cord injury. A review and classification of 22 new cases with details from a case of chronic cord compression with extensive focal demyelination. Adv Neurol. 1993; 59:75–89

[37] Fleming JC, Norenberg MD, Ramsay DA, et al. The cellular inflammatory response in human spinal cords after injury. Brain. 2006; 129(Pt 12):3249–3269

[38] Tator CH, Koyanagi I. Vascular mechanisms in the pathophysiology of human spinal cord injury. J Neurosurg. 1997; 86(3):483–492

[39] Dusart I, Schwab ME. Secondary cell death and the inflammatory reaction after dorsal hemisection of the rat spinal cord. Eur J Neurosci. 1994; 6(5):712–724

[40] Anderson DK, Hall ED. Pathophysiology of spinal cord trauma. Ann Emerg Med. 1993; 22(6):987–992

[41] Fitch MT, Silver J. CNS injury, glial scars, and inflammation: Inhibitory extracellular matrices and regeneration failure. Exp Neurol. 2008; 209(2):294–301

[42] Kroemer G, Petit P, Zamzami N, Vayssière JL, Mignotte B. The biochemistry of programmed cell death. FASEB J. 1995; 9(13):1277–1287

[43] Lipton SA, Rosenberg PA, Rosenberg PA. Excitatory amino acids as a final common pathway for neurologic disorders. N Engl J Med. 1994; 330(9):613–622

[44] Hall ED, Braughler JM. Free radicals in CNS injury. Res Publ Assoc Res Nerv Ment Dis. 1993; 71:81–105

[45] Siesjö BK. Pathophysiology and treatment of focal cerebral ischemia. Part II: Mechanisms of damage and treatment. J Neurosurg. 1992; 77(3):337–354

[46] Kurihara M. Role of monoamines in experimental spinal cord injury in rats. Relationship between Na + -K + -ATPase and lipid peroxidation. J Neurosurg. 1985; 62(5):743–749

[47] Bracken MB, Shepard MJ, Hellenbrand KG, et al. Methylprednisolone and neurological function 1 year after spinal cord injury. Results of the National Acute Spinal Cord Injury Study. J Neurosurg. 1985; 63(5):704–713

[48] Bracken MB, Shepard MJ, Collins WF, Jr, et al. Methylprednisolone or naloxone treatment after acute spinal cord injury: 1-year follow-up data. Results of the second National Acute Spinal Cord Injury Study. J Neurosurg. 1992; 76(1):23–31

[49] Bracken MB, Shepard MJ, Collins WF, et al. A randomized, controlled trial of methylprednisolone or naloxone in the treatment of acute spinal-cord injury. Results of the Second National Acute Spinal Cord Injury Study. N Engl J Med. 1990; 322(20):1405–1411

[50] Hall ED, Braughler JM. Glucocorticoid mechanisms in acute spinal cord injury: a review and therapeutic rationale. Surg Neurol. 1982; 18(5):320–327

[51] Hall ED, Wolf DL, Braughler JM. Effects of a single large dose of methylprednisolone sodium succinate on experimental posttraumatic spinal cord ischemia. Dose-response and time-action analysis. J Neurosurg. 1984; 61(1):124–130

[52] Hall ED, Yonkers PA, Horan KL, Braughler JM. Correlation between attenuation of posttraumatic spinal cord ischemia and preservation of tissue vitamin E by the 21-aminosteroid U74006F: evidence for an in vivo antioxidant mechanism. J Neurotrauma. 1989; 6(3):169–176

[53] Hayashi N, Green BA, Gonzalez-Carvajal M, Mora J, Veraa RP. Local blood flow, oxygen tension, and oxygen consumption in the rat spinal cord. Part 2: Relation to segmental level. J Neurosurg. 1983; 58(4):526–530

[54] Hayashi N, Green BA, Gonzalez-Carvajal M, Mora J, Veraa RP. Local blood flow, oxygen tension, and oxygen consumption in the rat spinal cord. Part 1: Oxygen metabolism and neuronal function. J Neurosurg. 1983; 58(4):516–525

[55] Wolman L. The disturbance of circulation in traumatic paraplegia in acute and late stages: A pathological study. Paraplegia. 1965; 2(4):213–226

[56] Kwon BK, Tetzlaff W, Grauer JN, Beiner J, Vaccaro AR. Pathophysiology and pharmacologic treatment of acute spinal cord injury. Spine J. 2004; 4(4):451–464

[57] Koyanagi I, Tator CH, Theriault E. Silicone rubber microangiography of acute spinal cord injury in the rat. Neurosurgery. 1993; 32(2):260–268, discussion 268

[58] Emery E, Aldana P, Bunge MB, et al. Apoptosis after traumatic human spinal cord injury. J Neurosurg. 1998; 89(6):911–920

[59] Crowe MJ, Bresnahan JC, Shuman SL, Masters JN, Beattie MS. Apoptosis and delayed degeneration after spinal cord injury in rats and monkeys. Nat Med. 1997; 3(1):73–76

[60] Li GL, Brodin G, Farooque M, et al. Apoptosis and expression of Bcl-2 after compression trauma to rat spinal cord. J Neuropathol Exp Neurol. 1996; 55(3):280–289

[61] Norenberg MD, Smith J, Marcillo A. The pathology of human spinal cord injury: defining the problems. J Neurotrauma. 2004; 21(4):429–440

[62] Kakulas BA. Neuropathology: the foundation for new treatments in spinal cord injury. Spinal Cord. 2004; 42(10):549–563

[63] Galluzzi L, Kroemer G. Necroptosis: a specialized pathway of programmed necrosis. Cell. 2008; 135(7):1161–1163

[64] Wang Y, Wang J, Yang H, et al. Necrostatin-1 mitigates mitochondrial dysfunction post-spinal cord injury. Neuroscience. 2015; 289:224–232

[65] Liu M, Wu W, Li H, et al. Necroptosis, a novel type of programmed cell death, contributes to early neural cells damage after spinal cord injury in adult mice. J Spinal Cord Med. 2015; 38(6):745–753

[66] Wang Y, Wang H, Tao Y, Zhang S, Wang J, Feng X. Necroptosis inhibitor necrostatin-1 promotes cell protection and physiological function in traumatic spinal cord injury. Neuroscience. 2014; 266:91–101

[67] Donnelly DJ, Popovich PG. Inflammation and its role in neuroprotection, axonal regeneration and functional recovery after spinal cord injury. Exp Neurol. 2008; 209(2):378–388

[68] Popovich PG, Wei P, Stokes BT. Cellular inflammatory response after spinal cord injury in Sprague-Dawley and Lewis rats. J Comp Neurol. 1997; 377(3):443–464

4 Initial Assessment (Including Imaging) of Cervical Spinal Cord Injury

Justin Iorio and Todd J. Albert

Abstract

The initial management of cervical spinal cord injuries includes following the ABCDEs: evaluation of airway, breathing, and circulation, followed by an assessment for disability/neurological deficits, and exposure of the patient. Immobilization should be performed in all patients with a spinal injury to prevent further neurological injury. A neurological examination as outlined by the American Spinal Injury Association (ASIA) must be performed. ASIA requires a detailed examination of 28 dermatomes (C2–S5) and 10 myotomes (C5–T1 and L2–S1) on each side of the body. An examination of upper extremity, lower extremity, and bulbocavernosus reflexes must be performed. Imaging of the spinal column is done to identify the location(s) of injury, fracture morphology, presence of dislocation, spinal instability, soft-tissue abnormalities, epidural hematoma, and neurological injury. Computed tomography (CT) and magnetic resonance imaging (MRI) are the most commonly utilized imaging modalities. Radiography, although less sensitive and specific than advanced techniques, has traditionally been used as the initial imaging in the awake patient. However, radiography is not necessary if CT imaging is available. In addition, a newer MRI technique known as diffusion tensor imaging has demonstrated improved ability to characterize spinal cord injury by providing detailed information about white matter tracts, which are responsible for the functional deficits following spinal cord injury. Early recognition of cervical spine injuries by thorough history, examination, and imaging may prevent neurological decline, improve outcomes, and mitigate the risk of delayed diagnosis and treatment.

Keywords: trauma, examination, assessment, cervical spine, fracture, spinal cord injury, imaging, MRI, CT

4.1 Introduction

Approximately 150,000 cervical spine injuries and 12,000 spinal cord injuries (SCIs) occur each year in the United States. Nearly half to three-fourths of SCIs are due to cervical spine trauma,[1] with incomplete quadriplegia being the most common diagnosis.[2,3] The majority of cervical injuries are sustained in the subaxial region with about 65% of fractures and more than 75% of dislocations occurring below C2.[4] Fractures and dislocations at the occipitocervical junction (OCJ) are more likely to result in death than subaxial trauma. Early recognition of cervical spine injuries by thorough history-taking, examination, and imaging may prevent neurological decline, improve outcomes, and mitigate the risk of delayed diagnosis and treatment, which occurs in nearly 33% of cervical spine patients.[5,6]

4.2 Initial Assessment

A systematic evaluation is performed on all trauma patients. The initial management is guided by the protocol set forth by the American College of Surgeons Advanced Trauma Life Support. The primary survey follows the ABCDEs: evaluation of airway, breathing, and circulation, followed by an assessment for disability/neurological deficits, and exposure of the patient. Spinal immobilization is applied in the field and strict adherence to spinal precautions (immobilization and log rolling) is required until mechanical spinal stability can be assured by clinical and radiographic evaluation. Immobilization should be performed in all patients with a spinal injury, or if a patient sustains an injury which has the potential to result in SCI. However, immobilization is not required for penetrating cervical trauma because of the risk of mortality from delayed resuscitation,[7] relatively low incidence of spinal instability, and high risk of airway compromise.[8] In unique situations, preexisting conditions, such as ankylosing spondylitis, will affect the position of the spine during immobilization. In such conditions, extension of the cervical spine can cause neurological deficits because it produces an opening wedge osteotomy in a normally kyphotic cervicothoracic spine.[9] Maintaining the normal cervicothoracic kyphosis is recommended during immobilization and imaging which can be done with the use of pillows or other supports.

A thorough history should be obtained from the patient, if possible, or from family members or witnesses to the injury. A detailed history involving medical comorbidities, prior surgeries, description of the injury, time of occurrence, presence and location of pain, severity and description of pain, neurological symptoms in the trunk and extremities (both transient or sustained), and prior spinal pathology is relevant to the management of the patient. A determination of underlying cardiopulmonary comorbidities including chronic obstructive pulmonary disease and heart disease is crucial, especially in the setting of chest wall or lung injury. Respiratory compromise may indicate the level of SCI. However, if family members or witnesses are not available to supplement the history of an unconscious patient, then the evaluation relies primarily on physical examination and imaging studies.

The physical examination begins with a visual inspection of the spine for malalignment, swelling, bruising, lacerations, and other lesions. Palpation of the spine from the skull to sacrum is performed for identifying tenderness, step-offs, gapped spinous processes, and other significant findings. Pain at the affected area is the most common presenting symptom after cervical trauma.[10] The International Spinal Cord Injury Pain Basic Data Set (ISCIPBDS) is a reliable and valid measure of SCI-related pain and should be used in conjunction with the ASIA scoring system.[11,12] The ISCIPBDS contains several domains for assessing pain related to the musculoskeletal and visceral systems, at and below the level of cord injury, and pain unrelated to SCI or without any identifiable etiology. An examination for other nonspinal musculoskeletal and nonorthopedic injuries is routinely completed as part of a thorough clinical analysis.

A neurological examination as outlined by the ASIA must be performed. The ASIA impairment scale is a standardized assessment for SCI patients to determine the neurological level. ASIA requires a detailed examination of 28 dermatomes (C2–S5) and 10 myotomes (C5–T1 and L2–S1) on each side of the body. Identifying a nerve root injury versus SCI can be difficult. Generally, multiple myotomal involvement suggests an SCI whereas unilateral, single myotome weakness represents a nerve root injury. However, high-energy injuries with unilateral, multiple myotomal involvement can result from brachial plexopathy. The sensory examination includes evaluation of light touch and pin prick and is categorized as absent (0), impaired (1), or normal (2). Myotomes in the extremities are graded as total paralysis (0), palpable or visible contractions (1), movement with gravity eliminated (2), movement against gravity only (3), movement against gravity with some resistance (4), and normal strength (5). The assessment of sacral sensation at the perianal area and deep sensation with digital rectal examination is a critical aspect of the physical examination because of its prognostic significance. Sacral sparing, which is the retention of sacral sensation, in the setting of absent motor indicates an incomplete injury.

Patients should also be evaluated for disproportionate weakness of the extremities because central cord syndrome is the most common SCI.[13] Hyperextension injuries have been traditionally associated with central cord syndrome, but fracture-dislocations and acute disc herniations can also result in upper extremity weakness with relative sparing of the bilateral lower extremities. Sensory loss and bladder dysfunction are variable after traumatic central cord syndrome. However, if the patient develops progressive neurological deficits after a stable interval, then an epidural hematoma must be ruled out with an MRI. Signs of an epidural hematoma include progression of ascending weakness and weakness within hours of an injury.[14] Other spinal cord syndromes include: Brown-Séquard, anterior spinal cord, posterior spinal cord, conus medullaris, and cauda equina syndromes.

An examination of upper extremity, lower extremity, and bulbocavernosus reflexes is critical. Initial flaccid paralysis, complete loss of sensation, and absent reflexes after a traumatic injury is referred to as spinal shock. In the absence of spinal shock, reflexes in the extremities are useful for differentiating a nerve root injury from a cord injury. Motor weakness in the presence of reflexes is common in SCI whereas weakness and areflexia is indicative of nerve root lesion. Altered reflexes occur in approximately 20% of injuries to the proximal cervical spine.[10] A critical reflex is the bulbocavernosus reflex because it is useful for the determination of spinal cord shock. The maneuver is performed by pinching the glans penis (clitoris in females) or tugging the Foley catheter and monitoring for involuntary contraction of the anal sphincter. An absent response indicates spinal shock. In contrast, contraction of the anal sphincter indicates the end of spinal shock. If the bulbocavernosus reflex does not return after 72 hours, the patient is presumed to be out of spinal shock. Clinical examination at the end of spinal shock is pertinent to the determination of incomplete versus complete SCI: presence of the bulbocavernosus reflex in the setting of complete motor and sensory loss indicates a complete SCI and poor prognosis for neurological recovery.

Cranial nerve function may provide additional information regarding the level of injury. The incidence of cranial nerve dysfunction is low after occipitocervical trauma (3.6%)[10] but aids in the localization of the lesion during clinical assessment. Occipital condyle fractures, for instance, may result in hypoglossal nerve dysfunction because the hypoglossal canal is positioned medially and superiorly to the condyles. Occipitocervical fractures can cause injury to the brainstem in which the nuclei of cranial nerves three to eight are located. Injury to the medulla can produce dysfunction of cranial nerves nine through twelve.

An evaluation for a source of hemorrhagic shock is warranted because both hemorrhagic and neurogenic shock may be present. Neurogenic shock occurs in patients who have sustained SCI to the cervical or upper thoracic region (above T6). Autonomic dysfunction inhibits the normal physiologic responses to blood loss: tachycardia and peripheral vasoconstriction. Patients with cervical SCI have lower baseline heart rates, systolic blood pressures, and mean arterial pressures while supine compared to patients without cervical SCI; blood pressure and mean arterial pressure may not increase during upright posture as expected.[15] The lack of sympathetic response to hypotension does not correlate with the severity of cervical SCI (i.e., incomplete vs. complete).

Vertebral artery injuries (VAIs) may occur during cervical trauma. Many VAIs are clinically silent, but symptomatic injuries have a wide range of manifestations. Patients may present with vertebrobasilar insufficiency (dizziness, ataxia, and vision changes), dysphagia, facial numbness, vertigo, Horner syndrome, or signs of anterior spinal cord ischemia (complete motor paralysis, loss of pain and temperature, autonomic dysfunction, areflexia, urinary retention, and retained proprioception and vibratory sensation). The screening protocol for VAI is controversial with some authors recommending an investigation in all cervical trauma patients,[16,17] and others recommending screening for patients with high-risk injuries. Guidelines by Biffl et al[18] proposed screening for VAIs in the setting of midface fractures, basilar skull fractures, cervical hematomas, neurological changes, Glasgow coma scale scores of less than 6 or 8, facet subluxations, cervical fractures between C1 and C3, fractures through the foramen transversarium, vertebral body fractures, or fractures causing ligamentous injury.[19] Members of the Cervical Spine Research Society (CSRS) have advocated for screening in patients with cervical injuries who have neurological symptoms reflective of a vascular etiology.[20] A significant, positive correlation between the incidence of VAI and ASIA grade has been reported.[21] In a study of 632 cervical fracture patients with or without SCI, 59% of vertebral artery thrombosis patients had an SCI. The incidence of VAI was significantly different between motor complete (20%) and neurologically intact patients (11%), but not between motor-incomplete (10%) and intact patients.[21]

4.3 Imaging

Imaging of the spinal column after a suspected injury is performed to identify the location(s) of injury, fracture morphology, presence of dislocation, spinal instability, soft tissue abnormalities, epidural hematoma, and neurological injury. Computed tomography (CT) and magnetic resonance imaging (MRI) are the two most commonly utilized imaging modalities. Radiography, although less sensitive and specific than the advanced techniques, has traditionally been used for initial imaging in awake patients. Radiographic assessment of symptomatic patients includes X-rays supplemented with CT to better define areas that are not easily visualized, such as the occipito-cervical and cervicothoracic junctions. However, plain radiographs are not currently required in the awake, symptomatic patient if CT imaging is available. If CT imaging is not readily available, a 3-view radiographic series should be performed and supplemented with CT imaging when available. Obtunded patients should similarly undergo CT imaging of the cervical spine; radiographs are not necessary in this situation. In addition, a newer MRI technique known as diffusion tensor imaging (DTI) has demonstrated an improved ability to characterize SCI.

4.3.1 Radiography

The standard radiographs for the initial evaluation of cervical trauma are the anteroposterior, lateral, and open-mouth odontoid views. Dynamic views have been advocated in the awake, cooperative, symptomatic patient with normal static X-rays to exclude discoligamentous injuries.[22] However, dynamic views in the setting of fractures or dislocations are not recommended and may place the obtunded patient at risk of neurological injury. The occipitocervical and subaxial spine is assessed for occipitocervical injury, atlantoaxial fractures and instability, facet dislocations, vertebral body fractures, listhesis, and post-traumatic kyphosis, among other injuries. Injury to the OCJ is often fatal at the time of injury. Radiographs can be used to identify atlanto-occipital dissociation; however, the sensitivity for identifying pathology is poor.[23]

Visualization of the midcervical region is superior to the upper and lower segments because parallax and mastoid air cells affect the identification of anatomy in the upper cervical region and the shoulder girdle obscures the lower cervical spine.[24] Important information about the vertebral bodies, pedicles, facets, canal diameter, and spinous processes can be gathered from lateral radiography. Vertebral bodies should be analyzed for radiolucencies indicating fracture lines, height loss, subluxation, facet pathology, and angulation. Distraction of spinous processes on lateral radiographs indicates a hyperflexion mechanism. Soft-tissue injury anterior to the cervical spine is represented by prevertebral soft-tissue swelling, which is measured between the anterior surface of the vertebral bodies and the air shadow of the airway. Various limits of normal have been reported from approximately 3 to 10 mm between C2 and C4.[25,26]

Anteroposterior views of vertebral bodies are similarly inspected for radiolucencies, height loss, interpedicular widening, and lateral listhesis. In addition to traumatic injuries, underlying degenerative changes and congenital stenosis of the cervical spine are important to recognize because of their contribution to cord injuries, such as central cord syndrome.[27] Approximately 50% of patients with traumatic central cord syndrome do not sustain fractures or dislocations.[27] Severe congenital stenosis is a risk factor for SCI.[28] In a study of 52 patients who sustained acute SCI, a disc-level canal diameter of ≤ 8 mm was the greatest risk factor for SCI after minor cervical trauma.[29]

However, radiographs are not required for the evaluation of SCI. Instead, CT imaging should be used as the initial screening method supplemented with MRI. Compared to advanced techniques, X-rays have not been found to identify additional fractures[30] due to their lower sensitivity and specificity.[31,32,33,34] Plain radiography has a sensitivity of 60% for detecting cervical spine fractures in a patient with blunt trauma,[35] and is insufficient for the screening of spine trauma patients.[36,37,38]

4.3.2 Computed Tomography

CT is the imaging modality of choice for evaluating bony anatomy. CT is accurate, efficient, and cost effective. Cervical CT imaging provides optimal evaluation of fracture location (i.e., vertebral body, pedicle, pars interarticularis, facet, lamina, and/or spinous process), injury morphology, vertebral translation, angulation, bony canal compromise, and facet dislocation (▶ Fig. 4.1). In addition, soft-tissue pathology and presence of a hematoma can be evaluated with the use of soft-tissue windows. Multidetector CT imaging permits the simultaneous acquisition of multiple sections of the spine and increases the speed of the study compared to conventional CT imaging. The advantages of CT imaging are, therefore, the rapid procurement of information and the ability to characterize bony injuries to a greater extent than plain radiography.[39] A Level II study of cervical trauma patients found that CT had a sensitivity of 100% for identifying bony and ligamentous injuries.[40]

An assessment of the entire cervical spine from the occipito-cervical to the cervicothoracic junction must be performed after cervical spine trauma. Visualization of the OCJ is important because of the high incidence of upper cervical injuries in cervical trauma patients. In a study of 34,069 trauma patients,

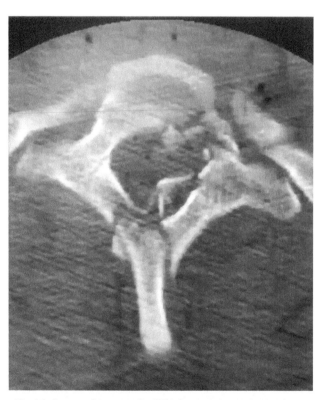

Fig. 4.1 Computed tomography (CT) of penetrating trauma to the cervicothoracic junction. The morphology of the fractured lamina and left pedicle is well visualized, as well as protrusion of bony fragments into the spinal canal.

2.4% sustained cervical spine injuries and 34% of these injuries occurred at the OCJ; the axis was the most commonly fractured cervical vertebra.[41] Injuries to the upper cervical spine that can be identified by CT imaging include atlanto-occipital dissociations, occipital condyle fractures, atlas and axis fractures, traumatic spondylolisthesis of the axis, and combinations of these injury patterns. The condyle–C1 interval has the highest sensitivity and specificity for atlanto-occipital dissociation among all measurement parameters.[7] Fracture, translation, and angulation of the C2 pars interarticularis is visualized in the coronal and sagittal planes. Atypical hangman's fractures involve the posterior vertebral body, either unilaterally or bilaterally, rather than the neural arch. Spinal cord compression against the posterior cortex of C2 and a high rate of neurological injury[42] occurs after these atypical fractures. Disc space widening and signal hyperintensity can often be seen on supplemental MRI. It is important to note that OCJ parameters (basion–dens interval, atlantodental interval, and atlanto-occipital interval) on CT imaging differ significantly from those measured on radiographs.[43]

Subaxial injuries are well-visualized by CT imaging. Fracture patterns are evaluated with sagittal and axial imaging to characterize the amount of retropulsion, translation, angulation, and canal compromise (▸ Fig. 4.2). Coronal imaging is useful for identifying horizontal fracture lines. Burst fractures with retropulsion may cause spinal cord or nerve root injury. In flexion-distraction injury patterns, axial CT imaging reveals a gradual loss of definition of the pedicles secondary to horizontal fracture lines.[44] Translation or rotation of one vertebral body on another occurs with facet dislocation or fracture. Uncovering of facets on axial imaging is the result of vertical distraction (▸ Fig. 4.3). Fractures of the pars interarticularis can cause instability and SCI. Widening of the spinous processes is indicative of posterior element disruption.

In addition to delineating bony pathology, traumatic disc herniations and epidural hemorrhage can be identified by soft tissue and lung windows. CT imaging identifies all unstable cervical injuries in the cervical spine[30] with negative predictive values of 98.9 and 100% for ligament injuries and unstable fractures, respectively.[45] Despite excellent evaluation of bony architecture and canal dimension, CT does have its disadvantages; it is less suitable than MRI for measuring cord compression.[46]

4.3.3 Magnetic Resonance Imaging

MRI identifies injuries to the neural elements, ligaments, and discs, provides evidence of injury mechanisms and spinal instability, and offers prognostic information.[47] Information about the integrity of soft-tissue structures including the posterior musculature, supra- and interspinous ligaments, ligamentum flavum, anterior longitudinal ligament, posterior longitudinal ligament, and facet capsules is well visualized. Knowledge of nerve root, spinal cord, and bony pathology is also gathered from MRI. In the pediatric population, the assessment of soft-tissue injury on MRI is especially useful after blunt trauma-induced SCI without radiographic abnormality. Adult patients without cervical fractures who present with neural deficits are likely to have underlying degenerative conditions or disc herniations (▸ Fig. 4.4).[48]

Quantitative measurements include the area of maximum spinal cord compression, bony canal compromise, and lesion length.[49] Assessment of intraspinal edema is performed on mid-sagittal T2-weighted imaging and the craniocaudal length has been found to correlate with the severity of neural deficits at the time of injury. Flanders et al[50] reported that craniocaudal length of edema and high cervical lesions correlated with poor functional outcomes. A study of cervical SCI patients concluded that intramedullary edema longer than 36 mm was associated with lack of neurological improvement at final follow-up regardless of initial neurological status.[1]

The standard MRI protocol includes sagittal and axial T1- and T2-weighted imaging, and fat-suppressed short tau inversion recovery (STIR) sequences. Sagittal T2-weighted images are critical for the evaluation of the spinal cord and are the only sequences which have prognostic value, but axial images also provide detail about the amount of spinal cord compression, canal compromise, and location of disc herniation. The various MRI sequences are critical for determining the severity of spinal cord parenchymal injury that varies from cord edema to contusion, hemorrhage, and transection (▸ Fig. 4.5). Neurological recovery is expected in the setting of cord edema. Spinal cord contusion and transection are associated with incomplete and complete SCIs, respectively, and neural recovery is less likely.[34] T2-weighted and STIR imaging are the most useful sequences for determining the amount of cord compression, hemorrhage, or edema at the site of injury (▸ Fig. 4.6). Hemorrhage or edema

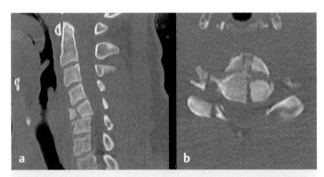

Fig. 4.2 Sagittal (*left*) and axial (*right*) computed tomography (CT) images of a C5 vertebral body fracture with bony canal compromise and focal kyphosis. Prevertebral soft-tissue swelling is seen up to the body of C3.

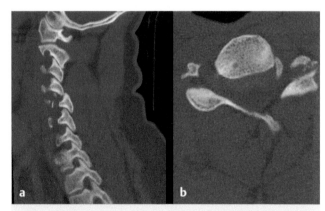

Fig. 4.3 Sagittal and axial computed tomography (CT) images of left unilateral C4–C5 facet dislocation (*left*) and fracture (*right*).

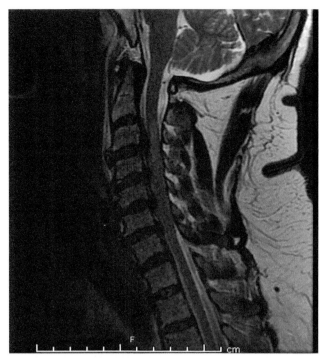

Fig. 4.4 T2-weighted magnetic resonance imaging (MRI) of patient with congenital stenosis who sustained a low-energy fall and central cord syndrome. Spinal cord signal abnormality is seen behind the C3 vertebral body.

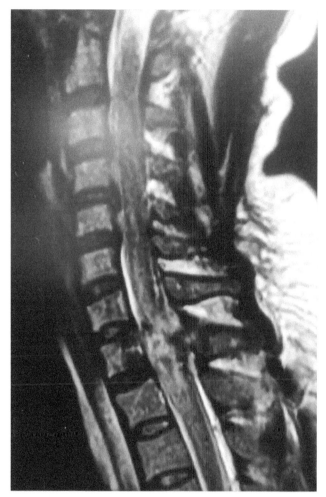

Fig. 4.5 T2-weighted magnetic resonance imaging (MRI) of complete cord transection at C7–T1 after a gunshot wound.

in the cord can be from single or multilevel injuries. In addition, cord infarction, subdural hematoma, intradiscal pathology, bony edema, and soft-tissue injury are well visualized on T2 and STIR sequences. In a study of spinal fractures, Lee et al[51] reported that T2-weighted MRI was highly sensitive, specific, and accurate for identifying posterior ligamentous complex injury. Cord swelling is identified by focal widening in the sagittal and axial planes. T1-weighted images, in contrast, provide excellent delineation of anatomic structures including the major ligaments of the spine. Spinal cord pathology can also be assessed on T1 imaging despite the traditional use of T2 signal abnormalities for routine clinical assessment. Edema, hyperacute hemorrhage, and infarction appear dark on T1-weighted imaging whereas subacute hemorrhage may be viewed as a bright signal.

Hemorrhage in the spinal cord is identified by hypointensity on T2-weighted imaging. Hemorrhage commonly occurs in the nuclei of the spinal cord and represents the point of maximum impact. In the cervical spine, intraspinal hemorrhage reflects a complete neurological injury.[47,52] Epidural hemorrhage can be difficult to identify acutely after trauma because it is isointense to the spinal cord on T1 and isointense to cerebrospinal fluid (CSF) on T2-weighted MRI.[34] Neural methemoglobin may take more than 7 days before it can be identified on T2-weighted imaging whereas extraneural methemoglobin appears within hours of injury. The appearance of hemorrhage on T1- and T2-weighted imaging is dependent on the presence of deoxyhemoglobin and methemoglobin, as well as the size of the hemor-

rhage. In the case of a larger hemorrhage, more time is required for deoxyhemoglobin to be converted into methemoglobin. Hemorrhage during spinal trauma contains oxyhemoglobin which is converted to deoxyhemoglobin within a few hours and is hypointense on T2-weighted MRI.[53] Intracellular methemoglobin is produced from deoxyhemoglobin after 3 to 8 days and is hyperintense on T1-weighted MRI and hypointense on T2, whereas extracellular methemoglobin is hyperintense on T1 and T2 imaging.[53] Gradient echo MR images detect the breakdown products of hemoglobin; in the acute phase, hemorrhage appears as hypointense around an isodense center.[54]

Facet widening and fluid-filled facets on T2 and STIR sequences represent facet capsular injury. Facet dislocation is a prognostic factor for poor neurological outcome.[1] Identification of a posttraumatic disc herniation is imperative because further displacement into the spinal canal can occur if closed reduction is performed. A systematic review of SCIs reported 36% incidence of disc herniations associated with cervical trauma, although the authors were unable to correlate herniations with neurological deficits based on the studies available.[47] Identification of

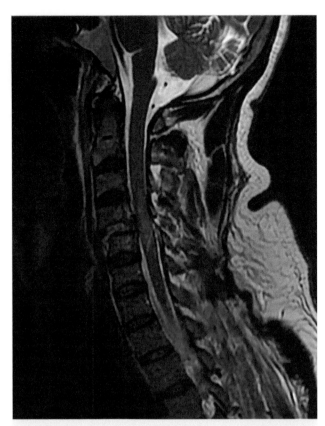

Fig. 4.6 Sagittal T2-weighted magnetic resonance image (MRI) demonstrating hyperintensity of interdiscal space and spinal cord edema. Uncovering of the posterior disc is seen.

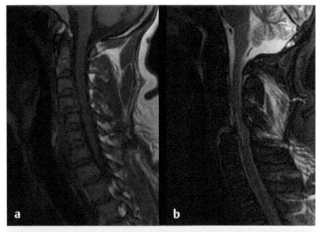

Fig. 4.7 T1-weighted magnetic resonance image (MRI) depicting injury to anterior and posterior longitudinal ligaments at C4–C5 (*left*). Injury to the interspinous ligament and posterior soft tissues is represented by hyperintensity on short tau inversion recovery MRI. Interdiscal injury and cord edema are also seen (*right*).

traumatic disc herniations is difficult if the patient has cervical spondylosis, but signal abnormality, asymmetric disc space widening, and listhesis may indicate an underlying traumatic disc herniation.

A thorough evaluation of anterior and posterior ligamentous structures is imperative especially in the setting of vertebral subluxation or dislocation. The ligamentous anatomy of the upper cervical spine maintains spinal alignment and stability. Disruption of the upper cervical soft-tissue structures, which include the cruciate, alar, apical, and transverse ligaments, and tectorial membrane,[55] can cause spinal instability and SCI.[10] Ligamentous structures in the middle to lower cervical spine include the anterior and posterior longitudinal ligaments, supraspinous ligament, interspinous ligament, and ligamentum flavum. The failure of all anterior structures or all posterior plus two anterior structures is a risk factor for cervical instability. The evaluation of ligamentous injury on MRI is critical. Ligaments are hypointense on all sequences; however, hyperintensity on T2 and STIR imaging indicates distention or injury. In contrast, the presence of a hypo- or hyperintense signal surrounding an absence of signal represents tissue disruption as can be seen in the anterior longitudinal ligament following a hyperextension injury (▶ Fig. 4.7). Posterior ligamentous complex injuries can affect the supraspinous ligament, interspinous ligament, and ligamentum flavum. Supra- and interspinous ligament injuries may be identified by T2 hyperintensity and wid-

ening of the distances between spinous processes (▶ Fig. 4.7). Ligamentum flavum injury can be seen as discontinuity or displacement into the thecal sac. In a study of cervical spine trauma, the incidence of SCI on MRI was 71% and MRI was found to be highly sensitive for disc (93%), posterior longitudinal ligament (93%), and interspinous ligament injuries (100%).[56] The sensitivity of MRI for detecting anterior longitudinal ligament (71%) and ligamentum flavum (67%) injuries was significantly less, and the correlation between abnormal ligament signal intensity and intraoperative findings was poor ($k = 0.029$–0.13). The association between soft-tissue injury and extent of SCI is inconclusive. Studies have failed to relate soft-tissue injury to the severity of SCI,[57] while others have reported an association between tissue injury and intramedullary lesion length.[58]

The requirement for MRI in obtunded or neurologically injured patients who have undergone CT imaging has been debated. Menaker et al[59] found that 25% of symptomatic patients with normal CT imaging had an abnormal MRI which affected the treatment plan. Schoenfeld et al[60] performed a meta-analysis of patients who had negative CTs after blunt cervical trauma and were then evaluated with MRI. Additional injuries were identified in 12% of patients, which included ligamentous injuries, fractures, and dislocations. Levitt and Flanders[61] compared CT imaging and MRI in cervical trauma patients and concluded that MRI identified SCI in 26% of patients compared to zero percent on CT imaging. However, CT imaging better identified bony pathology. Therefore, combined use of MRI and CT imaging is recommended in patients with cervical spine trauma and associated neurological exam findings.

4.3.4 Vertebral Artery Injury

Imaging is also useful for the evaluation of VAIs that may occur in up to 15% of traumatic SCI patients.[47] As expected, the majority of VAIs occur in the setting of cervical fractures because of the position of the vertebral artery in the cervical spine.[20] Injuries are most commonly identified in the foraminal segment of the artery and present as occlusions, stenosis, intimal injuries, or dissections. Subluxation, transverse foramen fractures, and cervical injuries between C1 and C3 are the most commonly cited risk factors for arterial injury.[20] If a VAI is suspected, CT angiography is the study of choice because of its high sensitivity (40–96%) and specificity (90–97%).[19] However, MRIs should be performed in patients with VAIs and complete SCIs or vertebral subluxations.[7] A VAI is identified on MRI by a lack of flow voids, crescentic high signal intensity, or a pseudoaneurysm (▶ Fig. 4.8). Magnetic resonance angiography (MRA) is an alternative option. In this study, intramural hematomas are seen on T1 imaging as a hyperintense rim surrounding a flow void. An increase in arterial diameter compared to the contralateral artery is another indicator of injury. However, the T1 signal representative of bleeding is not observed within the first several hours after injury. Disadvantages, such as length of imaging time, undefined effectiveness of imaging additional body areas in the acutely injured patient with this modality, and low specificity and sensitivity, limit its use in the trauma setting.[62] CT angiography, meanwhile, is cost effective, noninvasive, widely available, and can be used for three-dimensional imaging.[19] Imaging findings that support a VAI include blood extravasation into the arterial wall and a false lumen, vessel wall expansion with compromise of the lumen, an extravascular hematoma, arterial occlusion, and/or transection.[20]

Nondisplaced fractures through the vertebrae, facets, laminae, and spinous processes may be difficult to observe on MRI. Fracture lines are represented by T2 hyperintensity and T1 hypointensity. Marrow edema from trabecular microfractures indicates vertebral body fracture but edema is less likely to occur in the bony posterior elements. A study of acute spine fractures concluded that only vertebral compression fractures reliably generated marrow edema, whereas distraction injuries and fractures without bony compression did not result in edema.[63] Therefore, knowledge of the injury mechanism is important because some injury patterns do not produce edema and this may result in a false-negative MRI reading. Additional limitations of MRI in the trauma setting include difficulties with patient transport and/or monitoring, limited access in some centers, and longer imaging time as compared with CT. Moreover, patient positioning for the MRI can result in neurological deterioration. Lastly, standard MRI sequences do not provide a direct measurement of axonal integrity; quantitative assessment of neuronal injury is provided by DTI.[64]

Despite the utility of MRI, subtle changes in spinal cord integrity may be missed with conventional techniques. In addition, the clinical examination may not correlate with MRI pathology[65] and signal changes may fail to predict functional outcome.[66] This is because MRI displays changes in signal intensity (secondary to the relaxation of protons) but the physiological state and functionality of nerve fiber tracts remains unclear.[67] Therefore, T2 hyperintensity does not predict functional outcome because it does not provide information regarding the integrity of nerve tracts responsible for clinical deficits after SCI.[68] Evaluating white matter tracts is suboptimal on MRI

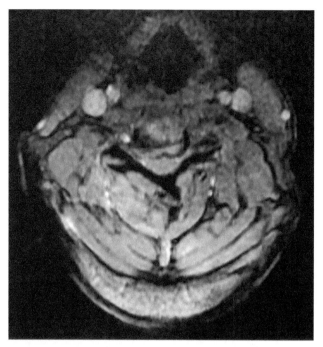

Fig. 4.8 Axial magnetic resonance image (MRI) demonstrating loss of normal flow void within left vertebral artery from acute vertebral artery injury.

because edema and hemorrhage blur the boundaries between gray and white matter; therefore, an imaging modality capable of providing information about the integrity of white matter tracts is clinically relevant.

4.3.5 Diffusion Tensor Imaging

DTI is an MRI technique that is more sensitive at detecting SCI compared to conventional MRI. While MRI relies on changes in signal intensity, DTI measures changes in the rate of water diffusion within white matter tracts of the spinal cord. DTI relies on anisotropic diffusion, which is the restricted movement of water molecules within tubular structures secondary to biological barriers. This imaging technique measures speed and directionality of water molecules along linear structures, such as nerve fibers, and identifies abnormalities of linear molecular movement.[67] DTI parameters that are useful in the assessment of SCI include fractional anisotropy and apparent diffusion coefficient (ADC). Fractional anisotropy is a commonly referenced parameter that ranges from 0 (representing isotropic diffusion or movement in a sphere) to 1 (representing anisotropic diffusion in a cylinder). Fractional anisotropy normally approximates the value "1" because intact nerve fibers are long, thin cylinders. If an injury occurs, the diffusion of water molecules becomes unrestricted (isotropic) and approaches "0".[67] A low ADC, which represents the magnitude of diffusion of water molecules, indicates neuronal integrity and a high value correlates with fiber tract injury. Therefore, high ADC values within the spinal cord represent axonal injury and discontinuity of myelin sheaths which may be from the impact of trauma, spinal cord ischemia, or swelling within the cord. The ability to detect abnormal molecular movement prior to structural changes makes DTI the most sensitive imaging study. Changes in diffusion occur prior to major structural alterations (as seen on MRI) and thus provide information about neural damage to white matter tracts, which are responsible for the functional deficits following SCI.

DTI has shown efficacy in detecting white matter injury in the hyperacute phase (within 6 hours) of SCI. In a mouse model, DTI identified mild, moderate, and severe SCI at 3 hours with histologic confirmation of white matter injury.[68] DTI provided clear distinction between gray and white matter within edematous regions of the spinal cord that is often obscured on T2-weighted imaging. One potential benefit of DTI is, therefore, the ability to measure the functional integrity of the cord in the early posttraumatic timeframe when the patient is in spinal shock. In a study of patients who sustained acute cervical trauma, ADC and fractional anisotropy were significantly different for injured areas as compared to healthy controls, and correlated with injury severity.[69] In addition, abnormalities on DTI were observed in the presence of normal conventional MRI sequences. Therefore, DTI may more precisely record the extent of SCI and potentially correlate clinical presentation with advanced imaging. D'Souza et al[70] evaluated 20 acute cervical trauma patients and 30 age and sex matched controls with DTI. Quantitative measurements via fractional anisotropy and ADC were found to significantly correlate with white matter integrity and functional outcome. Compared to controls, FA and ADC were decreased and increased, respectively, even in patients with neurological deficits in the setting of a negative conventional MRI.

Currently, DTI is not widely available for clinical use because of several challenges in humans, which include the effect of CSF on diffusion anisotropy indices, consequences of physiologic motion on imaging, and low spatial resolution and artifacts on echo planar diffusion imaging from magnetic susceptibility effects.[64,67] Different imaging techniques such as line-scan diffusion imaging have been used in pediatric spinal cord imaging without degradation of imaging quality from cardiac pulsations or respiratory motion,[71] but the scanning time required for this sequence makes it impractical for cervical SCI patients.[69]

4.4 Imaging in Patients with Ankylosing Conditions

Ankylosing spondylitis and diffuse idiopathic skeletal hyperostosis are unique conditions in which fractures of the spinal column occur after low-energy injuries. Fractures commonly occur through the vertebral bodies and disc spaces because of ossification, osteoporosis, kyphosis, and ultimately a brittle spinal column. Cervical fractures are often secondary to hyperextension and are unstable, three-column injuries. As a result, the risk of neurological injury after cervical injury is three times greater than the general population.[72] In a study of 939 ankylosing spondylitis patients, 53% of fractures occurred in the cervical region, 27.5% were associated with SCI, and 13.1% of patients had noncontiguous fractures.[73] In the cervical spine, the lower vertebral bodies are most likely to fracture (▶ Fig. 4.9).[14] Cervical radiography is insufficient for identifying pathology because the shoulders obscure the lower cervical spine and cervicothoracic junction, an abnormal anatomy precludes a detailed analysis of fracture morphology, and osteopenia affects visualization of the bones. In a review of ankylosing spondylitis patients with cervical fractures, radiography when used alone was unable to visualize the entire cervical spine in 92% of patients, and only 48% of fractures could be identified.[74] CT imaging and MRI should be routinely performed in all ankylosing spondylitis patients who sustain minor trauma.

A CT scan of the entire spinal column provides superior definition of bony pathologies and noncontiguous fractures. Fractures typically occur through the disc spaces in early ankylosing spondylitis, and through the vertebral bodies in latter stages because the vertebrae, adjacent to the fused disc spaces, become osteopenic (▶ Fig. 4.10). MRI is recommended in conjunction with CT imaging because of the high rate of SCI in these patients, the frequent presence of epidural hematomas, and the increased sensitivity of this imaging modality for detecting soft-tissue injuries. Moreover, Wang et al[75] found that MRI identified posterior column injuries in AS patients that were not detected via CT imaging.

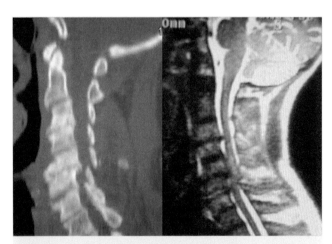

Fig. 4.9 Patient with diffuse idiopathic skeletal hyperostosis. Anterior gapping at C6–C7 is seen on computed tomography (CT) with hyperintensity on T2-weighted magnetic resonance imaging (MRI) through the disc space indicative of acute disruption.

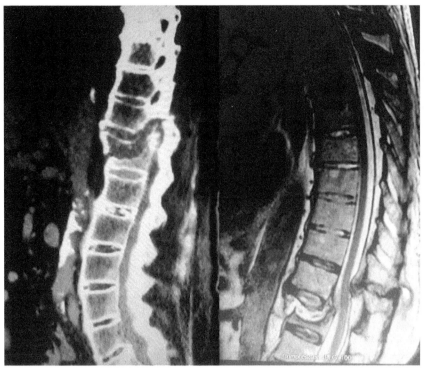

Fig. 4.10 Sagittal computed tomography (CT) and T2-weighted magnetic resonance imaging (MRI) of ankylosing spondylitis. Fracture through the vertebral body is well visualized on CT. Three-column injury with epidural component is seen on MRI.

References

[1] Martínez-Pérez R, Cepeda S, Paredes I, Alen JF, Lagares A. MRI prognostication factors in the setting of cervical spinal cord injury secondary to trauma. World Neurosurg. 2017; 101:623–632

[2] Silva OT, Sabba MF, Lira HI, et al. Evaluation of the reliability and validity of the newer AOSpine subaxial cervical injury classification (C-3 to C-7). J Neurosurg Spine. 2016; 25(3):303–308

[3] Gupta R, Bathen ME, Smith JS, Levi AD, Bhatia NN, Steward O. Advances in the management of spinal cord injury. J Am Acad Orthop Surg. 2010; 18(4):210–222

[4] Formby P, Helgeson MD. Nonoperative management of cervical spine Trauma. In: Oner FC, Vacarro AR, Vialle LR eds. AOSpine Masters Series, Volume 5: Cervical Spine Trauma. New York, NY: Thieme; 2015:79–97

[5] Bohlman HH. Acute fractures and dislocations of the cervical spine. An analysis of three hundred hospitalized patients and review of the literature. J Bone Joint Surg Am. 1979; 61(8):1119–1142

[6] Anderson PA, Gugala Z, Lindsey RW, Schoenfeld AJ, Harris MB. Clearing the cervical spine in the blunt trauma patient. J Am Acad Orthop Surg. 2010; 18(3):149–159

[7] Hadley MN, Walters BC. Introduction to the guidelines for the management of acute cervical spine and spinal cord injuries. Neurosurgery. 2013; 72(2) Suppl 2:5–16

[8] Jakoi A, Iorio J, Howell R, Zampini JM. Gunshot injuries of the spine. Spine J. 2015; 15(9):2077–2085

[9] Papadopoulos MC, Chakraborty A, Waldron G, Bell BA. Lesson of the week: exacerbating cervical spine injury by applying a hard collar. BMJ. 1999; 319(7203):171–172

[10] Martinez-Del-Campo E, Turner JD, Kalb S, et al. Occipitocervical fixation: a single surgeon's experience with 120 patients. Neurosurgery. 2016; 79(4):549–560

[11] Jensen MP, Widerström-Noga E, Richards JS, Finnerup NB, Biering-Sørensen F, Cardenas DD. Reliability and validity of the International Spinal Cord Injury Basic Pain Data Set items as self-report measures. Spinal Cord. 2010; 48(3):230–238

[12] Widerström-Noga E, Biering-Sørensen F, Bryce TN, et al. The International Spinal Cord Injury Pain Basic Data Set (version 2.0). Spinal Cord. 2014; 52(4):282–286

[13] Seecharan DJ, Arnold PM. Spinal cord injuries and syndromes. In: Samartzis D, Fessler RJ eds. Textbook of the Cervical Spine. Missouri: Saunders, 2014:192–196

[14] Thumbikat P, Hariharan RP, Ravichandran G, McClelland MR, Mathew KM. Spinal cord injury in patients with ankylosing spondylitis: a 10-year review. Spine. 2007; 32(26):2989–2995

[15] Claydon VE, Krassioukov AV. Orthostatic hypotension and autonomic pathways after spinal cord injury. J Neurotrauma. 2006; 23(12):1713–1725

[16] Kaye D, Brasel KJ, Neideen T, Weigelt JA. Screening for blunt cerebrovascular injuries is cost-effective. J Trauma. 2011; 70(5):1051–1056, discussion 1056–1057

[17] Miller PR, Fabian TC, Croce MA, et al. Prospective screening for blunt cerebrovascular injuries: analysis of diagnostic modalities and outcomes. Ann Surg. 2002; 236(3):386–393, discussion 393–395

[18] Biffl WL, Cothren CC, Moore EE, et al. Western Trauma Association critical decisions in trauma: screening for and treatment of blunt cerebrovascular injuries. J Trauma. 2009; 67(6):1150–1153

[19] Grabowski G, Robertson RN, Barton BM, Cairns MA, Webb SW. Blunt cerebrovascular injury in cervical spine fractures: are more-liberal screening criteria warranted? Global Spine J. 2016; 6(7):679–685

[20] Fassett DR, Dailey AT, Vaccaro AR. Vertebral artery injuries associated with cervical spine injuries: a review of the literature. J Spinal Disord Tech. 2008; 21(4):252–258

[21] Torina PJ, Flanders AE, Carrino JA, et al. Incidence of vertebral artery thrombosis in cervical spine trauma: correlation with severity of spinal cord injury. AJNR Am J Neuroradiol. 2005; 26(10):2645–2651

[22] Assaker R, Zairi F, Demondion X. Evaluation of an injured cervical spine. In: Oner FC, Vacarro AR, Vialle LR eds. AOSpine Masters Series, Volume 5: Cervical Spine Trauma. New York, NY: Thieme, 2015:56–78

[23] Gregg S, Kortbeek JB, du Plessis S. Atlanto-occipital dislocation: a case study of survival with partial recovery and review of the literature. J Trauma. 2005; 58(1):168–171

[24] Bellabarba C, Bransford RJ, Chapman JR. Occipitocervical and upper cervical spine fractures. In: Samartzis D, Fessler RJ, eds. Textbook of the Cervical Spine. Missouri: Saunders, 2014:168–183

[25] Templeton PA, Young JW, Mirvis SE, Buddemeyer EU. The value of retropharyngeal soft tissue measurements in trauma of the adult cervical spine. Cervical spine soft tissue measurements. Skeletal Radiol. 1987; 16(2):98–104

[26] Song KJ, Choi BW, Kim HY, Jeon TS, Chang H. Efficacy of postoperative radiograph for evaluating the prevertebral soft tissue swelling after anterior cervical discectomy and fusion. Clin Orthop Surg. 2012; 4(1):77–82

[27] Aarabi B, Koltz M, Ibrahimi D. Hyperextension cervical spine injuries and traumatic central cord syndrome. Neurosurg Focus. 2008; 25(5):E9

[28] Rao SC, Fehlings MG. The optimal radiologic method for assessing spinal canal compromise and cord compression in patients with cervical spinal cord

injury. Part I: An evidence-based analysis of the published literature. Spine. 1999; 24(6):598–604

[29] Aebli N, Rüegg TB, Wicki AG, Petrou N, Krebs J. Predicting the risk and severity of acute spinal cord injury after a minor trauma to the cervical spine. Spine J. 2013; 13(6):597–604

[30] Harris TJ, Blackmore CC, Mirza SK, Jurkovich GJ. Clearing the cervical spine in obtunded patients. Spine. 2008; 33(14):1547–1553

[31] Diaz JJ, Jr, Gillman C, Morris JA, Jr, May AK, Carrillo YM, Guy J. Are five-view plain films of the cervical spine unreliable? A prospective evaluation in blunt trauma patients with altered mental status. J Trauma. 2003; 55(4):658–663, discussion 663–664

[32] Griffen MM, Frykberg ER, Kerwin AJ, et al. Radiographic clearance of blunt cervical spine injury: plain radiograph or computed tomography scan? J Trauma. 2003; 55(2):222–226, discussion 226–227

[33] Holmes JF, Akkinepalli R. Computed tomography versus plain radiography to screen for cervical spine injury: a meta-analysis. J Trauma. 2005; 58(5): 902–905

[34] Shah LM, Ross JS. Imaging of spine trauma. Neurosurgery. 2016; 79(5): 626–642

[35] Berne JD, Velmahos GC, El-Tawil Q, et al. Value of complete cervical helical computed tomographic scanning in identifying cervical spine injury in the unevaluable blunt trauma patient with multiple injuries: a prospective study. J Trauma. 1999; 47(5):896–902, discussion 902–903

[36] Acheson MB, Livingston RR, Richardson ML, Stimac GK. High-resolution CT scanning in the evaluation of cervical spine fractures: comparison with plain film examinations. AJR Am J Roentgenol. 1987; 148(6):1179–1185

[37] Grogan EL, Morris JA, Jr, Dittus RS, et al. Cervical spine evaluation in urban trauma centers: lowering institutional costs and complications through helical CT scan. J Am Coll Surg. 2005; 200(2):160–165

[38] Ross SE, Schwab CW, David ET, Delong WG, Born CT. Clearing the cervical spine: initial radiologic evaluation. J Trauma. 1987; 27(9):1055–1060

[39] Antevil JL, Sise MJ, Sack DI, Kidder B, Hopper A, Brown CV. Spiral computed tomography for the initial evaluation of spine trauma: a new standard of care? J Trauma. 2006; 61(2):382–387

[40] Vanguri P, Young AJ, Weber WF, et al. Computed tomographic scan: it's not just about the fracture. J Trauma Acute Care Surg. 2014; 77(4):604–607

[41] Goldberg W, Mueller C, Panacek E, Tigges S, Hoffman JR, Mower WR, NEXUS Group. Distribution and patterns of blunt traumatic cervical spine injury. Ann Emerg Med. 2001; 38(1):17–21

[42] Al-Mahfoudh R, Beagrie C, Woolley E, et al. Management of typical and atypical Hangman's fractures. Global Spine J. 2016; 6(3):248–256

[43] Rojas CA, Bertozzi JC, Martinez CR, Whitlow J. Reassessment of the craniocervical junction: normal values on CT. AJNR Am J Neuroradiol. 2007; 28(9):1819–1823

[44] Bernstein MP, Mirvis SE, Shanmuganathan K. Chance-type fractures of the thoracolumbar spine: imaging analysis in 53 patients. AJR Am J Roentgenol. 2006; 187(4):859–868

[45] Hogan GJ, Mirvis SE, Shanmuganathan K, Scalea TM. Exclusion of unstable cervical spine injury in obtunded patients with blunt trauma: is MR imaging needed when multi-detector row CT findings are normal? Radiology. 2005; 237(1):106–113

[46] Lammertse D, Dungan D, Dreisbach J, et al. National Institute on Disability and Rehabilitation. Neuroimaging in traumatic spinal cord injury: an evidence-based review for clinical practice and research. J Spinal Cord Med. 2007; 30(3):205–214

[47] Bozzo A, Marcoux J, Radhakrishna M, Pelletier J, Goulet B. The role of magnetic resonance imaging in the management of acute spinal cord injury. J Neurotrauma. 2011; 28(8):1401–1411

[48] Dreizin D, Kim W, Kim JS, et al. Will the real SCIWORA please stand up? Exploring clinicoradiologic mismatch in closed spinal cord injuries. AJR Am J Roentgenol. 2015; 205(4):853–860

[49] Miyanji F, Furlan JC, Aarabi B, Arnold PM, Fehlings MG. Acute cervical traumatic spinal cord injury: MR imaging findings correlated with neurologic outcome–prospective study with 100 consecutive patients. Radiology. 2007; 243(3):820–827

[50] Flanders AE, Spettell CM, Friedman DP, Marino RJ, Herbison GJ. The relationship between the functional abilities of patients with cervical spinal cord injury and the severity of damage revealed by MR imaging. AJNR Am J Neuroradiol. 1999; 20(5):926–934

[51] Lee HM, Kim HS, Kim DJ, Suk KS, Park JO, Kim NH. Reliability of magnetic resonance imaging in detecting posterior ligament complex injury in thoracolumbar spinal fractures. Spine. 2000; 25(16):2079–2084

[52] Ramón S, Domínguez R, Ramírez L, et al. Clinical and magnetic resonance imaging correlation in acute spinal cord injury. Spinal Cord. 1997; 35(10):664–673

[53] Grabb PA, Pang D. Magnetic resonance imaging in the evaluation of spinal cord injury without radiographic abnormality in children. Neurosurgery. 1994; 35(3):406–414, discussion 414

[54] Copenhaver BR, Shin J, Warach S, Butman JA, Saver JL, Kidwell CS. Gradient echo MRI: implementation of a training tutorial for intracranial hemorrhage diagnosis. Neurology. 2009; 72(18):1576–1581

[55] Martin MD, Bruner HJ, Maiman DJ. Anatomic and biomechanical considerations of the craniovertebral junction. Neurosurgery. 2010; 66(3) Suppl:2–6

[56] Goradia D, Linnau KF, Cohen WA, Mirza S, Hallam DK, Blackmore CC. Correlation of MR imaging findings with intraoperative findings after cervical spine trauma. AJNR Am J Neuroradiol. 2007; 28(2):209–215

[57] Flanders AE, Schaefer DM, Doan HT, Mishkin MM, Gonzalez CF, Northrup BE. Acute cervical spine trauma: correlation of MR imaging findings with degree of neurologic deficit. Radiology. 1990; 177(1):25–33

[58] Martínez-Pérez R, Paredes I, Cepeda S, et al. Spinal cord injury after blunt cervical spine trauma: correlation of soft-tissue damage and extension of lesion. AJNR Am J Neuroradiol. 2014; 35(5):1029–1034

[59] Menaker J, Stein DM, Philp AS, Scalea TM. 40-slice multidetector CT: is MRI still necessary for cervical spine clearance after blunt trauma? Am Surg. 2010; 76(2):157–163

[60] Schoenfeld AJ, Bono CM, McGuire KJ, Warholic N, Harris MB. Computed tomography alone versus computed tomography and magnetic resonance imaging in the identification of occult injuries to the cervical spine: a meta-analysis. J Trauma. 2010; 68(1):109–113, discussion 113–114

[61] Levitt MA, Flanders AE. Diagnostic capabilities of magnetic resonance imaging and computed tomography in acute cervical spinal column injury. Am J Emerg Med. 1991; 9(2):131–135

[62] Berne JD, Reuland KS, Villarreal DH, McGovern TM, Rowe SA, Norwood SH. Sixteen-slice multi-detector computed tomographic angiography improves the accuracy of screening for blunt cerebrovascular injury. J Trauma. 2006; 60(6):1204–1209, discussion 1209–1210

[63] Brinckman MA, Chau C, Ross JS. Marrow edema variability in acute spine fractures. Spine J. 2015; 15(3):454–460

[64] Kim JH, Loy DN, Wang Q, et al. Diffusion tensor imaging at 3 hours after traumatic spinal cord injury predicts long-term locomotor recovery. J Neurotrauma. 2010; 27(3):587–598

[65] Kerkovský M, Bednařík J, Dušek L, et al. Magnetic resonance diffusion tensor imaging in patients with cervical spondylotic spinal cord compression: correlations between clinical and electrophysiological findings. Spine. 2012; 37(1):48–56

[66] Matsumoto M, Toyama Y, Ishikawa M, Chiba K, Suzuki N, Fujimura Y. Increased signal intensity of the spinal cord on magnetic resonance images in cervical compressive myelopathy. Does it predict the outcome of conservative treatment? Spine. 2000; 25(6):677–682

[67] Rajasekaran S, Kanna RM, Shetty AP. Diffusion tensor imaging of the spinal cord and its clinical applications. J Bone Joint Surg Br. 2012; 94(8):1024–1031

[68] Loy DN, Kim JH, Xie M, Schmidt RE, Trinkaus K, Song SK. Diffusion tensor imaging predicts hyperacute spinal cord injury severity. J Neurotrauma. 2007; 24(6):979–990

[69] Shanmuganathan K, Gullapalli RP, Zhuo J, Mirvis SE. Diffusion tensor MR imaging in cervical spine trauma. AJNR Am J Neuroradiol. 2008; 29(4): 655–659

[70] D'souza MM, Choudhary A, Poonia M, Kumar P, Khushu S. Diffusion tensor MR imaging in spinal cord injury. Injury. 2017; 48(4):880–884

[71] Robertson RL, Maier SE, Mulkern RV, Vajapayam S, Robson CD, Barnes PD. MR line-scan diffusion imaging of the spinal cord in children. AJNR Am J Neuroradiol. 2000; 21(7):1344–1348

[72] Sapkas G, Kateros K, Papadakis SA, et al. Surgical outcome after spinal fractures in patients with ankylosing spondylitis. BMC Musculoskelet Disord. 2009; 10:96

[73] Lukasiewicz AM, Bohl DD, Varthi AG, et al. Spinal fracture in patients with ankylosing spondylitis: cohort definition, distribution of injuries, and hospital outcomes. Spine. 2016; 41(3):191–196

[74] Koivikko MP, Kiuru MJ, Koskinen SK. Multidetector computed tomography of cervical spine fractures in ankylosing spondylitis. Acta Radiol. 2004; 45(7):751–759

[75] Wang YF, Teng MM, Chang CY, Wu HT, Wang ST. Imaging manifestations of spinal fractures in ankylosing spondylitis. AJNR Am J Neuroradiol. 2005; 26(8):2067–2076

5 Cranioskeletal Traction for the Management of Trauma to the Cervical Spine

Robert F. Heary, Raghav Gupta, and Sanford E. Emery

Abstract

Cranioskeletal traction is a treatment modality by which traumatic cervical fractures or dislocations can be reduced allowing reconstitution of the normal cervical spine alignment. In doing so, the neural elements are freed of any ongoing compression from displaced vertebral or disc material. This method was reportedly first used by the Greeks in the 4th century B.C. for the management of thoracic dislocations. Multiple devices have since been invented which can be used to apply traction to the cervical spine; the two most commonly utilized devices are the Gardner–Wells tongs and the halo apparatus. In the present chapter, we consider the primary indications for use of these two devices. We further describe how these devices are applied and the common complications encountered in the clinical setting when using either of these devices. Finally, we summarize data from previous studies delineating the clinical outcomes in patients who underwent closed reduction and/or cervical spine stabilization with either of these two devices.

Keywords: cranioskeletal traction, Gardner–Wells tongs, halo fixation, cervical spine trauma, indications, clinical outcomes

5.1 Introduction and Origins of Cervical Traction

Cranioskeletal traction is a treatment modality that can be used for the reduction and stabilization of cervical spine fractures or dislocations. It may also be used for immobilization of the cervical spine following trauma. When used alone, or in conjunction with surgery, it promotes normal spinal cord alignment, decompression of the nerves and spinal cord, protection of soft tissues, and bone healing. The initial use of skeletal traction for the treatment of spinal fractures has been attributed to Hippocrates and the Greeks in the 4th century B.C., though the use was limited to thoracic dislocations at that time.[1] In the mid-17th century, toward the end of the Renaissance Period, Fabricius Hildanus developed the first device specifically designed to reduce cervical spine fracture-dislocations, though it was not widely adopted. The device consisted of forceps which were spread apart and affixed to the back of the neck. A needle was threaded in between its ends and inserted below the spinous process. Traction was then placed using the forceps.[1,2]

It was not until the early 20th century, however, that the importance of treating cervical spinal cord injuries (SCIs) became apparent. Citing the increasing number of automobile accidents and hyperflexion injuries, Alfred Taylor outlined a method by which skin traction could be used to stabilize the cervical spine. This became known as halter traction. It utilized the mandible and inion for support and was used successfully in the management of pediatric atlantoaxial rotatory subluxations and cervical radiculopathy in adult patients.[3,4,5] However, only limited force could be applied using this technique and several complications could result from its use including temporomandibular dysfunction and pressure ulcers. Its use was also contraindicated in patients with mandibular fractures. As a result, its role in the long-term reduction of cervical spine injuries has since been limited.[6]

The largest increase in the number of cervical skeletal traction devices occurred during the period immediately preceding World War II.[1] In 1933, W.G. Crutchfield reported the use of modified Edmonton extension tongs (later termed Crutchfield tongs), which could be inserted into the skull above both ears, for the reduction of a cervical fracture dislocation.[1,6] Today, Gardner–Wells tongs, which were first described in the medical literature in 1973, are the most frequently used iteration of the cranial tong design (Fig. 5.1a). These allow for application of greater traction forces compared to previous designs and contain a C-shaped bow that is affixed to the skull through two pins.[7,8] The typical fixation point is 2 cm above the superior aspect of the pinna of the ear in line with the external auditory meatus. Traction can be gradually maintained through the addition of weights attached to a rope and pulley system which is attached to the bow.

Similarly, Perry and Nickel, in 1959, reported using a "halo skeletal apparatus" for the management of poliomyelitis-induced cervical spine instability.[9] The cranial halo consists of a metal ring that is anchored to the skull using a four-pin fixation system, utilizing two anterior and two posterior pins secured in the outer table of the cortical bone. For pediatric patients with thinner skulls, six or eight points of fixation at lower insertion torques are utilized to secure the halo to the skull to decrease the risk of penetrating the skull proper. As is the case with Gardner–Wells tongs, weights can also be hung from a rope and pulley system to maintain traction. Alternatively, the halo ring can be attached to adjustable rods and a fleece-lined vest to allow for rigid fixation/immobilization of the cervical spine and maintenance of cervical spine stability following successful closed reduction. The device is indicated in the outpatient setting where patient mobility is necessary.

5.2 Indications for Use

Cervical traction is indicated in the context of facet dislocations (Fig. 5.2a–c), certain types of occipital condyle and C1 fractures, C2 hangman and odontoid fractures (particularly type II), rotatory atlantoaxial subluxations, lateral mass fractures, subaxial compression fractures, burst fractures, and in patients with kyphotic/scoliotic deformities.[10,11,12,13] However, cranioskeletal traction is contraindicated in patients with skull fractures and bone density disorders such as Paget disease. Relative contraindications may include occipitocervical dislocations and subluxations, intracranial pathologies requiring open surgical management (i.e., hemorrhage, neoplasms, etc.), cervical distraction-extension injuries, in cases where there is evidence of

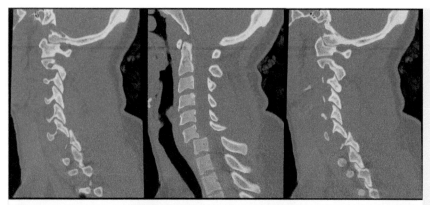

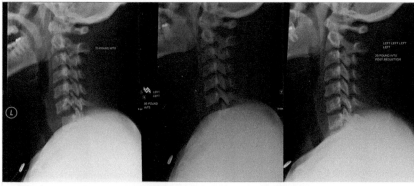

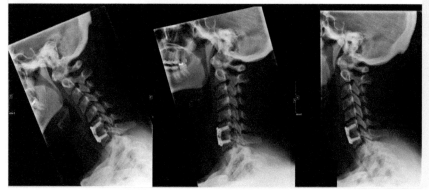

Fig. 5.1 A 33-year-old woman fell down stairs on her birthday and was brought emergently to the emergency room. She had neck pain, an inability to move her lower extremities, and weakness and numbness in her hands. A detailed neurological assessment confirmed an American Spinal Injury Association A spinal cord injury at the C7 level. Plain films were normal to the C6 level and C7 was not able to be visualized. A STAT computed tomography (CT) scan was obtained. **(a)** CT scan sagittal reconstructions—Bilateral jumped facets with the subluxation just short of completely burying the facets (partially perched). **(b)** Patient was taken immediately to Radiology suite and placed in traction. No reduction was achieved at 70 lb. At 90 lb, reduction occurred with a palpable "clunk." Immediately, the weights were reduced to 20 lb and alignment was maintained. **(c)** Patient was taken from Radiology suite directly to the operating room for an anterior cervical discectomy and fusion (ACDF) at C6–C7. This surgery was performed in less than 1 hour from when the fall occurred. Six-month post-operative images show solid fusion with bridging trabecular bone and no motion between the spinous processes on flexion/extension views. The patient regained motor and sensory functions in the initial 48 hours following surgery. At her 6-month evaluation, she had only numbness in the left C7 dermatome. The rationale for going immediately to traction was the complete injury and the perceived need to reduce the subluxation as soon as possible. In this setting, our opinion was that magnetic resonance imaging would delay the treatment and could lessen the chance of a neurological recovery.

disc or bone displaced within the spinal canal (▶ Fig. 5.3),[10] and in young patients without fused cranial plates (less than 3 years of age). Caution must be exercised when applying traction in patients with decreased consciousness and in patients who are not stable and/or alert, as obtaining neurological assessments both prior to and following the application of weighted traction, may not be possible.

5.3 Gardner–Wells Tongs

5.3.1 Tong Placement

As had been previously discussed, the Gardner–Wells tongs consist of a stainless steel or graphite-based C-shaped rod attached via two-point pin fixation to the skull (▶ Fig. 5.2a). Once a thorough history has been taken and a detailed neurological assessment (including analysis of sensation and motor responses) of the patient has been performed, he or she is placed in the supine position on a hard surface. The sites where the two pins are to be inserted should be cleaned with an anti-

septic solution. A local anesthetic can then be applied to these regions. The pins are positioned 2 cm superior to the pinna in line with the external auditory meatus while being inferior to the equator of the calvarium to prevent slippage. They can be placed anterior to, in line with, or posterior to the external auditory meatus depending on the degree of neck flexion or extension required to achieve spinal cord decompression and cervical alignment. This may be done with the aid of imaging. Once the pins are secured to the outer table of the skull (at which point the unmarked indicator stems protrude approximately 1 mm and indicate that 25 pounds of force have been applied), nuts should be secured lateral to the tong proper to prevent pin detachment (▶ Fig. 5.2b).[14] The pins should be retightened only once within the first 24 hours. A rope-and-pulley system can be then attached to the center of the rod for the application of weighted traction that is in line with the axial skeleton. Manipulation of the height of the rope-and-pulley system allows for control of the degree of flexion or extension of the cervical spine. Traction is typically applied in 5 to 10 lb increments (over 15- to 20-minute time intervals), between

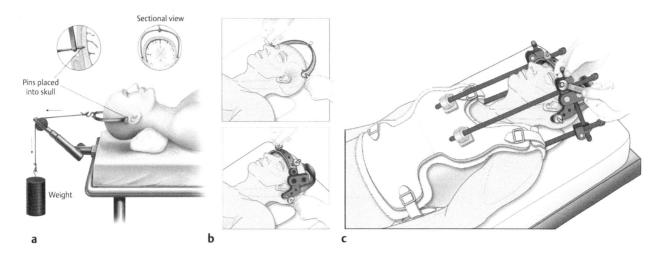

Fig. 5.2 **(a)** Gardner–Wells tongs in place with traction. **(b)** Procedural steps:
(1) Gardner–Wells tongs: Place pins through the tongs into scalp and pericranium. Tighten both pins simultaneously until torque indicator on one pin protrudes approximately 1 to 2 mm, indicating adequately tightened screws.
(2) Halo ring: Tighten two diametrically opposed screws simultaneously until "finger tight." Then tighten the other two screws simultaneously until "finger tight." At this point, use torque wrench to adequately and safely secure pin tightness to preset maximal torque (8 inch-lb for adults).
Pearls:
• Pay attention to eyes and eyebrows to avoid pinning eyes open or closed.
For children: Use lower final torque for tightening (4–8 inch-lb for children aged 3–10 years, 2–4 inch-lb for children under age 3 years). Use multiple (6–10) pins in order to distribute pressure evenly circumferentially and avoid fracture or excessive skull penetration. Also, use specially supplied pediatric pins with short tips and wide flange, if available. **(c)** Procedural steps: Select correct vest size for the patient. Connect posterior ring to posterior vest with upright post. Connect anterior ring to anterior vest with upright posts. Connect anterior/posterior halves of vest to each other. Once in place, secure the ring to the posts at each point with torque wrench, maintaining head in correct alignment. Check post-placement X-rays immediately after placement and when upright day 1 and day 3.
Pearls:
• Important note: Every brand and style of halo vest and head ring comes with a detailed set of instructions for application. It is recommended to review these instructions carefully prior to applying the apparatus.
• Incorrect sizing of vest can lead to loss of alignment.
• If posterior vest has not been "preplaced," patient can be logrolled, or elevated 30 degrees while head held in gentle manual traction.
• Tape wrench to anterior vest for easy access in emergency.
• Watch for pressure ulcers at sites of excess pressure on shoulders, back, and chest.
(Fig. 5.2a reproduced from An HS, Singh K. Synopsis of Spine Surgery. New York, NY: Thieme; 2016. Fig. 5.2b, c reproduced from Ullman JS, Raskin PB. Atlas of Emergency Neurosurgery. New York, NY: Thieme; 2015.)

which serial neurological and radiological examinations are performed in order to identify changes in neurological status, and/or any evidence of overdistraction injury.[15] Much variability exists regarding the ideal weight to use for traction. Some surgeons have used 5 lb per level as the maximum amount of weight applied, while other prior studies have recommended traction weights of 45 to 80 pounds be applied.[16,17,18,19] Adjuvant muscle relaxants can also be administered to prevent muscle spasm.[20] Once closed reduction is achieved, traction weights can be reduced and the patient can be placed. Typically, upon reduction of a subluxation, a traction weight between 15 and 20 lb is adequate to maintain the reduction.

5.3.2 Clinical Outcomes Following Closed Reduction of the Cervical Spine with Gardner–Wells Tongs

Gardner–Wells tongs are utilized to provide temporary (rather than long-term) craniocervical traction for the restoration of anatomic alignment of the spine and, thereby, achieve spinal cord decompression.[19] The most common indications for their use include unilateral or bilateral cervical facet joint disloca-

tions (▶ Fig. 5.2 and ▶ Fig. 5.3).[14] Star et al reported on their use of the Gardner–Wells tongs in 1990 for the closed reduction of cervical facet dislocations in a series of 53 patients. They found that 68% of patients in their cohort had an improvement in neurological status following the application of traction. Based upon a cadaveric analysis, they advised that the tongs could support traction weights of up to 100 lb.[8] In 1993, Cotler et al reported on a series of 24 patients with C4–C7 facet joint dislocations who underwent successful reduction via weighted traction of up to 140 lb and subsequent posterior fusion procedures. Of note, these "high-weight" reductions were performed under continuous direct observation by the treatment team who immediately decreased the weight upon achieving reduction. The authors did not note any instances of deterioration in neurological status.[21] Gardner–Wells tongs have been used for the application of cranioskeletal traction following isolated cervical facet fractures as well. In a systematic review performed by Kepler et al, the authors documented that 63.8% of patients with cervical facet fractures underwent successful closed reduction with tongs.[22] Successful closed reduction has also been reported in a series of 121 patients with cervical compressive burst fractures, extension injuries, or fractures with subluxations. The average time taken to achieve reduction in these

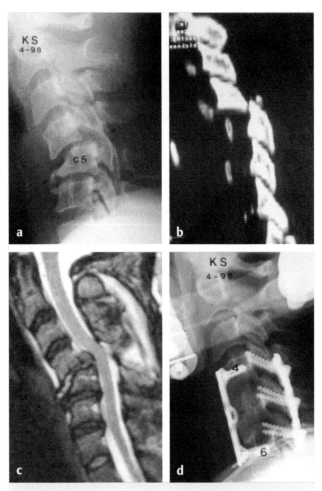

Fig. 5.3 A 45-year-old woman was assaulted by her boyfriend and she sustained a cervical spine injury. She was brought to the emergency room, awake and coherent, and a neurological examination demonstrated only a right sided C5 nerve deficit. Spinal cord function was preserved. **(a)** Plain radiograph demonstrated perched facets at the C4–C5 level. **(b)** A CT scan with sagittal reconstructions showed that the perched facets were actually partially jumped (high-riding facets). **(c)** A magnetic resonance imaging (MRI) study showed a large herniated disc located behind the C4 vertebral body with a significant C4–C5 subluxation and cord compression but no abnormal cord signal in the spinal cord proper. Abnormal signal traversed the C4–C5 disc space and there was splaying of the spinous processes of C4–C5 with abnormal signal in the interspinous ligaments. **(d)** One-year postoperative plain film demonstrating successful fusion (C4–C6) following an AP treatment including a C5 corpectomy followed by posterior lateral mass fusions from C4–C6. The patient was taken to an MRI study because her neurological examination demonstrated only minor nerve root symptomatology, and she was wide awake and able to cooperate with serial neurological examinations. Upon noting the large disc herniation at C4–C5, the decision was made to not utilize traction (out of concern for inducing a cord deficit); rather, an immediate operation was performed which decompressed the cord anteriorly and then stabilized posteriorly. At 1 year postoperatively, she was neurologically intact.

patients was 2.1 hours.[20] Subsequent open surgical reduction was required in two (2.4%) patients.

The exact time point following injury at which closed reduction should be performed remains unclear. Cotler and colleagues have observed greater neurological recovery if reduction is attempted within the initial 8-hour period immediately following injury. This would suggest that a neuroprotective effect may be present for a short period of time following injury.[23] In neurologically intact patients, the relative role of timing the decompression is poorly understood. In patients with neurological injuries with radiographic evidence of canal compromise, our practice has been the immediate application of traction in the emergency department. Prospective randomized control studies evaluating the optimal time point at which closed reduction for spinal cord decompression should be attempted would be ideal.

5.3.3 Timing of MRI and Traction Reduction

A debate exists among spine surgeons regarding magnetic resonance imaging (MRI) before versus after traction reduction of cervical dislocations or fracture-dislocations. There is a small but real risk of displacing or dragging disc material posteriorly into the spinal canal with any method of reduction, possibly causing neurological compromise.[24] Obtaining an MRI scan before reduction can identify a disc herniation that may be behind the dislocated vertebra and thus guide the surgeon to a pre-emptive anterior operative approach to first clean out the disc herniation, and then reduce and stabilize the dislocation. However, logistically obtaining an MRI in the setting of an acute injury takes time, and cord compression from the vertebral displacement can be most rapidly corrected with traction reduction. Thus, there is potential benefit or mitigation of risk with either pathway for any given patient.

Recommendations for this scenario depend on the specifics of the patient's condition, including neurological status (SCI vs. normal neurologically) and mental status (awake and communicative vs. obtunded/noncommunicative). In a patient without neurological deficit and a dislocation, it seems prudent to obtain an MRI to rule out a disc herniation that might cause deficit with reduction. However, an argument can be made to reduce this patient promptly, in case they are awake and alert. Any neurological symptoms during or after reduction can be immediately acted on such as halting the reduction, although if necessary, getting an emergent MRI and proceeding to the operating room in this situation takes valuable time. For patients with known SCI, prompt traction reduction to realign the canal seems paramount to quickly relieve as much compression as possible. Obtunded or intubated patients with an unknown neurological status require a choice. Severe dislocations with obvious canal compromise and suspected SCI probably warrant immediate reduction, whereas less severe injuries where the cord might have escaped injury could be imaged first to look for disc material. One clue to disc disruption is a narrowed disc space on plain films or CT scans compared to the other levels, as that nucleus pulposus/annulus possibly extruded into the canal.

5.3.4 Complications Associated with Use of the Gardner–Wells Tongs

Complications associated with use of the Gardner–Wells tongs include infection at the site of pin insertion (which can lead to osteomyelitis of the skull),[14] pin perforation of the inner table of the calvarium and subsequent intracranial trauma,[15] and pin pull-out/migration with resultant scalp lacerations. Patients can also develop pressure ulcers over the occiput if craniocervical traction is maintained for prolonged periods of time. A prior cadaveric study has demonstrated that the pullout strength of the Gardner–Wells tongs is dependent on the materials used to make the pins, with MRI-compatible titanium pins and graphite tongs more likely to undergo mechanical deformation leading to tong slippage as compared to stainless steel pins and tongs.[25] An advantage of graphite tongs is the ability to obtain MR images while in traction; however, the downside is the higher likelihood of pin pullout (particularly at higher weights). Consequently, traction weights greater than 50 lb should be applied with caution when MRI-compatible tongs are being used. Lerman et al posit that the pullout strength also decreases in heavily used tongs due to wear-and-tear on the pins/pin springs. In such cases, replacement or recalibration of the tongs may be indicated to prevent device failure and/or detachment from occurring.[26] To prevent infection of the pin insertion sites, they should be cleaned daily with an antiseptic solution.

Indicator stem protrusion less than 0.25 mm has been associated with a pullout strength of less than 60 lb, suggesting that the pins should be adequately tightened prior to application of weighted traction.[27] Overtightening and/or frequent retightening of the pins, however, can lead to pin penetration through the inner table and subsequent intracranial injury or hemorrhage.

5.4 Halo Fixation

5.4.1 Halo Application

The halo ring (or cranial halo) is secured to the skull via four-point fixation in adults. This allows for higher traction weights to be applied and, by design, results in an increase in the pullout force needed for the device to detach.[14] The ring is typically made of a composite of carbon fiber and titanium, and can also be attached to a fleece-lined vest (via rods) for the rigid immobilization of the cervical spine in the outpatient setting. This brace is collectively referred to as the halo vest. Application of the fixator requires selection of a halo ring of the appropriate size. A ring, which leaves 1 to 2 cm gap between the scalp and the ring when placed at the circumference of the equator of the skull, is appropriate. Prior to insertion of the pins that hold the device in place, the pin sites should be cleaned with an antiseptic solution. A local anesthetic can then be injected into each of the four planned pin sites (which must be carefully selected prior to pin insertion).

The anterior pin sites should be located 1 cm above the orbital rims (i.e., above the eyebrow to prevent damage to the supraorbital and/or trochlear nerves), and superior to the lateral two-thirds of the orbit. The posterior pins should be inserted behind the ears, below the equator of the calvarium, and diagonally across from the anterior pins. Once both anterior and posterior pin sites have been determined, the pins can be inserted perpendicular to the surface of the scalp provided that the patient's head is kept immobilized by a separate member of the treatment team and the patient has been placed in the supine position. Caution must be exercised to ensure that the pins do not perforate the temporalis muscle or the squamous part of the temporal bone (which is appreciably thinner than the parietal bone). A torque wrench is used to tighten the pins to a force no greater than 10 inch-lb to prevent penetration of the inner table.[28] The usual insertion torques in our practice have been 8 inch-lb for adults and 4 to 6 inch-lb for pediatric patients. The pins should be tightened in an alternating fashion (i.e., first the anterior followed by the contralateral posterior pins) to keep tension among the pins and to minimize the risk of perforation (▶ Fig. 5.1b). The pins should be retorqued after 24 hours. Hexagonal lock nuts, which are threaded onto the ends of the pins, are used to prevent pin loosening and detachment. Traction can be applied in a similar manner to Gardner–Wells tongs. In pediatric patients, additional pin sites may be used to increase the distribution of the traction weight. A halo vest affixed to the cranial halo via posts may be used to maintain stabilization of the c-spine and to promote bony union on a longer-term outpatient basis (▶ Fig. 5.1c).

5.4.2 Clinical Outcomes Following Halo Fixation of the Cervical Spine

The halo apparatus is commonly used to reduce and stabilize axial odontoid and hangman fractures, ring fractures of the atlas, and, less commonly, subaxial (C3–C7) burst fractures.[19,29,30,31,32,33] Fixation to the halo vest provides a greater degree of immobilization of the cervical spine compared with other orthotic devices (it restricts up to 75% of flexion or extension of the upper cervical spine[34]). It also allows for control of the spine in three different planes and can be used successfully following reduction with the halo ring as a substitute for surgical decompression. It can also be used as an adjunct following open reduction and internal surgical cervical fixation.[10,35,36]

Prior studies have demonstrated that immobilization of the cervical spine with the halo apparatus can achieve outcomes comparable to those following open surgical fusion procedures. Bucholz et al reported on 109 patients who underwent fixation for C1–C2 injuries (including atlantoaxial subluxations, hangman fractures, axial body fractures, and arch fractures of the atlas) and C3–T1 injuries. They documented an 85% success rate, but cautioned against the use of halo fixation in patients with locked or "perched" facets.[35] In a larger cohort of 188 patients with traumatic cervical spine injuries, who underwent fixation with the halo apparatus, Chan and colleagues reported that cervical alignment and stability was maintained in 89% of patients at follow-up. The mean time for bony union was 11.5 weeks. However, in a subset of 40 patients from this study who underwent halo immobilization for locked facets, halo fixation alone was unsuccessful in 32.5% of cases as compared to 0% when patients had previously undergone open cervical fusion procedures. In another study, Cooper et al reported that 85% of patients with cervical spine fractures or subluxations treated with the halo apparatus obtained restoration of spinal stability at radiographic follow-up.[10] Finally, Ekong and colleagues noted an increased rate of bone nonunion in elderly patients and in patients with type 2 odontoid fractures.[37]

5.4.3 Complications Associated with Use of the Cranial Halo and/or Halo Vest

Complications observed when reducing and/or stabilizing the cervical spine with the cranial halo are similar to those previously discussed in the context of Gardner–Wells tongs. Briefly, these can include but are not limited to pin penetration of the inner table of the calvarium, infection at a pin insertion site (which can lead to osteomyelitis or subdural abscess formation in severe cases), periorbital edema, pressure ulcers, and nerve palsies.[38] Halo vest immobilization has been found to be less effective in the lower cervical spine as compared with the upper cervical spine due to the phenomenon of "snaking" described originally by Johnson et al.[39,40] "Snaking" refers to the combination of flexion at one cervical level and extension at an adjacent cervical level that can occur when the halo apparatus is utilized. This results in significant motion of the cervical spine at individual vertebral levels that can lead to loss in reduction.[41] Other orthoses may be indicated in patients presenting with lower cervical spine injuries.

5.5 Conclusion

Controversy exists regarding the ideal timing of decompression following fracture-subluxations of the cervical spine. While recent reports of the Surgical Timing in Acute Spinal Cord Injury Study (STASCIS) trial favor surgical reduction within 8 hours, it is not clear where reduction with traction fits into this algorithm.[42,43] Our treatment philosophy has been to attempt to achieve reduction with traction as soon as possible in emergency trauma situations. This typically is done within 2 to 4 hours from the injury. Once the spine has been reduced and the neural elements are no longer compressed, the exact timing for definitive surgical stabilization remains controversial and is currently not well established. It has been our consistent belief that relieving the pressure on the spinal cord is the essential feature of treating SCI victims and whether this should be done with traction or immediate surgery is debatable. If traction is not able to decompress the spinal canal in a reasonable time frame (within 2–4 hours), our treatment algorithm calls for prompt operative intervention to achieve decompression of the spinal cord.

References

[1] Loeser JD. History of skeletal traction in the treatment of cervical spine injuries. J Neurosurg. 1970; 33(1):54–59

[2] Hildanus F. Opera (1672). 1 History of Neurological Surgery. New York, NY: Hatner Publishing Company; 1967:366

[3] Taylor AS. Fracture dislocation of the cervical spine. Ann Surg. 1929; 90(3):321–340

[4] Park SW, Cho KH, Shin YS, et al. Successful reduction for a pediatric chronic atlantoaxial rotatory fixation (Grisel syndrome) with long-term halter traction: case report. Spine. 2005; 30(15):E444–E449

[5] Olivero WC, Dulebohn SC. Results of halter cervical traction for the treatment of cervical radiculopathy: retrospective review of 81 patients. Neurosurg Focus. 2002; 12(2):ECP1

[6] Crutchfield WG. Skeletal traction in treatment of injuries to the cervical spine. J Am Med Assoc. 1954; 155(1):29–32

[7] Gardner WJ. The principle of spring-loaded points for cervical traction. Technical note. J Neurosurg. 1973; 39(4):543–544

[8] Star AM, Jones AA, Cotler JM, Balderston RA, Sinha R. Immediate closed reduction of cervical spine dislocations using traction. Spine. 1990; 15(10):1068–1072

[9] Perry J, Nickel VL. Total cervicalspine fusion for neck paralysis. J Bone Joint Surg Am. 1959; 41-A(1):37–60

[10] Cooper PR, Maravilla KR, Sklar FH, Moody SF, Clark WK. Halo immobilization of cervical spine fractures. Indications and results. J Neurosurg. 1979; 50(5):603–610

[11] Hsu LC. Halo-pelvic traction: a means of correcting severe spinal deformities. Hong Kong Med J. 2014; 20(4):358–359

[12] Morton J, Malins P. The correction of spinal deformities by halo-pelvic traction. Physiotherapy. 1971; 57(12):576–581

[13] Twomey MR. Halo pelvic traction. A new method of correcting deformities of the spine. Nurs Times. 1970; 66(39):1225–1228

[14] Medress ZA, Veeravagu A, Ratliff JK, Grant GA. Spinal traction. In: Steinmetz MP, Benzel EC, eds. Benzel's Spine Surgery: Techniques, Complication Avoidance, and Management. Vol 2. Philadelphia, PA: Elsevier; 2017:1196–1201

[15] Campe C, Hilibrand A. Closed skeletal traction techniques. In: Vaccaro A, Anderson P, eds. Cervical Spine Trauma. Philadelphia, PA: Lippincott, Williams and Wilkins; 2009

[16] Yashon D, Tyson G, Vise WM. Rapid closed reduction of cervical fracture dislocations. Surg Neurol. 1975; 4(6):513–514

[17] Norrell H. The treatment of unstable spinal fractures and dislocations. Clin Neurosurg. 1978; 25:193–208

[18] Cotler HB, Miller LS, DeLucia FA, Cotler JM, Davne SH. Closed reduction of cervical spine dislocations. Clin Orthop Relat Res. 1987(214):185–199

[19] Eskander MS, Brooks DD. Cervical orthoses and cranioskeletal traction. In: Benzel EC, ed. The Cervical Spine. 5th ed. Philadelphia, PA: Lippincott Williams and Wilkins; 2012 104–115

[20] Grant GA, Mirza SK, Chapman JR, et al. Risk of early closed reduction in cervical spine subluxation injuries. J Neurosurg. 1999; 90(1) Suppl:13–18

[21] Cotler JM, Herbison GJ, Nasuti JF, Ditunno JF, Jr, An H, Wolff BE. Closed reduction of traumatic cervical spine dislocation using traction weights up to 140 pounds. Spine. 1993; 18(3):386–390

[22] Kepler CK, Vaccaro AR, Chen E, et al. Treatment of isolated cervical facet fractures: a systematic review. J Neurosurg Spine. 201 6; 24:347–354

[23] Rizzolo SJ, Vaccaro AR, Cotler JM. Cervical spine trauma. Spine. 1994; 19(20):2288–2298

[24] Eismont FJ, Arena MJ, Green BA. Extrusion of an intervertebral disc associated with traumatic subluxation or dislocation of cervical facets. Case report. J Bone Joint Surg Am. 1991; 73(10):1555–1560

[25] Blumberg KD, Catalano JB, Cotler JM, Balderston RA. The pullout strength of titanium alloy MRI-compatible and stainless steel MRI-incompatible Gardner-Wells tongs. Spine. 1993; 18(13):1895–1896

[26] Lerman JA, Haynes RJ, Koeneman EJ, Koeneman JB, Wong WB. A biomechanical comparison of Gardner-Wells tongs and halo device used for cervical spine traction. Spine. 1994; 19(21):2403–2406

[27] Krag MH, Byrt W, Pope M. Pull-off strength of Gardner-Wells tongs from cadaveric crania. Spine. 1989; 14(3):247–250

[28] Botte MJ, Byrne TP, Abrams RA, Garfin SR. Halo skeletal fixation: techniques of application and prevention of complications. J Am Acad Orthop Surg. 1996; 4(1):44–53

[29] Apuzzo ML, Heiden JS, Weiss MH, Ackerson TT, Harvey JP, Kurze T. Acute fractures of the odontoid process. An analysis of 45 cases. J Neurosurg. 1978; 48(1):85–91

[30] Ewald FC. Fracture of the odontoid process in a seventeen-month-old infant treated with a halo. A case report and discussion of the injury under the age of three. J Bone Joint Surg Am. 1971; 53(8):1636–1640

[31] Lyddon DW, Jr. Experience with the halo and body cast in the ambulatory treatment of cervical spine fractures. Ill Med J. 1974; 146(5):458–461, 490

[32] Prolo DJ, Runnels JB, Jameson RM. The injured cervical spine. Immediate and long-term immobilization with the halo. JAMA. 1973; 224(5):591–594

[33] Zimmerman E, Grant J, Vise WM, Yashon D, Hunt WE. Treatment of Jefferson fracture with a halo apparatus. Report of two cases. J Neurosurg. 1976; 44(3):372–375

[34] Lauweryns P. Role of conservative treatment of cervical spine injuries. Eur Spine J. 2010; 19 Suppl 1:S23–S26

[35] Bucholz RD, Cheung KC. Halo vest versus spinal fusion for cervical injury: evidence from an outcome study. J Neurosurg. 1989; 70(6):884–892

[36] Kostuik JP. Indications for the use of the halo immobilization. Clin Orthop Relat Res. 1981(154):46–50

[37] Ekong CE, Schwartz ML, Tator CH, Rowed DW, Edmonds VE. Odontoid fracture: management with early mobilization using the halo device. Neurosurgery. 1981; 9(6):631–637

[38] Hayes VM, Silber JS, Siddiqi FN, Kondrachov D, Lipetz JS, Lonner B. Complications of halo fixation of the cervical spine. Am J Orthop. 2005; 34(6):271–276

[39] Johnson RM, Owen JR, Hart DL, Callahan RA. Cervical orthoses: a guide to their selection and use. Clin Orthop Relat Res. 1981(154):34–45

[40] Johnson RM, Hart DL, Simmons EF, Ramsby GR, Southwick WO. Cervical orthoses. A study comparing their effectiveness in restricting cervical motion in normal subjects. J Bone Joint Surg Am. 1977; 59(3):332–339

[41] Glaser JA, Whitehill R, Stamp WG, Jane JA. Complications associated with the halo-vest. A review of 245 cases. J Neurosurg. 1986; 65(6):762–769

[42] Fehlings MG, Vaccaro A, Wilson JR, et al. Early versus delayed decompression for traumatic cervical spinal cord injury: results of the Surgical Timing in Acute Spinal Cord Injury Study (STASCIS). PLoS One. 2012; 7(2):e32037

[43] Jug M, Kejžar N, Vesel M, et al. Neurological recovery after traumatic cervical spinal cord injury is superior if surgical decompression and instrumented fusion are performed within 8 hours versus 8 to 24 hours after injury: a single center experience. J Neurotrauma. 2015; 32(18):1385–1392

6 Atlanto-occipital Injuries

Derrick Sun and Paul A. Anderson

Abstract

Injuries to the upper cervical spine are common after high-energy trauma and are associated with high morbidity and mortality. Rapid diagnosis and appropriate treatment of these injuries lead to improved mortality and patient outcomes. Injuries to the atlas, occipital condyles, and the craniocervical junction, including the atlanto-occipital articulation, are the focus of this chapter. The relevant anatomy, diagnosis, classification systems, and treatment options are discussed.

Keywords: atlas fracture, occipital condyle fracture, Jefferson fracture, atlanto-occipital dissociation, craniocervical dissociation

6.1 Introduction

Injuries between the occiput and C2 constitute "upper cervical spine injuries," and these are common after high-energy trauma. The magnitude and the direction of the impact force may vary, from direct axial loading, to bending in the sagittal and coronal plane, or rarely, in rotation. The complex anatomy of the craniocervical junction and the variable mechanism of injury lead to a wide spectrum of injuries. The upper cervical spine allows for approximately 50% of the total cervical spine rotation, and 20% of the anterior, posterior, and lateral bending.

This chapter will focus on injuries of the atlas, the occipital condyle, and the craniocervical junction. Injuries to the axis and the atlantoaxial articulation will be discussed elsewhere. These areas are anatomically and biomechanically related, and injury to one area may occur concomitantly with injury to another.

6.2 Anatomy

6.2.1 Occiput

The occipital bone forms the foramen magnum. The occipital condyles are semilunar projections from the inferior surface of the occiput that lie within the concavities of the lateral masses of the atlas, forming a shallow ball-and-socket configuration. The atlanto-occipital joint articulation is stabilized by the alar ligaments, which are paired, cord-like structures that project laterally from the tips of the odontoid process to the inner aspect of each occipital condyle, and by the tectorial membrane, which is the cranial continuation of the posterior longitudinal ligaments to the anterior aspect of the foramen magnum. The tectorial membrane and the paired alar ligaments are crucial for craniocervical stability.[1] The alar ligaments are slack when the head is in mid position. As the head rotates toward one direction, the alar ligament contralateral to the direction of rotation tightens, while the ipsilateral ligament slackens. Together with the tectorial membrane, the alar ligaments also limit flexion, but play no role in limiting extension.

Anteriorly, the well-developed atlanto-occipital membrane, an extension of the anterior longitudinal ligament, limits extension. Structures such as the apical ligaments, the occipitocervical membrane, and the atlanto-occipital joint capsules provide little intrinsic stability. Normally, the atlanto-occipital joints have a congruous relationship, and more than 2 mm of diastasis suggests a ligamentous disruption and unstable injury[2] (▶ Fig. 6.1c).

6.2.2 Atlas

The atlas is a ring-shaped structure with large lateral masses and thin anterior and posterior connecting arches (▶ Fig. 6.1a). The lateral masses of the atlas articulate superiorly with the occipital condyles, and inferiorly with the lateral masses of the axis (▶ Fig. 6.1b). In the coronal plane, the atlas lateral masses are trapezoid in shape. The articulation of atlanto-occipital joint is sloped from inferior medially to superior laterally. The articulation of the atlantoaxial joint is sloped from superior medially to inferior laterally. This configuration results in transferring of axial loading forces onto the atlas lateral masses to be directed laterally, causing the typical "burst" pattern of injury.

The cruciate ligament lies behind the dens and consists of the transverse ligament and fibers that attach cranially to the basion and caudally to the axis. The transverse ligament, which passes around the dens at its waist, attaches to the tubercles on the medial side of each atlas lateral mass (▶ Fig. 6.1d). The atlantoaxial articulation allows for 45 degrees of axial rotation in each direction, limited in part by tightening of the opposite alar ligament. It accounts for 50% of the rotation of the cervical spine and allows for 20 to 30 degrees of flexion-extension.[3,4] Werne et al have shown the atlanto-occipital articulation allows for 15 degrees of flexion-extension, 8 degrees of lateral bending, and 0 degrees of axial rotation.[5,6]

Steel's "rule of thirds" states that at the level of the atlas, the odontoid process takes up one-third of the total space, the spinal cord takes up one-third of the space, and the cerebrospinal fluid space constitutes the remaining one-third.[7]

6.2.3 Axis

The axis has a large projection, called the dens or odontoid process. The dens lies behind the anterior arch of the atlas, and the transverse ligament wraps behind the dens, providing stability and prevents anterior-to-posterior atlantoaxial shear.

6.2.4 Vertebral Arteries

The vertebral arteries are paired vessels that typically arise from the right and left subclavian arteries. Rarely, the vertebral artery could arise directly from the aortic arch itself.[39] The vertebral arteries ascend cephalad to enter the transverse foramina typically at the C6 vertebral segment. In 12% of the cases, the

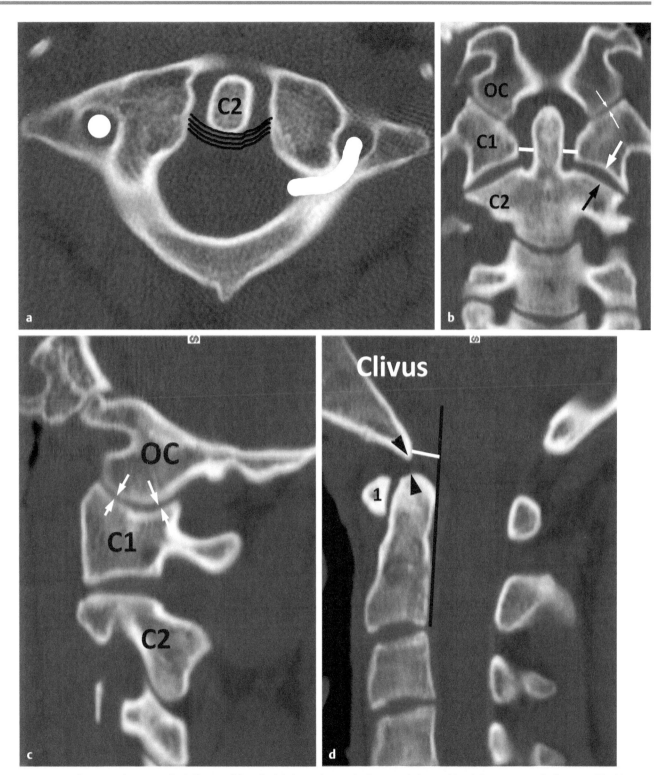

Fig. 6.1 Axial computed tomography (CT) scan of the atlas (**a**) shows the vertebral arteries (*white circle*) and the transverse alar ligament (*black lines*). Coronal image (**b**) shows the relationship of the occipital condyles (OC), atlas lateral masses, and axis. Parasagittal image (**c**) demonstrates the condyle–C1 interval (*thin white arrows*). Mid-sagittal view (**d**) shows the basion–dens interval (*black arrowheads*), the basion–axis interval (*white line*).

vertebral arteries enter the foramen at other vertebral levels. The vertebral artery is divided into following four segments:

1. The V1 (extraosseous) segment courses cephalad from the subclavian arteries to enter the transverse foramen of the C6 vertebra.
2. The V2 (foraminal) segment ascends vertically through the C6 to C3 transverse foramina, turns laterally to exit the C2 foramen, then turns medially once it exits above the C1 foramen.
3. The V3 (extraspinal) segment begins as the artery exits from the C1 foramen and ends when it penetrates the dura. The vertebral artery forms a prominent groove along the posterior arch of the atlas.
4. The V4 (intradural) segment courses anteromedially through the foramen magnum and joins the contralateral vertebral artery to form the basilar artery at the pontomedullary junction.

Burst fractures of the atlas with displacement could be associated with injuries to the V3 (extraspinal) segment of the vertebral artery. Ponticulus posticus is an osseous anomaly of the atlas, characterized by the presence of an arcuate foramen. This is a poorly recognized anatomic anomaly that is present in up to 15.5% of the patients; its proper recognition is important to avoid injury to the vertebral artery during exposure or placement of C1 lateral mass screws.[40]

6.3 Physical Exam

Upper cervical spine injuries often occur as result of high-energy trauma resulting in skull impaction. Partial or total loss of consciousness is often reported. Alert patients may complain of upper cervical pain to movement or palpation. Various neurological syndromes have been described in patients with upper cervical spine injuries, especially involving cranial nerve VI and the lower cranial nerves IX, X, XI, and XII. Full neurological assessment should be performed according to the American Spinal Injury Association (ASIA) guidelines.

6.4 Radiographic Exam

Upper cervical spine injuries are best evaluated with computed tomography (CT) imaging with sagittal and coronal reconstruction. CT scan has been shown to be timely, cost effective, and more sensitive and specific in high-risk trauma patients.[2] On CT imaging, the atlanto-occipital joint should be congruous, and greater than 2 mm of diastasis of the articulation should prompt concern for atlanto-occipital dissociation (AOD). Pang et al reported an average of 1.28 mm of condyle–C1 interval (CCI) in normal children, and none of the CCIs exceeded 1.95 mm.[8,37] The Harris' "rule of twelves" indicates that the distance from the tip of the dens to the basion (basion–dental interval) should be less than 12 mm, and the basion–axial interval, which is the distance from the basion to the posterior axial line, should also be less than 12 mm. Violation of this rule should prompt concern for AOD.[9,10]

The atlantodental interval (ADI) is the distance between the anterior atlas arch and the odontoid process. In adults, ADI less than 3 mm is considered normal, while in children, less than

5 mm is normal. ADI greater than this indicates potential disruption of the transverse ligament and potential atlantoaxial instability.

Magnetic resonance imaging (MRI) focused toward the skull base or the craniocervical junction may be useful to rule out ligamentous injury when diagnosis is not clear. Indicators of unstable injury include significant prevertebral soft-tissue edema or hematoma, increased joint edema in atlanto-occipital or atlantoaxial joints, tectorial membrane disruption, transverse ligament or alar ligament disruption, or subarachnoid hemorrhage.

6.5 Occipital Condyle Injury

6.5.1 Introduction

Traumatic occipital condyle fracture (OCF) was first described by Sir Charles Bell in 1817 based on autopsy of a patient from a fall.[11] Plain radiographs rarely visualize OCFs. Improvement in advanced imaging and more prevalent use of CT imaging over the past two decades have led to an increase in detection of this injury. Except when associated with craniocervical instability, OCFs are relatively benign and are usually managed conservatively. OCFs occur in 1 to 4% of patients with traumatic brain injury[12] (▶ Fig. 6.2).

The most common mechanisms of injury are from impaction of skull onto the cervical spine or rapid head deceleration. OCFs should be suspected in patients with high-energy head trauma, altered mental status, upper cervical spine tenderness, lower cranial nerve deficits, and retropharyngeal hematoma or edema. Cranial nerve XII, the hypoglossal nerve, travels in the hypoglossal canal superior to the occipital condyle and may be injured with OCF.

6.5.2 Classification

The most commonly utilized classification system was proposed in 1988 by Anderson and Montesano that classifies OCF into following three types:[13]

1. Type I fractures are comminuted fractures secondary to axial loading and impaction of the occipital condyle on the lateral masses of the atlas. These are stable (▶ Fig. 6.2).
2. Type II fractures are extension of a linear basilar skull base fracture.
3. Type III fractures are traumatic avulsion of a fragment via the tensile forces of the alar ligament. These may be potentially unstable and may be associated with craniocervical dissociation (CCD) (▶ Fig. 6.3).

Type I fractures are stable and cervical collar immobilization is recommended for these. Type II fractures are typically stable, except in the rare instance when the entire condyle is detached, making the atlanto-occipital articulation unstable. Cervical collar immobilization is recommended for stable type II fractures, whereas halo vest should be considered for unstable type II fracture with incompetent alar ligament and displacement of atlanto-occipital alignment. Type III fracture should prompt evaluation for possible AOD with MRI of the craniocervical junction. Evaluation of the atlanto-occipital articulation is

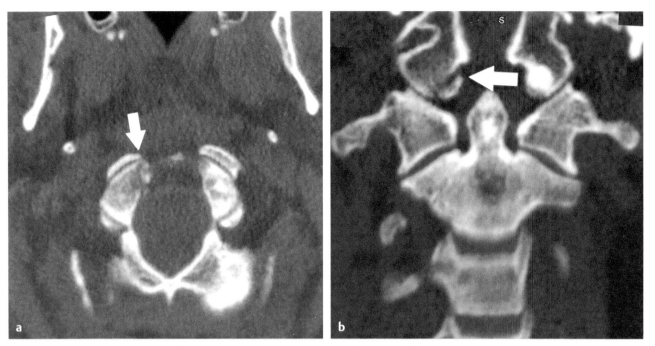

Fig. 6.2 Axial (**a**) and coronal (**b**) computed tomography (CT) scans show a type I right occipital condyle fracture in a 54-year-old male who was an unrestrained passenger in a motor vehicle crash. No ligamentous injury was noted on magnetic resonance imaging, and he was successfully treated with 6 weeks of hard cervical collar immobilization.

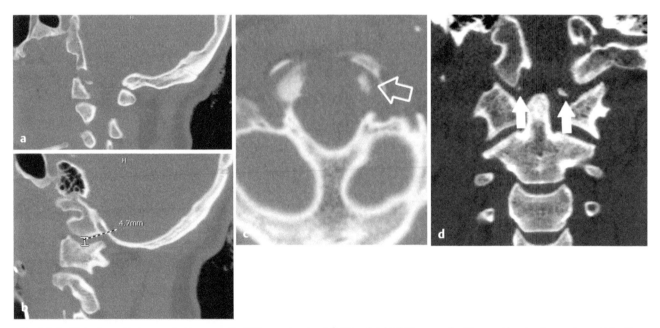

Fig. 6.3 Sagittal reformatted computed tomography (CT) scan showing left (**a**) and right (**b**) images of a 44-year-old male who was brought in after automobile-versus-pedestrian accident, demonstrating type III occipital condyle fractures, and increased condyle-to-C1 interval. Axial (**c**) and coronal (**d**) images demonstrate bilateral occipital condyle fractures. The patient remained comatose and succumbed to his concomitant brain injury.

essential to determine the integrity of the alar ligaments.[1] Presence of AOD should prompt consideration for occiput-cervical instrumented fusion. Otherwise, a stable type III fracture could be treated with cervical collar immobilization.

In a review of current literature, Theodore et al identified 415 patients with OCF, with 84 type I, 125 type II and 207 type II

unilateral OCFs, and 37 bilateral OCFs. They are relatively uncommon injuries, with various reports of 1 to 3% frequency in patients sustaining high-energy, blunt craniocervical trauma.[11,14,15]

OCFs are typically diagnosed with CT imaging, as plain radiographs typically have low sensitivity.[11] Of the 415 patients with

OCF described in the literature, clinical information was provided for 119 patients. Normal neurological exam was reported in 35 patients (30%). Loss of consciousness was reported in 36 patients (30%), and focal neurological deficit was reported in 48 patients (40%), which included cranial nerve deficits alone, cranial nerve deficit with limb weakness, mild to severe limb weakness without cranial nerve deficits, vertigo, hyperreflexia, and diplopia.

6.5.3 Treatment

Of the 415 patients with OCF reported in the literature, treatment information is offered on 259 patients. Of the 43 OCF patients who did not receive treatment, 9 patients developed cranial nerve deficits within days to weeks after injury. One hypoglossal nerve palsy resolved, two hypoglossal nerve deficits improved, three cranial nerve deficits persisted, and outcomes for three cases were not reported. Six additional patients were identified with untreated OCFs who developed delayed deficits or symptoms.[11]

One hundred ninety patients with OCF were initially treated with cervical collar immobilization. Sixty-eight of those patients had complete recovery at last follow-up. Outcome following the treatment is inconsistently reported, but one patient had modest reduction in neck rotation after treatment, one had hypoglossal nerve deficit at last follow-up, two patients had persistent mild dysphonia, and three had persistent neck pain. Thirty-two patients with OCF were treated with halo/Minerva immobilization devices. One had slight improvement of Collet–Sicard syndrome, another had persistent trapezius weakness, two had chronic neck pain, and two had complete recovery at last follow-up.[11]

Seventeen patients with OCF were treated with surgery. Fourteen of these underwent occiput-cervical internal fixation and fusion (1 unknown type, 2 type II, and 11 type III). Three of these patients underwent surgery for decompression of the brainstem (one type II and two type III injuries) in addition to internal fixation and fusion. One patient with delayed diplopia had symptom resolution after removal of fracture fragment, one patient with lower cranial nerve deficit and one with diplopia and hemiparesis remained unchanged several days after surgery.[11]

Hanson et al retrospectively reviewed 95 patients with 107 OCFs. Three patients had type I fractures, 24 fractures in 23 patients were type II fracture, and 69 patients had 80 type III fractures (11 were bilateral). Unilateral injury was present in 77% of the cases. Eight patients had craniocervical instability and were treated surgically with occiput-cervical fusion, and four patients were treated with halo vest. Sixty patients (63%) had evidence of diffuse head injury or focal intracranial hematoma. Long-term outcomes were more correlated to associated traumatic brain injury, rather than the OCF itself.[16]

Maserati et al reviewed their series of 100 patients with 106 OCFs. The incidence of OCF was 0.4%. Two patients who had AOD and one patient with C1–C2 fracture were treated surgically. The remaining patients were treated with rigid collar or counseling alone. No patients developed delayed craniocervical instability, nor delayed neural element compression, or cranial neuropathy. The authors conclude that further classification of OCFs is unnecessary, and that management should consist of occiput-cervical fusion or halo vest for cases demonstrating occipitocervical misalignment, and rigid collar immobilization for 6 weeks with radiographic and clinical follow-up for cases where misalignment is not present.[17]

Patient outcomes are correlated with the presence of concurrent craniocervical trauma, neural element compression from fragments, or associated AOD. Overall, nonoperative treatment with external cervical immobilization is usually sufficient to promote bony healing, and resolution or improvement in lower cranial nerve deficits. Isolated bilateral OCF should prompt consideration of more rigid external immobilization,[11] while OCF associated with atlanto-occipital injury should prompt consideration for surgical stabilization or halo vest immobilization.

6.5.4 Conclusion

OCF is a relatively uncommon injury that requires CT imaging to evaluate. CT scan of the craniocervical junction should be considered in anyone who presents with high-energy trauma to the craniocervical junction, particularly with clinical presentation of neck pain, lower cranial nerve deficits, or decreased level or loss of consciousness. Treatment with cervical collar immobilization is typically sufficient for almost all types of OCF. Untreated OCF may rarely develop acute or delayed lower cranial nerve palsies, which typically resolve with collar immobilization. Bilateral OCF should prompt consideration for more rigid immobilization. OCF with evidence of instability, such as atlanto-occipital or atlantoaxial dissociation, should prompt consideration for surgical fixation and fusion. Neural element compression from avulsed and displaced fracture fragment should also prompt consideration for surgical decompression, fixation, and fusion.

6.6 Atlas Fractures

6.6.1 Introduction

Atlas fractures account for 2 to 13% of acute injuries of the cervical spine and 1 to 2% of all spine injuries. Atlas fractures occur due to traumatic axial loading and 5 to 53% of these will have associated axial or other cervical spine injuries.[18] Approximately 21% of patients with an atlas fracture will also have an associated head injury. The majority of these fractures are a result of motor vehicle collisions and motorcycle collisions. However, diving into shallow waters, fall, and assault can also be the reasons for these injuries.

Atlas fractures are rarely associated with neurological deficit, and it is generally believed to be due to the large diameter of the spinal canal at this level and the orientation of the atlas lateral masses. Axial loading forces the lateral masses out laterally, away from the spinal cord, with resultant increase in the size of the spinal canal.

The mechanisms of injury are usually due to axial loading forces from blows to the cranium and hyperextension. The forces are resisted first by the anterior and posterior arches, then by the transverse ligament, and finally by the alar ligaments.

6.6.2 Classification

Because of the ringed anatomy of C1, a single fracture is highly unlikely. Displacement of the ring structure of the atlas requires at least a minimum of two fractures. Atlas fractures can be divided into several patterns based on location of the injury, mechanism of injury, and the integrity of the transverse ligament.

Type I injuries are isolated fractures of the posterior arch and are the most common injuries. This is typically due to hyperextension, with the posterior atlas arch being caught between the occiput and the axis arch. Fracture occurs at the weakest portion of the posterior arch at its attachment to the lateral masses. Note that the vertebral arteries course over the grooves on the posterior arch of the atlas, therefore a displaced fracture may cause vertebral artery injury.

Type II injuries are burst fractures of the atlas ring, classically referred to as "Jefferson fracture." First described in 1920 by Sir Geoffrey Jefferson, this injury typically presents with four bony fractures, with two fractures through the anterior arch and two fractures through the posterior arch.[19] Jefferson described the mechanism of injury as direct vertical compression of the atlas between the occipital condyles and the axis lateral masses with the neck in neutral position. Fracture occurs at the weakest areas of the anterior and posterior rings: at their attachments to the lateral masses. The axial loading vector, along with the sloped orientation of the atlas lateral masses, force the C1 lateral masses laterally (i.e., away from the spinal cord). The transverse ligament, which is attached to the tubercles in the medial lateral masses, is progressively tensioned and fails secondary to midsubstance tear or avulsion from the bony tubercle (▶ Fig. 6.4).

Type III injuries are fractures of unilateral lateral mass, with breaks in the atlas ring just anterior and posterior to the lateral mass. This is thought to occur due to axial loading with the

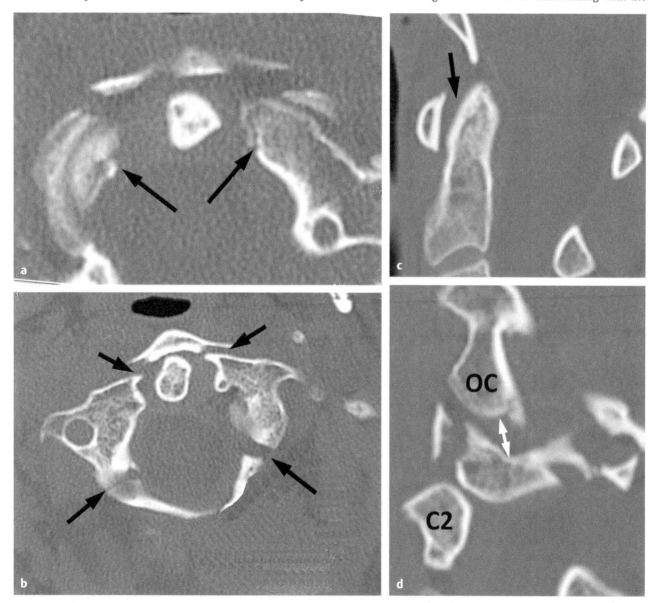

Fig. 6.4 Axial computed tomography (CT) scans of a 25-year-old female who suffered occipital condyle fractures (**a**) and Jefferson burst fracture of the atlas (**b**). Sagittal (**c**) and right parasagittal (**d**) images show increased atlas–dens interval, ADI (*black arrow*), and increased condyle–C1 interval (*white arrow*). (*continued*)

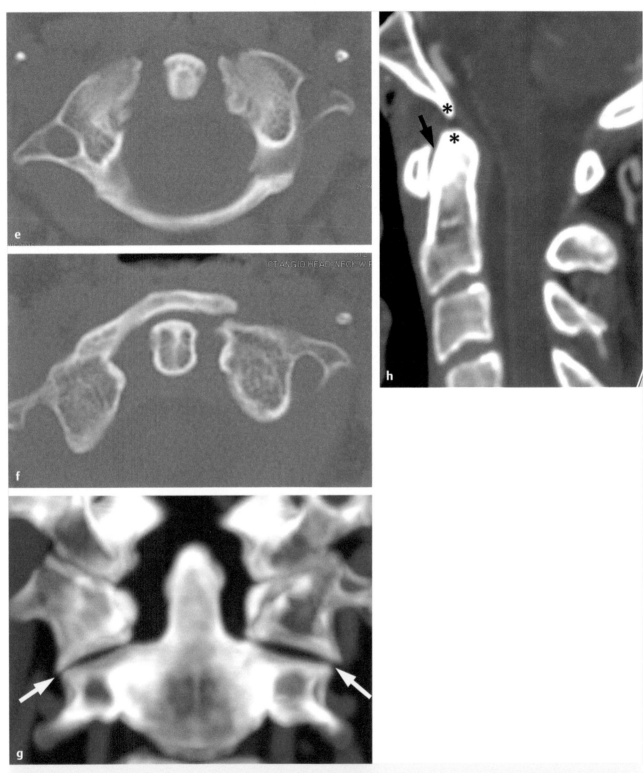

Fig 6.4 (*continued*) She was treated with halo vest immobilization for 12 weeks. Axial CT scan at 6 months post injury shows healing of the atlas ring (**e**, **f**). Coronal (**g**) and sagittal (**h**) images show satisfactory healing of the atlas and preserved basion–dens interval (*asterisks*).

head in lateral bending or axial rotation, thus transmission of the force is directed toward the ipsilateral lateral mass. Significant lateral mass displacement could occur with the disruption of the capsular structures (▶ Fig. 6.5).

Another type of atlas fracture involves a break to the transverse process of the atlas and it is a stable injury. These frac-

tures could be associated with injuries to the vertebral artery, which courses through the transverse foramina. A final type of atlas fracture is fracture through the anterior arch and it represents an avulsion by the longus colli muscle. This injury is typically stable, as it represents an avulsion and not failure through the entire anterior arch or the dens. This should be

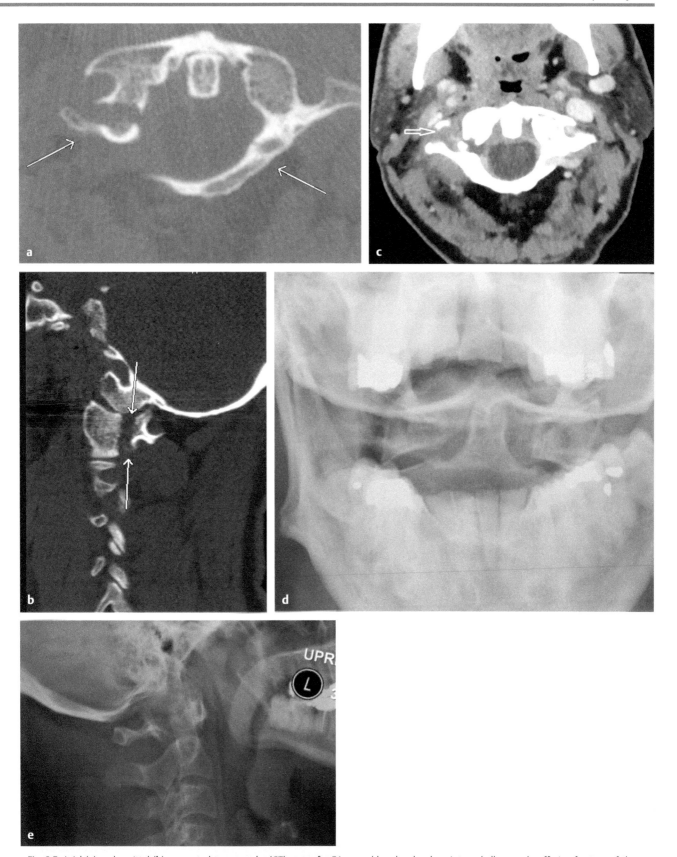

Fig. 6.5 Axial (**a**) and sagittal (**b**) computed tomography (CT) scan of a 51-year-old male who dove into a shallow pool, suffering fracture of the right atlas lateral mass and left posterior arch. Axial CT angiogram (**c**) shows occlusion of the right vertebral artery from C3 to C1. Upright open-mouth odontoid (**d**) and lateral (**e**) plain radiographs show satisfactory cervical alignment. After consultation with endovascular neurosurgeon, he was treated conservatively with hard cervical collar immobilization and daily aspirin for his vertebral artery occlusion.

distinguished from the more serious plough fracture. A plough fracture is an unstable anterior arch fracture due to the posterior or shear force that causes the dens to plough through the anterior atlas, causing a posterior atlantoaxial dislocation. These are unstable fractures (▶ Fig. 6.6).

The rule of Spence indicates that the transverse ligament is "probably torn" when the combined displacement of the lateral masses (LMD) relative to the axis is at least 6.9 mm.[20] Further displacement of the lateral masses could occur during immobilization if the transverse ligament is disrupted. His study utilized cadaveric specimens and the findings were confirmed by Fielding et al.[20,21] Heller et al reported their observation on 35 open-mouth odontoid films using calibration markings to assess radiographic magnification. They found an 18% magnification factor on open-mouth odontoid films. Applying this to the rule of Spence suggests that the LMD measured on open-mouth odontoid radiographs should be raised from 6.9 to 8.1 mm[22] (▶ Fig. 6.7, ▶ Fig. 6.8).

Dickman et al described two types of transverse ligament injuries based on MRI findings.[23] Type I injuries involve an intrasubstance tear of the ligament without associated fracture. Type II injuries involve avulsion fracture at the insertion site of the transverse ligament. The authors concluded that type I injuries are inherently unstable and unlikely to heal without inter-

nal fixation. Type II injuries had higher chance of healing and should be treated with rigid external immobilization. In his series of 39 patients, those with type II injuries were managed nonoperatively with a Philadelphia collar or halo vest for 13 weeks and 74% of these patients were healed.[23,24] His series did not include patients with atlas fractures, so it is unclear whether their conclusions could be extrapolated to the management of atlas fractures.

6.6.3 Treatment

Treatment of isolated atlas fractures is guided by the integrity of the transverse ligament and the presence of other associated cervical spine injuries. There are no prospective randomized trials evaluating the various treatment modalities for atlas fractures. All of the available evidence is based on case series, retrospective reviews, and expert opinions.

A stable injury could be treated with cervical collar immobilization for 6 to 12 weeks. The treatment of a stable type II burst (Jefferson) fracture with no displacement or minimal displacement is more controversial, and some authors recommend treatment with rigid collar immobilization or halo vest for 12 weeks. Serial upright cervical radiographs with open-mouth odontoid views should be followed and closely analyzed for

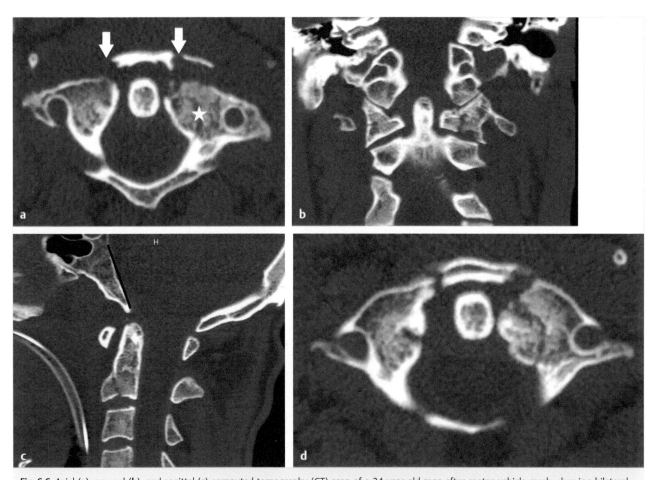

Fig. 6.6 Axial (**a**), coronal (**b**), and sagittal (**c**) computed tomography (CT) scan of a 34-year-old man after motor vehicle crash, showing bilateral anterior arch fractures (*white arrows*) and nondisplaced left atlas lateral mass fracture (*white star*), and C2 anterior vertebral body fracture. He refused treatment, including hard cervical collar, and presented 4 weeks later to the emergency department complaining of severe neck pain and arm paresthesia. CT scan showed progressive collapse of the left lateral mass (**d**). (*continued*)

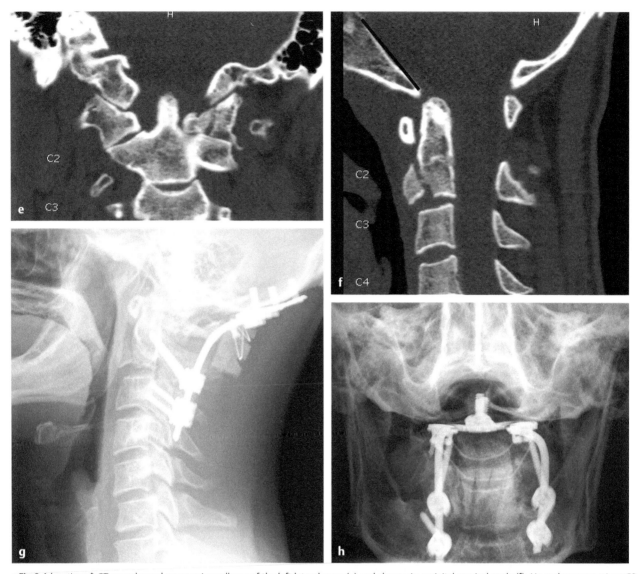

Fig 6.4 (*continued*) CT scan showed progressive collapse of the left lateral mass (**e**) and change in occipital-cervical angle (**f**). He underwent occiput-C3 posterior instrumented fusion. At 3 months follow-up, his paresthesia resolved and his neck improved significantly; upright lateral (**g**) and anteroposterior (**h**) radiographs show preserved cervical alignment.

displacement during immobilization. In a series of 29 patients with nondisplaced atlas fracture, treatment with halo vest resulted in 96% healing.[25]

Treatment for unstable Jefferson fractures with greater than 7 mm of combined LMD has been debated in the literature. Treatment options include rigid cervical immobilization, cervicothoracic brace, halo vest, posterior fusion, and osteosynthesis (anterior or posterior). Osteosynthesis sounds appealing in theory, as bony reduction is achieved, and no fusion is necessary. However, the indications are debated, and its superiority over other treatment options is not studied. Some experts recommend initial traction to reduce the fracture, followed by 12 weeks of halo vest immobilization. Atlantoaxial stability is then assessed with flexion-extension radiographs, and if instability is still present, then C1–C2 instrumented fusion is recommended.[1] Another treatment option includes immediate C1–C2 posterior instrumented fusion. This offers the advantage

of avoiding prolonged immobilization in a halo vest. However, a comminuted atlas lateral mass fracture may preclude adequate screw purchase into C1. Occiput–C2 fusion may be indicated for cases with displaced fractures, excessive comminution, subluxation, or when spinal cord or brainstem compression is present. Efforts should be taken to avoid extension of fusion to the occiput if possible, due to the morbidity of fusing the entire craniocervical junction.

Hadley et al evaluated 32 patients with atlas fractures; 5 of these had unstable Jefferson fractures. These five patients underwent 12 to 16 weeks of halo vest treatment. The rest of the patients underwent 8 to 12 weeks of either rigid collar or Sternal Occipital Mandibular Immobilizer (SOMI) brace. No patients developed signs of instability or nonunion and none required subsequent surgical fixation.[26]

Fowler et al evaluated 48 patients with atlas fractures; 30 of these had Jefferson fractures. All patients with greater than

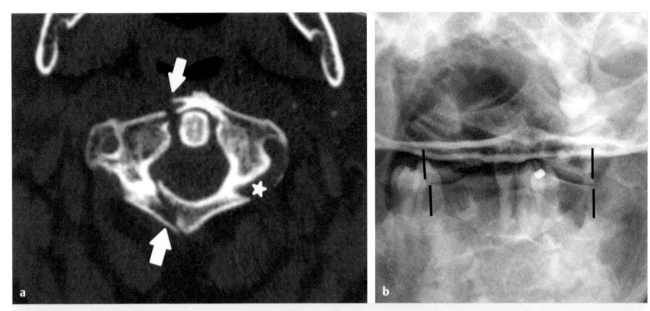

Fig. 6.7 Axial computed tomography (CT) scan (**a**) of a 67-year-old male who suffered an automobile-versus-pedestrian accident, showing anterior and posterior arch fractures. (*White star* marks the groove made by the left vertebral artery). Upright open-mouth odontoid view plain radiograph (**b**) shows that the rule of Spence is not violated (*black lines*), and his C1 fracture was treated successfully with hard cervical collar immobilization.

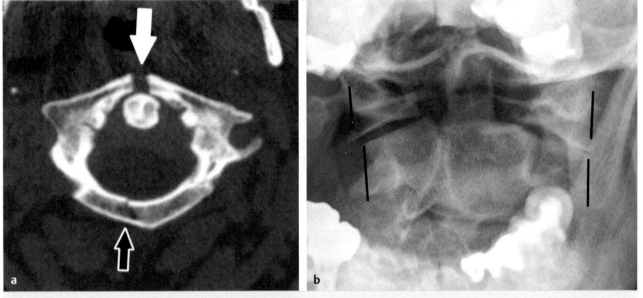

Fig. 6.8 Axial computed tomography (CT) scan (**a**) of a 70-year-old male who fell 12 feet from a deck. He suffered C1 anterior and posterior arch fractures *(arrows)*, as well as T7–8 fracture with epidural hematoma and spinal cord compression, and underwent thoracic spine decompression and fusion. Upright open-mouth odontoid view plain radiograph (**b**) shows that the rule of Spence is not violated (*black lines*), and his C1 fracture was treated successfully with hard cervical collar immobilization.

7 mm of LMD were treated with 4 to 6 weeks of cranial traction, followed by placement in halo. All of these patients had bony union and none required surgery.[27]

6.6.4 Conclusion

The majority of fractures involving the atlas are stable and not associated with neurological deficits. CT imaging is the most sensitive method for detecting these injuries. Initial management involves placement in rigid cervical immobilization which is sufficient for stable fractures such as isolated posterior arch fractures, transverse process fractures, anterior tubercle fractures, and nondisplaced lateral mass fractures.

Upright cervical spine radiograph with open-mouth odontoid views is useful in inferring the integrity of the transverse ligament. MRI may also be used to assess the integrity of the transverse ligament. Even select patients with burst fractures with greater than 7 mm of combined displacement can be treated with halo vest for 12 weeks. Careful analysis of flexion-extension radiographs must be done following immobilization to rule out persistent atlantoaxial instability. C1–C2 posterior instrumented fusion can be performed, with C1–C2 transarticular screws or C1 lateral mass screws and C2 pars/pedicle screws construct as the preferred methods.

6.7 Craniocervical Dissociation

6.7.1 Introduction

CCD (including atlanto-occipital and atlantoaxial dissociations) is a leading cause of death in as many as 8 to 25% of fatal injuries from motor vehicle crashes.[28,29,30,31] CCD represents a spectrum of injuries with varying degrees of stability.

Increasing awareness of these injuries and the more prevalent use of CT imaging has resulted in earlier detection of these injuries, earlier treatment, and thus improved mortality for these patients. Nearly 20% of patients with acute traumatic CCD will have normal neurological examination on presentation, and a high index of suspicion must be maintained.[37]

6.7.2 Mechanism of Injury

CCD is more common in children and young adults, likely due to flatter condyles in pediatric patients, the higher cranium-to-body-weight ratio and increased ligamentous laxity. It is caused by partial or complete disruption of the posterior longitudinal ligament and tectorial membrane, as well as the bilateral alar ligaments. Subluxation or dislocation could occur at the atlanto-occipital articulation, the atlantoaxial articulation, or both. It could be associated with lower cranial nerve deficits (cranial nerves IX, X, XI and XII), cranial nerve VI palsy (long intracranial course and therefore prone to stretch or avulsion injury), vertebral artery injury, and injury to the brainstem. Severity of neurological injury at the time of presentation is the most important predictor of outcome[32] (▶ Fig. 6.9).

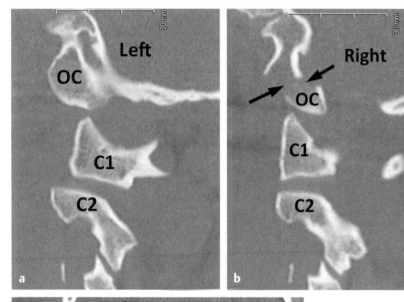
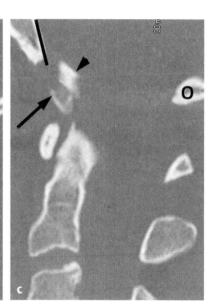
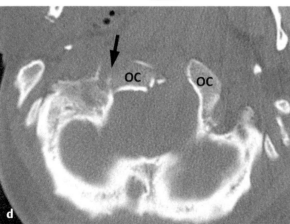

Fig. 6.9 Sagittal reformatted computed tomography (CT) scan showing left (a) and right (b) images of a 41-year-old male after helmeted motorcycle crash, demonstrating anteriorly displaced left occipital condyle and a fractured right occipital condyle. Midsagittal view (c) shows increased basion–axis interval, BAI and basion–dens interval, BDI. Axial CT (d) shows avulsion fracture of the right occipital condyle (*black arrow*). The patient underwent occiput-C2 posterior instrumented fusion. (*continued*)

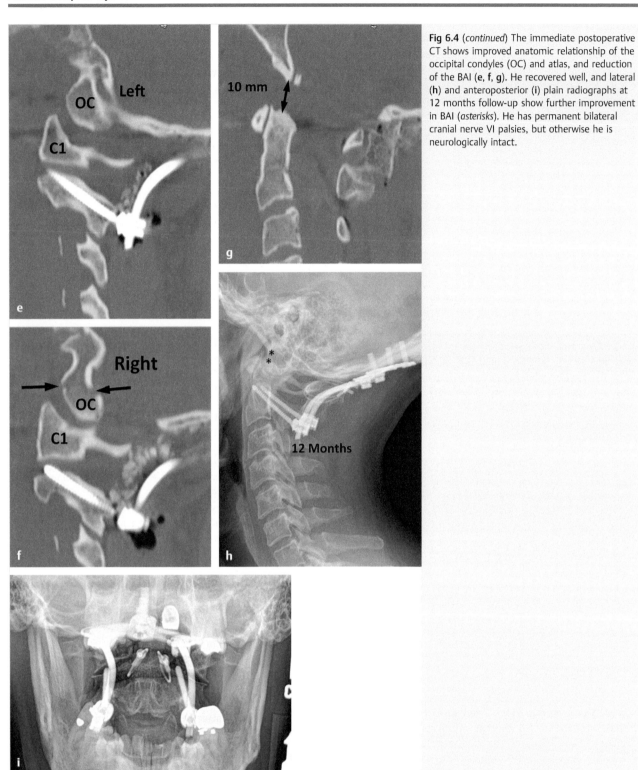

Fig 6.4 (*continued*) The immediate postoperative CT shows improved anatomic relationship of the occipital condyles (OC) and atlas, and reduction of the BAI (**e, f, g**). He recovered well, and lateral (**h**) and anteroposterior (**i**) plain radiographs at 12 months follow-up show further improvement in BAI (*asterisks*). He has permanent bilateral cranial nerve VI palsies, but otherwise he is neurologically intact.

6.7.3 Diagnosis

Diagnosis is commonly made with CT and/or MRI. Lateral plain radiographs have lower sensitivity but may pick up abnormal relationships among the basion, tip of the dens, and anterior atlas arch.[37] Prevertebral soft-tissue swelling on plain radiographs should prompt consideration of the diagnosis of CCD. The Harris "rule of twelves," and the CCI, which is the distance between the occipital condyle and the superior articular surface of C1, are recommended to rule out CCD. Typically, the basion (the tip of the clivus) should point toward the tip of the dens. Indirect signs on CT imaging include blood in the basilar cisterns, or, on thin-cut axial CT, one or more slices show no bone at all due to the distraction gap between the occipital condyle and C1.

The Powers ratio can be used to detect certain CCD. The ratio, BC/AO, represents the ratio between the distance from the basion (B) to the posterior C1 arch (C), to the distance between the anterior C1 arch (A) to the opisthion (O).[38] In normal adults, Powers ratio < 0.9 is normal and > 1.0 is abnormal, and ratio between 0.9 and 1.0 is considered indeterminate. The Powers ratio is most useful in anteriorly translated AOD and cannot be used when there is fracture in the anterior arch of C1 or of the dens.

The prevalence of vascular injuries is high, including vertebral or carotid artery vasospasm, intimal tears, thrombosis, dissection, and pseudoaneurysm. In a series of 39 patients with CCD, 28 patients were screened through CT angiography or catheter angiography and 50% of the patients screened had evidence of blunt cerebrovascular injuries.[33]

6.7.4 Classification

Traynelis classified AOD according to the direction of occiput dislocation: type I (occiput is translated anteriorly relative to the atlas), type II (longitudinal distraction), and type III (occiput is translated posteriorly relative to the atlas).[34] Most injuries are likely unstable in all directions, and thus this classification is not useful in determining the treatment course.

The Harborview craniocervical injury classification describes three types of injuries based on severity of dislocation.[35] Type I is described as MRI evidence of injury to craniocervical osseoligamentous stabilizers; the craniocervical alignment is within 2 mm of normal, and distraction of 2 mm or less on provocative cervical traction radiograph. These include unilateral type III OCFs or isolated alar ligament tears. Type II represents dynamic instability, with MRI evidence of injury to craniocervical osseoligamentous stabilizers; the craniocervical alignment is within 2 mm of normal, but distraction of more than 2 mm occurs on provocative cervical traction radiograph. In type III injury, imaging shows craniocervical malalignment of more than 2 mm on static radiographic studies. This represents complete disruption of all interconnecting ligaments with gross displacement. The authors recommend cervical traction challenge to differentiate patients with minimally displaced type I injuries (< 2 mm) who can be treated nonoperatively versus patients with highly unstable injuries that have been partially reduced (type II), who require operative stabilization despite well-aligned static radiographs.[2]

6.7.5 Treatment

If a patient has suspected CCD, immediate head immobilization with sandbags, tape, or specialized head holders should be utilized, and reverse Trendelenburg positioning is necessary. No attempt should be made to blindly apply cervical traction, as this may worsen the dislocation and cause further neurological injury.[1,2,37]

Conversely, if a patient's neurological status worsens after application of cervical traction, an immediate lateral plain radiograph must be done to rule out CCD.

Principles of Advanced Trauma Life Support (ATLS) apply, including appropriate fluid resuscitation and possible vasopressor support for neurogenic shock. All care team members are notified to minimize transferring of patients as much as possible. Halo vest immobilization can be considered initially to reduce gross malalignment and temporarily stabilize the cra-

niocervical junction, but anatomic alignment is difficult to maintain over time.[1,2]

Surgical fixation and fusion are the mainstay of treatment for CCD. Horn et al recommended that in cases with no abnormal CT criteria and only moderately abnormal MRI signals in the posterior ligaments or atlanto-occipital joints, external orthosis with halo or collar could be considered. Whereas in cases with one or more abnormal CT criteria or with grossly abnormal MRI findings in the atlanto-occipital joints, tectorial membranes, or alar or cruciate ligaments, surgical stabilization is recommended.[32] Surgical stabilization is performed as soon as medically possible in polytrauma patients to prevent further neurological deterioration.

Bellabarba et al recommend cervical collar immobilization for Harborview type I injuries and surgical stabilization for type II and III injuries. Treatment in a halo vest may be satisfactory for some type II injuries, especially in the pediatric population.[36]

The most important predictor of outcome is the severity of neurological injuries at the time of presentation.[32]

In a review of the available literature on AOD, Theodore et al identified that out of 84 patients in whom treatment data was reported, 13 patients did not receive initial treatment for AOD. Of this group of untreated patients, two died, two improved neurologically, four had unchanged deficits, and five worsened neurologically. Of 29 patients initially treated with external immobilization, 17 were immobilized in anticipation of internal fixation and fusion and none worsened during the presurgical interval. The remaining 12 were treated with external immobilization alone, of which 4 worsened transiently and underwent surgery. Three were unstable after 6 to 22 weeks of immobilization and underwent surgery. Only five patients with AOD described in the literature were successfully treated with external immobilization alone. The authors caution against external immobilization alone for treatment of AOD.

6.7.6 Conclusion

CCD is caused by high-energy trauma. Timely diagnosis and treatment are critical in reducing mortality and neurological deficits. Patients with preserved craniocervical alignment and < 2 mm of displacement who are stable on cervical traction challenge may be treated nonoperatively. Patients with > 2 mm of displacement should undergo posterior occiput-cervical instrumented fusion. Blind traction is not recommended in cases of AOD. Patients who survive CCD injuries often have neurological impairment including cranial nerve deficits, unilateral or bilateral paresis, or even quadriplegia.

References

[1] Anderson PA. Upper cervical spine injuries. In: Rao RD, Smuck M, eds. Orthopaedic Knowledge Update: Spine 4. AAOS; 2012:209–220

[2] Bransford RJ, Manoso M, Bellabarba C. Occipital-cervical spine injuries. In: Browner BD, Jupiter JB, Krettek C, Anderson PA, eds. Skeletal Trauma, 5th ed. Elsevier, Philadelphia, PA, 2015:813–829

[3] Panjabi M, Dvorak J, Crisco J, III, Oda T, Hilibrand A, Grob D. Flexion, extension, and lateral bending of the upper cervical spine in response to alar ligament transections. J Spinal Disord. 1991; 4(2):157–167

[4] Panjabi MM, Oxland TR, Parks EH. Quantitative anatomy of cervical spine ligaments. Part I. Upper cervical spine. J Spinal Disord. 1991; 4(3):270–276

[5] Werne S. Studies in spontaneous atlas dislocation. Acta Orthop Scand Suppl. 1957; 23:1–150

[6] Dvorak J, Panjabi M, Gerber M, Wichmann W. CT-functional diagnostics of the rotatory instability of upper cervical spine. 1. An experimental study on cadavers. Spine. 1987; 12(3):197–205

[7] Steel HH. Anatomical and mechanical consideration of the atlantoaxial articulation. J Bone Joint Surg Am. 1968; 50:1481–1482

[8] Pang D, Nemzek WR, Zovickian J. Atlanto-occipital dislocation–part 2: The clinical use of (occipital) condyle-C1 interval, comparison with other diagnostic methods, and the manifestation, management, and outcome of atlanto-occipital dislocation in children. Neurosurgery. 2007; 61(5):995–1015, discussion 1015

[9] Harris JH, Jr, Carson GC, Wagner LK. Radiologic diagnosis of traumatic occipitovertebral dissociation: 1. Normal occipitovertebral relationships on lateral radiographs of supine subjects. AJR Am J Roentgenol. 1994; 162(4):881–886

[10] Harris JH, Jr, Carson GC, Wagner LK, Kerr N. Radiologic diagnosis of traumatic occipitovertebral dissociation: 2. Comparison of three methods of detecting occipitovertebral relationships on lateral radiographs of supine subjects. AJR Am J Roentgenol. 1994; 162(4):887–892

[11] Theodore N, Aarabi B, Dhall SS, et al. Occipital condyle fractures. Neurosurgery. 2013; 72(3) Suppl 2:106–113

[12] Anderson PA. Upper cervical injuries. In: Bulstrode CJK, ed. Oxford Textbook of Trauma and Orthopaedics. 2nd ed. Oxford University Press; 2011: 1200–1212

[13] Anderson PA, Montesano PX. Morphology and treatment of occipital condyle fractures. Spine. 1988; 13(7):731–736

[14] Leone A, Cerase A, Colosimo C, Lauro L, Puca A, Marano P. Occipital condylar fractures: a review. Radiology. 2000; 216(3):635–644

[15] Noble ER, Smoker WR. The forgotten condyle: the appearance, morphology, and classification of occipital condyle fractures. AJNR Am J Neuroradiol. 1996; 17(3):507–513

[16] Hanson JA, Deliganis AV, Baxter AB, et al. Radiologic and clinical spectrum of occipital condyle fractures: retrospective review of 107 consecutive fractures in 95 patients. AJR Am J Roentgenol. 2002; 178(5):1261–1268

[17] Maserati MB, Stephens B, Zohny Z, et al. Occipital condyle fractures: clinical decision rule and surgical management. J Neurosurg Spine. 2009; 11(4): 388–395

[18] Haynes NG, Gust TD, Arnold PM. Atlas injuries: atlas fractures. In: Vaccaro A, Anderson P, eds. Cervical Spine Trauma. Rothman Institute; 2010;317–321

[19] Jefferson G. Fracture of the atlas vertebra: report of 4 cases and a review of those previously recorded. Br J Surg. 1920; 7:407–422

[20] Spence KF, Jr, Decker S, Sell KW. Bursting atlantal fracture associated with rupture of the transverse ligament. J Bone Joint Surg Am. 1970; 52(3): 543–549

[21] Fielding JW, Cochran Gv, Lawsing JF, III, Hohl M. Tears of the transverse ligament of the atlas. A clinical and biomechanical study. J Bone Joint Surg Am. 1974; 56(8):1683–1691

[22] Heller JG, Viroslav S, Hudson T. Jefferson fractures: the role of magnification artifact in assessing transverse ligament integrity. J Spinal Disord. 1993; 6(5):392–396

[23] Dickman CA, Mamourian A, Sonntag VK, Drayer BP. Magnetic resonance imaging of the transverse atlantal ligament for the evaluation of atlantoaxial instability. J Neurosurg. 1991; 75(2):221–227

[24] Dickman CA, Greene KA, Sonntag VK. Injuries involving the transverse atlantal ligament: classification and treatment guidelines based upon experience with 39 injuries. Neurosurgery. 1996; 38(1):44–50

[25] Kontautas E, Ambrozaitis KV, Kalesinskas RJ, Spakauskas B. Management of acute traumatic atlas fractures. J Spinal Disord Tech. 2005; 18(5):402–405

[26] Hadley MN, Dickman CA, Browner CM, Sonntag VK. Acute traumatic atlas fractures: management and long term outcome. Neurosurgery. 1988; 23(1):31–35

[27] Fowler JL, Sandhu A, Fraser RD. A review of fractures of the atlas vertebra. J Spinal Disord. 1990; 3(1):19–24

[28] Alker GJ, Jr, Oh YS, Leslie EV. High cervical spine and craniocervical junction injuries in fatal traffic accidents: a radiological study. Orthop Clin North Am. 1978; 9(4):1003–1010

[29] Bucholz RW, Burkhead WZ, Graham W, Petty C. Occult cervical spine injuries in fatal traffic accidents. J Trauma. 1979; 19(10):768–771

[30] Adams VI. Neck injuries: I. Occipitoatlantal dislocation—a pathologic study of twelve traffic fatalities. J Forensic Sci. 1992; 37(2):556–564

[31] Cooper Z, Gross JA, Lacey JM, Traven N, Mirza SK, Arbabi S. Identifying survivors with traumatic craniocervical dissociation: a retrospective study. J Surg Res. 2010; 160(1):3–8

[32] Horn EM, Feiz-Erfan I, Lekovic GP, Dickman CA, Sonntag VK, Theodore N. Survivors of occipitoatlantal dislocation injuries: imaging and clinical correlates. J Neurosurg Spine. 2007; 6(2):113–120

[33] Kazemi N, Bellabarba C, Bransford R, Vilela M. Incidence of blunt cerebrovascular injuries associated with craniocervical distraction injuries. Evid Based Spine Care J. 2012; 3(4):63–64

[34] Traynelis VC, Marano GD, Dunker RO, Kaufman HH. Traumatic atlanto-occipital dislocation. Case report. J Neurosurg. 1986; 65(6):863–870

[35] Chapman JR, Bellabarba C, Newell DW, et al. Craniocervical injuries: atlanto-occipital dissociation and occipital condyle fractures. Semin Spine Surg. 2001; 13(2):90–105

[36] Bellabarba C, Mirza SK, West GA, et al. Diagnosis and treatment of craniocervical dislocation in a series of 17 consecutive survivors during an 8-year period. J Neurosurg Spine. 2006; 4(6):429–440

[37] Theodore N, Aarabi B, Dhall SS, et al. The diagnosis and management of traumatic atlanto-occipital dislocation injuries. Neurosurgery. 2013; 72(3) Suppl 2:114–126

[38] Powers B, Miller MD, Kramer RS, Martinez S, Gehweiler JA, Jr. Traumatic anterior atlanto-occipital dislocation. Neurosurgery. 1979; 4(1):12–17

[39] Osborn AG, ed. Diagnostic Cerebral Angiography. 2nd ed. Philadelphia, PA: Lippincott Williams & Wilkins; 1999

[40] Young JP, Young PH, Ackermann MJ, Anderson PA, Riew KD. The ponticulus posticus: implications for screw insertion into the first cervical lateral mass. J Bone Joint Surg Am. 2005; 87(11):2495–2498

7 Odontoid and Hangman's Fractures

Megan M. Jack, Domenico A. Gattozzi, and Paul M. Arnold

Abstract

Fractures of the axis are common traumatic injuries of the cervical spine that present as challenging clinical problems for both patients and practitioners. In the setting of trauma, quick evaluation with physical examination and radiographic identification of axis fractures can help safely direct management including operative and nonoperative techniques and achieve successful functional outcomes for the patient. This chapter will review odontoid and hangman's fractures resulting from cervical trauma with a focus on clinical decision-making regarding definitive management.

Keywords: odontoid fractures, hangman fractures, C1–C2 fusion, external immobilization

7.1 Odontoid Fractures

7.1.1 Introduction

Due to the unique biomechanics of the C1 region, the upper cervical spine is highly susceptible to bony fractures and ligamentous injuries following trauma, which can lead to fracture of the dens. Odontoid fractures range from 10 to 20% of cervical spine fractures.[1] These most commonly occur in older adults and the prevalence is increasing substantially with the growth rate of the elderly population. Odontoid fractures more frequently affect men with a sex ratio of nearly 3:1. Odontoid fractures generally are classified based on their anatomical fracture patterns. While many types of odontoid fractures can be treated conservatively, surgical intervention including posterior C1–C2 fusion and anterior odontoid screws, are options for the management of unstable fractures or those unlikely to heal with external immobilization alone. Rates of mortality following odontoid fractures in the elderly population have been reported to be as high as 30%.[7]

7.1.2 Mechanism of Injury

Trauma accounts for majority of odontoid fractures. Motor vehicle accidents and low-velocity falls are the most frequent traumas associated with odontoid fractures for younger and older patients, respectively. The main forces that result in dens fractures are flexion, extension, lateral bending, and rotation forces, or a combination of these. The direction of the forces applied during trauma dictate the fracture pattern. It has been suggested that high-energy mechanisms account for fractures in younger patients, while low-energy impacts produce similar anatomic injuries in the geriatric population due to reduced bone density.[3,4,5]

7.1.3 Classification

The Anderson and D'Alonzo classification is the most frequently utilized classification scheme (▶ Fig. 7.1). It categorizes C2 dens

fractures based on their location within the odontoid: type I fractures are limited to avulsions of the odontoid tip, type II fractures occur through the neck, and type III fractures involve the odontoid base. Type I odontoid fractures are relatively rare in comparison to the other types of C2 fractures.[4] Type II and III fractures are frequently seen in busy trauma centers. Type II fractures are by far the most common of the three in young and elderly patients.[4] Based on this classification scheme, Hadley et al proposed the addition of the IIA communition fracture pattern, referring to chip-fracture fragments of the odontoid base.

While the Anderson and D'Alonzo classification is the most commonly used system, multiple other classification systems do exist. The Schatzker's, the Althoff's, and the Mourgues's classifications systems are based on the direction of the fracture. The Schatzker's classification distinguishes two fracture types based on their location either above or below the attachment of the accessory ligaments.[6] The Althoff classification also describes four types of fractures based on anatomic location including fractures at the neck, the superior body, the lateral masses, and the inferior body. The Mourgues classification proposes two fracture types based on fractures either through the

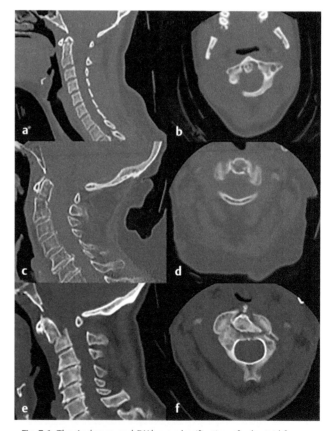

Fig. 7.1 The Anderson and D'Alonzo classification of odontoid fractures. Type I fractures (**a** and **b**) occur through the odontoid tip. Type II fractures (**c** and **d**) occur through the neck of the dens. Type III fractures (**e** and **f**) occur through the base of C2.

neck or through the base of the odontoid process. The Korres classification, on the other hand, is an anatomically based delineation of four fracture types that occur resulting from hyperflexion and produce teardrop formations. The Roy-Camille classification describes three types of fractures that are based on the direction of the fracture line through the odontoid, correlating with the biomechanical stress applied during the trauma. Each classification has been linked with prognosis of union or fracture healing.

7.1.4 Physical Exam

The primary and secondary trauma surveys help identify clinical features that are suggestive of underlying injuries. Particularly in the case of upper cervical fractures, such as odontoid fractures, patients may report tenderness to palpation, neck pain with motion, and exhibit ecchymosis indicative of underlying traumatic injury. Dysphagia may also indicate an odontoid fracture with the development of a large hematoma which compromises surrounding structures. Neurological examination is also key to determining the need for further cervical imaging. Though neurological compromise is rare following odontoid fractures, weakness or sensory changes may indicate a concomitant fracture at another spinal level.

7.1.5 Imaging

The choice of imaging following cervical trauma is influenced by numerous patient factors, including age, stability of the patient, the mechanism of injury, presence of neurological deficits, and the existence of confounding injuries. Cervical radiographs with odontoid views are preferred for patients that do not require advanced imaging or are too unstable for advanced imaging to be obtained, and for younger patients to reduce radiation exposure. Plain films that reveal asymmetry between the dens and lateral masses of C1 are indicative of transverse ligament injury. While routine films achieve the diagnosis, computed tomography (CT) scans allow for much more detailed classification of the fracture and remain the study of choice for traumatic odontoid fractures. Magnetic resonance imaging (MRI) of the cervical spine would be indicated if the patient has neurological compromise. Similarly, CT angiogram may be useful in determining the course of the vertebral artery for surgical planning, but it is typically unnecessary.

7.1.6 Treatment Considerations

Treatment of odontoid fractures begins with appropriate management following an acute trauma with principles of advanced trauma and life support. Following diagnostic imaging, the appropriate treatment varies depending on the classification of the odontoid fracture. There are numerous important factors that influence surgical considerations and patient outcomes which include the fracture pattern, age, degree of comminution, fracture displacement, angulation, and nonunion, as well as patient comorbidities.

Age is an important predictor of outcome following traumatic fracture of the dens. Elderly patients suffer higher rates of odontoid fractures; however, they also experience higher rates of complications depending on the type of treatment. Similarly,

they are at higher risk for nonunion, while younger patients with better bone quality are less likely to experience pseudarthrosis or fibrous nonunion. Thus, younger patients may be successfully treated with conservative measures, while elderly patients may require surgical intervention to achieve fracture healing.

The degree of angulation and/or displacement also influences clinical decision-making and treatment options. Greater than 5 mm of displacement may influence the decision to recommend surgical fixation of a type III fracture in order to reduce the risk of nonunion.[7] Nonunions are often considered treatment failure, however they are often clinically insignificant.[8] Type II fractures have an average rate of pseudarthrosis of 36%.[6] Pseudarthrosis is often a feared result, but rarely causes cervical myelopathy.[9] Similarly, fibrous union likely provides sufficient stability. However, nonunion remains a reason for delayed surgical intervention in approximately 20 to 30% of cases.

Finally, the fracture type greatly influences the decision to undergo surgical intervention. Based on the Anderson and D'Alonzo classification, type I and III fractures are known to be stable fractures and can be treated conservatively. The management of type II fractures, however, remains controversial. Generally, surgical intervention is reserved for type IIA fractures or those associated with transverse ligament injury or severe dens displacement.[10] Chapman et al reviewed 322 elderly patients with type II odontoid fractures and found nonoperative management was associated with a higher 30-day mortality risk.[11] On the other hand, other studies have found significant mortality indices and high rates of complications with surgical intervention in older adults.[9,11] This variability in outcome data has contributed to the controversy surrounding the optimum treatment of type II odontoid fractures.

7.1.7 Nonoperative Management

Cervical spine immobilization is a common treatment for type I and III odontoid fractures. Halo vests or hard cervical collars are rigid immobility techniques that allow for bony fusion to occur following injury. Pseudarthrosis can occur if limited mobility is not successfully preserved. Koller et al demonstrated comparable limitations in flexion and extension with either a halo vest or Philadelphia collar.[12] However, halo vests showed a superior ability to limit axial rotation and coronal bending compared to rigid collars.[13]

One systematic review compared failure rates of odontoid fractures following treatment with either halo placement or immobilization with a hard collar. Treatment failure was defined as the need for surgical intervention. There were no differences in failure rates between halo and collar treatment for type II odontoid fractures. However, halo treatment was associated with significantly higher rates of complications.[1] The most common complications included pin-site infections, hardware failure, pneumonia, and respiratory failure.[1] Other studies have demonstrated impaired swallowing and reduced mobilization with halo vest treatment.[14,15] It is important to note neurological decline is rarely reported. Halo vests are especially poorly tolerated in the elderly.

Type I and most type III fractures generally are managed conservatively or with external immobilization. Evidence has shown patients are able to achieve high fusion rates without neurological decline for these types of fractures. Type I fractures have a nearly 100% fusion rate independent of the specific immobilization device chosen.[7]

7.1.8 Operative Management

The patients' comorbidities and neurological function coupled with regional practice patterns are all considerations when determining the appropriate treatment course for individual patients with odontoid fractures as discussed above. The risk of nonunion must be weighed against potential surgical complications. Relative indications for surgical fixation include > 5 mm of fracture dislocation, > 10 mm of angulation, and the inability to reduce the fracture through conservative measures.[3] The rate of surgical intervention on elderly patients is near 15%.[9]

Type II fractures have significant controversy surrounding the appropriate management. There are no clear guidelines regarding which type II fractures necessitate surgery as both conservative and operative management techniques have proven effective.[16] Due to limited blood supply and poor bone quality, fractures through the base of the dens are at high risk for nonunion.[11] Thus, some advocate for surgical intervention due to the high rate of pseudarthrosis with nonoperative management. Others consider conservative management more appropriate, particularly in patients with significant medical comorbidities that are also associated with adverse outcomes following surgery. Therefore, due to the frail nature of those that suffer odontoid fractures, operative intervention is often viewed as too risky compared to nonoperative management. Low hemoglobin, neurological deficits on presentation, type III odontoid fractures, and elderly nursing home patients were all found to be independent predictors of mortality following traumatic odontoid fractures in older adults.[2] However, there remains evidence to suggest that patients, particularly the elderly, have improved 30-day and long-term survival following surgery compared with nonoperative management.[4]

Anterior odontoid screw placement is considered the treatment of choice for type II and certain rostral shallow type III fractures.[17] The benefits of anterior screw placement include immediate fracture stabilization, increased fusion rates compared to rigid collar treatment, and sparing of atlantoaxial rotation. The key to determining if anterior odontoid screws are the appropriate surgical approach is verifying the transverse ligament has not been ruptured resulting from the trauma. Anterior screw placement should be avoided in cases involving fractures with an oblique orientation or large gap, severe osteopenia, fractures older than 6 months, irreducible fractures, and in patients with large barrel chests that make the surgical approach difficult. Anterior odontoid screw placement is associated with higher failure rates than posterior cervical fusion.[18]

Posterior C1–C2 fusion should be considered for type III odontoid fractures at risk for nonunion and for type II fractures. Class II medical evidence supports early surgical fixation and fusion for elderly patients with type II odontoid fractures.[7] Other considerations for posterior atlantoaxial fusions include type IIA fractures with significant comminution that are unlikely to heal without operative management, and fractures in which the dens is significantly displaced. While an anterior approach may be considered, evidence of transverse ligament compromise, comminution of the fracture, or anteroinferior to posterosuperior type II fracture lines are clear indications that posterior C1–C2 fusion is the definitive treatment.

A variety of different techniques has been described to achieve C1–C2 fusion. All posterior fixation techniques achieve a high fusion rate.[7] While much more infrequently encountered in the modern management of spine fractures, wiring techniques may be used as rescue procedures or supplementation to other internal fixation methods to improve fusion outcomes.[7] Stereotactic navigation has been popularized in spinal surgery. The Harms technique has become popular in the past few years for managing these lesions and has largely supplanted the use of transarticular screws.[9] Stereotactic navigation has been utilized for anterior odontoid screw placement and for posterior C1–C2 fusions, with success.[19,20] This technique is purported to improve the safety of screw placement in the upper cervical spine. The use of stereotactic navigation following traumatic odontoid fractures may help improve outcomes particularly for elderly patients.

While posterior atlantoaxial fixation achieves high fusion rates, there remains some drawbacks to the procedure. Nearly 50% of axial rotation occurs at the atlantoaxial complex; thus, posterior C1–C2 fusion greatly limits movement of the head following fixation. This often drastically limits patients' activities of daily living and quality of life. This limited neck motion remains a consideration for posterior surgical stabilization, particularly in the elderly.

7.1.9 Conclusion

Odontoid fractures are a commonly occurring fracture following significant trauma. While they can occur at any age, elderly patients are at particular risk given their propensity to fall coupled with poor bone quality. The Anderson and D'Alonzo classification categorizes odontoid fractures based on the anatomical fracture pattern. It is generally agreed upon that type I and III fractures can be managed using noninvasive strategies such as rigid cervical collar or halo immobilization. There remains much clinical controversy surrounding the treatment of type II fractures. Surgical intervention including posterior C1–C2 fusion and anterior odontoid screws are options for unstable fractures or those unlikely to heal with conservative measures.

7.2 Hangman's Fractures

7.2.1 Introduction

Traumatic spondylolisthesis of the axis is the second most common C2 fracture after odontoid fractures. It comprises approximately 20% of C2 fractures that present for clinical attention, accounting for approximately 5% of all cervical spine fractures.[21] This type of fracture has been described historically in numerous studies. In 1913, a postmortem anatomical study of judicial hangings described bilateral pars fractures of the axis, and distraction as cause of injury and death. A series reported by Schneider et al in 1964 commented on traumatic spondylolisthesis of the C2 vertebra and paralleled the radiographic findings with the anatomical description of the hanging victims. It is from the title of this manuscript that the colloquial eponym of "hangman's fracture" for this type of injury is derived.[22]

With increasing awareness of the frequency of this injury, further studies were performed to classify this fracture into clinical grades for prognosis and for guidance on treatment.

7.2.2 Anatomy

Hangman's fractures of the C2 vertebra are classically described as bilateral pars interarticularis fractures of the ring of C2 with varying degrees of anterolisthesis of C2 on C3, and varying degrees of angulation of the odontoid process. The second cervical vertebra is often described as a "transitional vertebra" due to its location between the atlas and the subaxial spine.[23] The superior and inferior facets are not vertically in-line, due to the need for support to the atlas and occipital condyles above, and fixation in-line with the C3 facet joints and remainder of the cervical spine below. This creates a weak point, especially as axial loading from hyperextension creates a force to the superior articular processes of C2, driving force into the facets posteriorly and the disc space anteriorly.[22] This distributes the forces during axial loading from a lateral and posterior position at the occipital condyles to a medial and anterior position on the axis, through the C1–C2 lateral masses. Compression of the posterior elements leads to fracture at the relatively weaker pars interarticularis of C2 bilaterally, with anterior displacement of the C2 vertebral body.[21,24,25]

7.2.3 Mechanism of Injury

The mechanism of injury resulting in hangman's fractures is typically hyperextension with axial loading. It is important to note that this fracture can also occur with hyperflexion with rebound extension and axial loading as well.[21,26] The two most common traumatic events leading to this injury are falls and motor vehicle accidents. The key distinction between trauma as opposed to judicial hanging is that with traumatic injuries the mechanism of action does not include distraction, which is thought to be the key factor along with hyperextension resulting in fatality from hanging.[27] In fact, it was noted from early studies that the incidence of neurological deficits in isolated traumatic spondylolisthesis of the axis were low, and, when present, were often transient.[22,27,28] This effect has been attributed to the fact the spinal canal is wider in the high cervical spine, as well as the fact that the hangman's fractures widen the spinal canal after injury.[21,24,25,28,29] Examples of neurological symptoms can include paresthesias, hemiparesis, and occipital neuralgia. It is not uncommon for concurrent head, face, and/or chest trauma to be present.[30] Concomitant cervical fractures can occur in up to 34% of hangman's fracture cases, with a reported 5 to 6% rate of concurrent odontoid fractures.[30,31]

7.2.4 Imaging

Historically, due to ease of access, lateral cervical plain films were the initial imaging modality for diagnosing cervical spine fractures after trauma. While plain films provide information regarding anterolisthesis or odontoid angulation, and demonstrating bilateral C2 pars fractures, unilateral C2 pars fractures may be missed up to 40% of the time.[21] CT of the cervical spine has increased the sensitivity in identifying this lesion and can be used in the mid-sagittal plane to identify odontoid angula-

tion or anterolisthesis of C2 on C3. MRI is a useful tool for identifying disc retropulsion, longitudinal ligamentous disruption, or other soft-tissue injury. Dynamic studies, such as flexion-extension films, can identify laxity of the C2–C3 disc space in apparently stable fractures on static images. Vertebral artery injury may result from high cervical fractures, including hangman's fractures. The rate of radiographically identified vertebral artery injury can approach 27%.[21] Given that unilateral vertebral artery injury is usually asymptomatic it may be important to identify this comorbidity with vascular imaging such as magnetic resonance angiography (MRA) or computed tomography angiography (CTA).[32] Vertebral artery injury should be considered in patients with neurological symptoms referable to the brainstem or cerebellum or with fractures extending to the transverse foramen of C2, especially if comminuted.[33]

7.2.5 Classifications

There have been several grading scales proposed for hangman's fractures. Francis et al graded traumatic spondylolisthesis of the axis in 1981 on a scale from I to V, with increasing grade indicating increasing severity. The appearance on lateral radiographs was used to calculate anterior displacement of the C2 vertebral body on the C3 vertebral body, the angulation of the dens, and concern for disc disruption.[27] Effendi et al classified spondylolisthesis of the axis into a three-tiered grading system with a case series of 131 patients, and provided the basis for the most commonly used clinical classification today. Effendi Class I patients had ring fractures with a stable disc space at C2–C3, identified by minimal anterior displacement of C2 (▶ Fig. 7.2, ▶ Fig. 7.3, and ▶ Fig. 7.4).

Effendi Class II patients were determined to be unstable at the C2–C3 disc space, evidenced by flexion, extension, or obvious anterolisthesis of C2 on C3 coupled with fractures of the C2 ring (▶ Fig. 7.5). Effendi Class III patients had C2 ring fractures with severe enough anterolisthesis to result in locked C2–C3 facets and were also considered to be unstable (▶ Fig. 7.6).[28] The Effendi classification was further modified by Levine and Edwards in 1985 to include a Grade IIa fracture, which is severe anterior flexion of the odontoid without anterolisthesis, coupled with C2 ring fractures. The importance of this finding is that it indicates a hyperflexion-type mechanism with concomitant distraction, which is critical when deciding on whether to use cervical traction. This also can indicate compromise of the posterior longitudinal ligament.[24,25,26]

7.2.6 Treatment Considerations

The classification of hangman's fractures resulted from increasing awareness of the injury and the need for management guidelines for practitioners. Earlier medical literature on the topic proposed prolonged cervical traction alone or coupled with subsequent bracing after reduction, reserving surgical intervention for fractures that failed to reduce or nonunions after conservative therapy.[27,28] Conservative management with external immobilization remains a viable first course of treatment for appropriate fractures.[33,34,35] While surgery for hangman's fractures has become a possible first option in the management tree for certain fractures, external immobilization of the fracture still has a strong presence in the modern

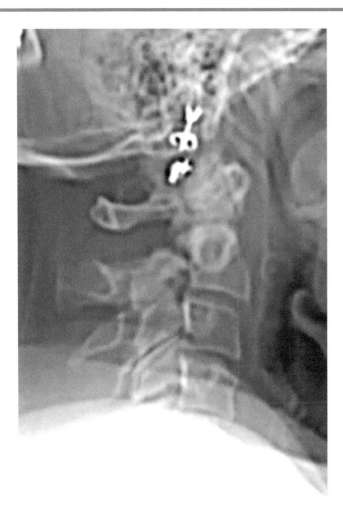

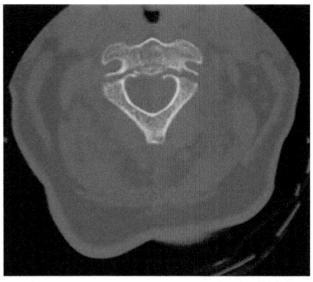

Fig. 7.3 Axial computed tomography of the cervical 2 vertebral arch demonstrating bilateral pars fractures in a Levine–Edwards type I hangman's fracture.

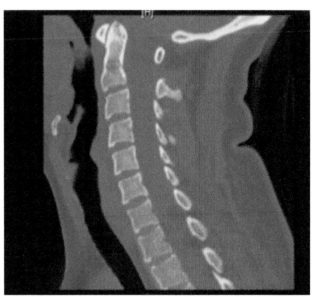

Fig. 7.2 A lateral radiograph demonstrating a bilateral C2 pars fracture with minimal odontoid angulation typical of a Levine–Edwards type I hangman's fracture.

Fig. 7.5 A mid-sagittal computed tomography image of a patient with a Levine–Edwards type I hangman's fracture. Note the minimal listhesis and angulation of the odontoid. Note also the relatively larger width of the cervical spinal canal at the level of the C2 vertebral body.

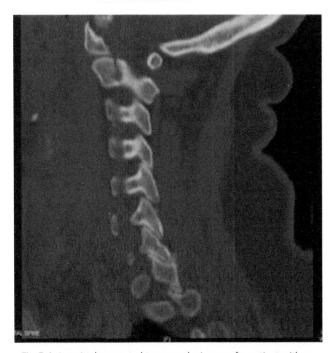

Fig. 7.4 A sagittal computed tomography image of a patient with a Levine–Edwards type I hangman's fracture with the fracture line involving the transverse foramen of C2.

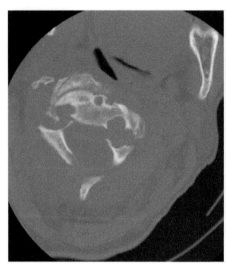
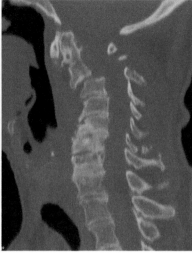

Fig. 7.6 Axial and sagittal computed tomography images of a patient with a Levine–Edwards type III hangman's fracture. Note the significant anterolisthesis of C2 on C3.

treatment algorithm. Most literature regarding treatment of traumatic spondylolisthesis of the axis is based on the Levine–Edwards modification of the Effendi classification system.[36]

7.2.7 Nonoperative Management

Most Levine–Edwards type I and II fractures can be successfully managed with collar or halo immobilization alone. Cervical traction using cranial tongs is a useful tool to reduce fractures before rigid immobilization with the cervical collar or halo device. This can be used safely for type II and III fractures with care not to exceed safe weight limits to prevent distraction at C2–3.[28] Care must be taken when applying traction to Levine–Edwards type IIa fractures, as worsening translation of the C2 body can result.[26] One study recommended flexion/extension films if anterolisthesis was < 6 mm, and to brace with a cervical collar if there was < 2 mm of movement on dynamic imaging. If there was > 2 mm of movement on flexion/extension films or the anterolisthesis was > 6 mm, they recommended a halo device, reserving surgery only for nonunions. Excellent fusion rates occurred, but the complication rate of the halo device was not insignificant.[23] The Halo device can have complications such as pin loosening, skin infection or breakdown at pin sites, subdural empyema, skull fracture, falls, transitory paresthesias, and pulmonary complications. In addition, patients often report discomfort from halo therapy.[23,34,37] One literature review noted that 62.5% of publications proposed nonoperative therapy for initial treatment for all hangman's fractures, with successful healing in type I and II fractures with rates of 100 and 60%, respectively.[35] This was likely due to good vascularization of the fractured bone. Another case series used collar or halo immobilization for type I, II, and IIa fractures and obtained good fusion in all cases without permanent neurological deficit.[29]

7.2.8 Operative Management

Primary surgical intervention has been increasing in popularity for the initial treatment of hangman's fractures (especially Levine–Edwards type II, IIa, and III fractures) and for cases with additional cervical fractures concerning for instability. Up to 50

to 60% of patients with Effendi II, IIa, and III axis fractures treated by conservative management demonstrate subsequent psudarthrosis, pain, continued angulation, or dislocation.[21,38] Surgical treatment can include anterior C2–C3 fusion, posterior C2–C3 fusion, more extensive posterior fixation of the C1, occiput, or lower subaxial vertebra, and both anterior and posterior fixation. Recent studies have discussed the use of C2 transpedicular screws for fracture reduction and preservation of lateral motion at the dens, but this fails to address C2–C3 disc instability and kyphosis; this should be reserved for fractures with minimal disc instability or ligamentous injury.[21,33,38] The advantages of an anterior approach are that it is the only approach that can address a retropulsed C2–C3 disc, it maintains C1–C2 joint mobility, and spine surgeons are familiar with this approach.[21,33,35] Advantages of posterior fusion include the ability to directly reduce kyphosis, address locked facets, and decompress the vertebral artery.[21,35]

7.2.9 Atypical Hangman Fractures

The category of "atypical" or "asymmetric" hangman's fractures includes fractures of the laminae, lateral masses, or facets, and coronal or oblique fractures of the C2 vertebral body. These fractures can arise from large impact trauma. No classification system or definitive management strategy exists. These fractures likewise have a low incidence of neurological deficit and when they are present, they are largely transient as in typical hangman's fractures. In the reported literature, majority of these fractures are treated satisfactorily with conservative therapy such as rigid collar or halo immobilization.[4,31]

7.2.10 Conclusions

Traumatic spondylolisthesis of the axis is a not uncommon cervical fracture occurring most commonly after motor vehicle trauma or falls and should be investigated in patients with neck pain even in the absence of neurological symptoms. The Levine–Edwards modification of the Effendi grading system can be used for direct management. Rigid collar immobilization may suffice for type I fractures, but a halo orthosis may be necessary for type II, IIa, and some type III fractures. Surgical management should not be discounted, especially if gross disc disruption, unreducible facet dislocations, or longitudinal ligamentous injury are identified on imaging. Surgery should aim at restoring stability at the C2–C3 disc level. Concomitant vertebral artery injury should be suspected in cases with vertebrobasilar symptoms or in fractures involving the transverse foramen of C2. Ultimately, there remains a lack of Class I or Class II evidence.[33] In the setting of a patient with a traumatic mechanism of injury to the cervical spine, prompt evaluation with physical examination and radiographic identification of a hangman fracture can give the prepared practitioner enough information to safely guide management and achieve optimal functional outcome for the patient.

References

[1] Waqar M, Van-Popta D, Barone DG, Sarsam Z. External immobilization of odontoid fractures: a systematic review to compare the halo and hard collar. World Neurosurg. 2017; 97:513–517

[2] Bajada S, Ved A, Dudhniwala AG, Ahuja S. Predictors of mortality following conservatively managed fractures of the odontoid in elderly patients. Bone Joint J. 2017; 99-B(1):116–121

[3] Torregrossa F, Grasso G. Conservative management for odontoid cervical fractures: halo or rigid cervical collar? World Neurosurg. 2017; 97:723–724

[4] Robinson AL, Möller A, Robinson Y, Olerud C. C2 fracture subtypes, incidence, and treatment allocation change with age: a retrospective cohort study of 233 consecutive cases. BioMed Res Int. 2017; 2017:8321680

[5] Kaesmacher J, Schweizer C, Valentinitsch A, et al. Osteoporosis is the most important risk factor for odontoid fractures in the elderly. J Bone Miner Res. 2017; 32(7):1582–1588

[6] Korres DS, Chytas DG, Markatos KN, Efstathopoulos NE, Nikolaou VS. The "challenging" fractures of the odontoid process: a review of the classification schemes. Eur J Orthop Surg Traumatol. 2017; 27(4):469–475

[7] Pryputniewicz DM, Hadley MN. Axis fractures. Neurosurgery. 2010; 66(3) Suppl:68–82

[8] Graffeo CS, Perry A, Puffer RC, et al. Odontoid fractures and the silver Tsunami: evidence and practice in the very elderly. Neurosurgery. 2016; 63 Suppl 1:113–117

[9] Guan J, Bisson EF. Treatment of odontoid fractures in the aging population. Neurosurg Clin N Am. 2017; 28(1):115–123

[10] Aldrian S, Erhart J, Schuster R, et al. Surgical vs nonoperative treatment of Hadley type IIA odontoid fractures. Neurosurgery. 2012; 70(3):676–682, discussion 682–683

[11] Chapman J, Smith JS, Kopjar B, et al. The AOSpine North America Geriatric Odontoid Fracture Mortality Study: a retrospective review of mortality outcomes for operative versus nonoperative treatment of 322 patients with long-term follow-up. Spine. 2013; 38(13):1098–1104

[12] Koller H, Zenner J, Hitzl W, et al. In vivo analysis of atlantoaxial motion in individuals immobilized with the halo thoracic vest or Philadelphia collar. Spine. 2009; 34(7):670–679

[13] Schneider AM, Hipp JA, Nguyen L, Reitman CA. Reduction in head and intervertebral motion provided by 7 contemporary cervical orthoses in 45 individuals. Spine. 2007; 32(1):E1–E6

[14] Morishima N, Ohota K, Miura Y. The influences of halo-vest fixation and cervical hyperextension on swallowing in healthy volunteers. Spine. 2005; 30(7):E179–E182

[15] Nemeth ZH, Difazio LT, Bilaniuk JW, et al. The incidence of severe dysphagia after odontoid fracture. Am Surg. 2017; 83(1):15–17

[16] Yang Z, Yuan ZZ, Ma JX, Ma XL. Conservative versus surgical treatment for type II odontoid fractures in the elderly: grading the evidence through a meta-analysis. Orthop Traumatol Surg Res. 2015; 101(7):839–844

[17] Guo Q, Wang L, Lu X, Guo X, Ni B. Posterior temporary fixation versus nonoperative treatment for Anderson-D'Alonzo type III odontoid fractures: functional computed tomography evaluation of C1-C2 rotation. World Neurosurg. 2017; 100:675–680

[18] Shen Y, Miao J, Li C, et al. A meta-analysis of the fusion rate from surgical treatment for odontoid fractures: anterior odontoid screw versus posterior C1-C2 arthrodesis. Eur Spine J. 2015; 24(8):1649–1657

[19] Smith JD, Jack MM, Harn NR, Bertsch JR, Arnold PM. Screw placement accuracy and outcomes following O-arm-navigated atlantoaxial fusion: a feasibility study. Global Spine J. 2016; 6(4):344–349

[20] Pisapia JM, Nayak NR, Salinas RD, et al. Navigated odontoid screw placement using the O-arm: technical note and case series. J Neurosurg Spine. 2017; 26(1):10–18

[21] Schleicher P, Scholz M, Pingel A, Kandziora F. Traumatic spondylolisthesis of the axis vertebra in adults. Global Spine J. 2015; 5(4):346–358

[22] Schneider RC, Livingston KE, Cave AJ, Hamilton G. "Hangman's fracture" of the cervical spine. J Neurosurg. 1965; 22:141–154

[23] Coric D, Wilson JA, Kelly DL, Jr. Treatment of traumatic spondylolisthesis of the axis with nonrigid immobilization: a review of 64 cases. J Neurosurg. 1996; 85(4):550–554

[24] Winn HR. Youman's Neurological Surgery. Vol 3. Philadelphia, PA: Elsevier Saunders; 2011:3192–3200

[25] Winn HR. Youman's Neurological Surgery. Vol 3. Philadelphia, PA: Elsevier Saunders; 2011:3177–3178

[26] Benzel EC. Spine Surgery: Techniques, Complication Avoidance, and Management. Vol 2. Philadelphia, PA: Elsevier Churchill Livingstone; 2005: 1911–1914

[27] Francis WR, Fielding JW, Hawkins RJ, Pepin J, Hensinger R. Traumatic spondylolisthesis of the axis. J Bone Joint Surg Br. 1981; 63-B(3):313–318

[28] Effendi B, Roy D, Cornish B, Dussault RG, Laurin CA. Fractures of the ring of the axis. A classification based on the analysis of 131 cases. J Bone Joint Surg Br. 1981; 63-B(3):319–327

[29] Ferro FP, Borgo GD, Letaif OB, Cristante AF, Marcon RM, Lutaka AS. Traumatic spondylolisthesis of the axis: epidemiology, management and outcome. Acta Ortop Bras. 2012; 20(2):84–87

[30] Greene KA, Dickman CA, Marciano FF, Drabier JB, Hadley MN, Sonntag VK. Acute axis fractures. Analysis of management and outcome in 340 consecutive cases. Spine. 1997; 22(16):1843–1852

[31] Al-Mahfoudh R, Beagrie C, Woolley E, et al. Management of typical and atypical hangman's fractures. Global Spine J. 2016; 6(3):248–256

[32] Ding T, Maltenfort M, Yang H, et al. Correlation of C2 fractures and vertebral artery injury. Spine. 2010; 35(12):E520–E524

[33] Ryken TC, Hadley MN, Aarabi B, et al. Management of isolated fractures of the axis in adults. Neurosurgery. 2013; 72 Suppl 2:132–150

[34] Benzel EC. Conservative treatment of neural arch fractures of the axis: computed tomography scan and X-ray study on consolidation time. World Neurosurg. 2011; 75(2):229–230

[35] Li XF, Dai LY, Lu H, Chen XD. A systematic review of the management of hangman's fractures. Eur Spine J. 2006; 15(3):257–269

[36] Levine AM, Edwards CC. The management of traumatic spondylolisthesis of the axis. J Bone Joint Surg Am. 1985; 67(2):217–226

[37] Shin JJ, Kim SJ, Kim TH, Shin HS, Hwang YS, Park SK. Optimal use of the halo-vest orthosis for upper cervical spine injuries. Yonsei Med J. 2010; 51(5):648–652

[38] Shin JJ, Kim SH, Cho YE, Cheshier SH, Park J. Primary surgical management by reduction and fixation of unstable hangman's fractures with discoligamentous instability or combined fractures: clinical article. J Neurosurg Spine. 2013; 19(5):569–575

8 Management of Traumatic Atlantoaxial Subluxations

Alexander D. Ghasem, Frank J. Eismont, Evan J. Trapana, and Joseph P. Gjolaj

Abstract

Most patients with type I (posterior C-1 arch) fractures and type III (C-1 lateral mass) atlas fractures will not have any C1–C2 subluxation. Type I fractures can be treated in a soft collar and type III fractures can be treated in a standard rigid cervical collar for 6 weeks. Most patients with traumatic atlantoaxial subluxation due to type II atlas fractures (Jefferson fractures) or transverse ligament injuries with a bony avulsion can be successfully treated with a rigid occipito-cervical-thoracic orthosis for 2 to 3 months. Surgery should be limited to patients with intrasubstance transverse ligament tears, patients with Jefferson fractures and C1–C2 instability after failure of appropriate bracing, and patients with bony avulsion transverse ligament injuries who do not heal after conservative care. C1-C2 posterior instrumented fusion is the usual type of surgery when surgery is indicated, but O–C2 fusion is sometimes necessary for treatment of patients with type II atlas fractures as described within the text of this chapter.

Keywords: atlas, facets, transverse ligament, apical ligament, alar ligament, atlantoaxial joint, atlanto-dens interval (ADI), posterior atlanto-dens interval (PADI), sum of lateral mass displacement, atlas fracture

8.1 Introduction

The upper cervical spine is composed of the occiput, atlas, and axis and is often described as the craniocervical junction (CCJ). The unique anatomical relationships within this osseoligamentous complex account for the injury patterns seen in the occipitoatlantoaxial spine. Unrecognized trauma to the upper cervical spine can result in devastating outcomes with injury to the brainstem and spinal cord. Nowadays, continually improving resuscitation protocols and lifesaving measures have increased the incidence of patients surviving high-energy trauma with concomitant atlantoaxial injury. Radiographs and advanced imaging techniques are utilized to assist surgeons in diagnosis and treatment planning. In this chapter, the authors discuss the diagnosis, anatomy, clinical evaluation, and surgical stabilization techniques for traumatic atlantoaxial subluxation.

8.2 Epidemiology and Associated Conditions

The etiologies for atlantoaxial instability are wide-ranging and include congenital (os odontoideum), infectious (Grisel syndrome), metabolic (Down syndrome), arthritic (rheumatoid arthritis), neoplastic, and traumatic causes. The focus of this chapter is on the traumatic causes of atlantoaxial subluxation and their respective management. Traumatic atlantoaxial instability is notably seen in a bimodal distribution in younger patients as well as those over the age of 60 years.[1] In pediatric patients, CCJ injury accounts for 56 to 73% of all cervical spine trauma.[2,3] Moreover in patients over the age of 60 years, C1-C2 injury accounts for 70% of all cervical trauma cases.[1] In both cohorts, atlantoaxial instability may result in unsatisfactory outcomes. Pediatric patients with cervical spine injuries and concomitant head injuries experience mortality rates as high as 41%.[4] Similarly, older patients with concomitant cervical spine injuries and neurological injuries have 2-year mortality rates of 41%.[5,6,7] Thoughtful consideration and a thorough understanding of upper cervical injury is crucial to the early recognition and appropriate management of atlantoaxial trauma.

8.3 Anatomy

Understanding the anatomy of the occipitoatlantoaxial complex is critical in evaluating upper cervical spine trauma and developing a treatment plan. The CCJ comprises the occiput, the atlas, and the axis, as well as their associated articulations and ligamentous attachments. There are six articular surfaces of the CCJ that allow for multiplanar motion. The conjoining surfaces between occiput–C1 and C1–C2 account for 50% of the total cervical flexion/extension and cervical rotation, respectively. The anterior atlanto-odontoid articulation is interposed between the posterior aspect of the anterior arch of the atlas and the anterior portion of the dens.

Conversely, the posterior atlanto-odontoid articulation is positioned between the posterior aspect of the dens and the anterior surface of the transverse ligament. The atlantoaxial joints are shallow, providing for increased rotation across C1–C2. Mechanical stability within the atlantoaxial complex is derived from the surrounding ligaments.

The ligaments spanning the CCJ include the transverse ligament, paired alar ligaments, the rudimentary apical ligament, the anterior longitudinal ligament, and the posterior longitudinal ligament (tectorial membrane). The transverse portion of the cruciform ligament is commonly referred to as the transverse ligament. The transverse ligament is attached to the tubercles on the medial aspect of each lateral mass of the atlas and is essential in maintaining atlantoaxial stability. Positioned anterior to the transverse ligament, the apical ligament extends from the tip of the dens to the basion. It is rudimentary and relatively weak. The paired alar ligaments connect the lateral aspect of the odontoid to the medial aspect of the occipital condyles and limit lateral bending forces as well as rotational forces.[8] They are strong and essential for stability. Barring vertebral artery anomalies, the paired arteries extend through the transversarium at the level of the axis and into a transverse groove above the superior articular facet of the atlas. Due to their proximity, the vertebral arteries, internal carotid vasculature, and cranial nerves are all vulnerable to injury and require special attention during examination.

8.4 Clinical Evaluation and Associated Conditions

Cervical spine injuries have been closely associated with high-energy accidents, focal neurological deficits, and severe head injury. As with any trauma evaluation, the airway must be secured first. In the setting of upper cervical spine injury, diaphragm and intercostal musculature may paralyze and result in respiratory failure. Large prevertebral hematomas may also produce airway obstruction. The remainder of the spine should also be evaluated as noncontiguous spine injuries are as high as 6% in trauma patients.

Patients often complain of suboccipital neck pain and a feeling of instability. It is difficult to assess focal injury since there is no dermatomal sensory or motor loss associated with this level. Posterior scalp sensation in the distribution of the greater occipital nerve may be diminished and cranial nerve injury is possible. Vaccaro et al demonstrated a 20% risk of vertebral artery injury in nonpenetrating cervical spine trauma.[9] This may result in severe sequelae such as blindness, quadriplegia, and death. However, many of these vascular injuries are clinically silent.

8.5 Imaging

A complete series of cervical radiographs is the principal means for evaluating cervical spine injuries and includes anteroposterior, lateral, and open-mouth odontoid views. Flexion-extension views are omitted due to risk of progressive neurological injury in the setting of instability as well as patient guarding.

8.5.1 Lateral X-ray

The lateral radiograph aids in evaluating prevertebral edema, sagittal balance, and instability. As a general rule for evaluating prevertebral swelling, soft-tissue shadows measured on the lateral radiograph should not exceed 10 mm at C1, 5 mm at C3, and 20 mm at C6. Sagittal balance is maintained in the cervical spine when lines drawn between the anterior border of the vertebral bodies, posterior border of the vertebral bodies, anterior aspect of the lamina, and spinous processes, are all continuous. Instability and potential spinal cord compression are assessed on the basis of following measurements:

1. Atlanto-dens interval (ADI): This is measured from the posterior border of the anterior arch of the atlas to the anterior border of the odontoid process. Accepted parameters for instability are ADIs measuring greater than 3.5 mm in adults and greater than 5 mm in children.[2,10]
2. Space available for the cord (SAC) and posterior ADI (PADI): This is measured from the anterior border of the posterior arch of the atlas to the posterior border of the odontoid process. Patients are at risk of neurological deterioration when the PADI is less than 14 mm and many consider this an indication for surgical intervention.[2]

8.5.2 Open-Mouth Odontoid X-ray

Sum of lateral mass displacement: Bilateral increased C1 lateral mass translation relative to the lateral mass of C2 indicates the presence of a bony fracture at C1 and possible transverse liga-ment disruption. In adults, when the sum of lateral mass displacement is greater than 6.9 mm, then a transverse ligament rupture is likely to be present, and this may be confirmed with magnetic resonance imaging (MRI) in equivocal cases.[11,12,13]

8.5.3 Advanced Imaging Modalities

Computed tomography (CT) has been shown to be cost effective and the most sensitive tool for detecting and delineating fracture patterns in the upper cervical spine.[14,15] MRI has been shown to be less cost effective and less accurate at detecting upper cervical spine fractures with a sensitivity ranging from 11 to 37%.[16,17,18] However, advantages of using MRI include further delineation of soft-tissue structures (including the intervertebral discs, the spinal cord, and ligaments such as the transverse ligament), as well as detection of compressive soft-tissues lesions such as hematomas.

8.6 Atlas Fractures

Most atlas fractures result from axial loading injuries and occur in the anterior and posterior arches. They account for an estimated 10% of all cervical spine fractures and 25% of injuries to the atlantoaxial complex.[3] The risk of having a spinal cord neurological injury caused by atlas fractures is low when occurring in isolation, although patients may have damage to the greater occipital nerve or to cranial nerves.[19] However, they are often observed in polytrauma patients with a multitude of injuries including other spine injuries which may have associated spinal cord injuries. Half of patients with atlas fractures have one or more other cervical spine fractures and 40% are associated with fractures of the axis.[20]

Atlas fractures are best visualized on thin-cut CT imaging and they are most commonly categorized according to Landells' fracture classification[21] which is as follows:

1. Type I: These fractures only include one arch, anterior or posterior, and do not cross the equator of the atlas. The two posterior arch fractures are usually due to hyperextension and abutment of the C1–arch against the occiput (▶ Fig. 8.1). The anterior arch fractures are due to abutment against the dens. Treatment usually consists of soft cervical collar immobilization for a short time since this is a stable injury. It is not necessary to wait for fracture union to occur.
2. Type II: Also known as a "Jefferson fracture." These fractures are the result of axial loading mechanisms of injury (▶ Fig. 8.2). This injury type produces bilateral anterior and posterior arch fractures and may cause C1–C2 instability depending on the integrity of the transverse ligament. If coronal displacement of the combined lateral masses exceeds 6.9 mm, then transverse ligament injury and resulting instability are present. In the setting of instability, C1–C2 or occiput–C2 fusion may be required for maintenance of neurological status and initiating early rehabilitation. However, the timing of any surgical fusion and the role for using a halo vest or other occipito-cervical-thoracic orthoses are not agreed upon.[20,21,22,23,24,25,26] The senior authors would recommend initial treatment with a rigid orthosis including either a halo vest or an occipito-cervical-thoracic brace for 2 to 3 months depending on the degree of instability present. The patient would then be reevaluated with X-rays and CT

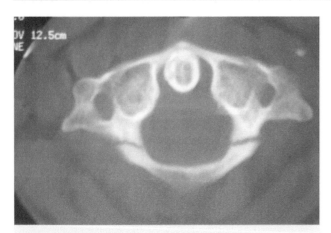

Fig. 8.1 This axial CT scan demonstrates a C1 posterior arch fracture that is minimally displaced, and this typically occurs at the vertebral artery groove. Provided there are no other associated injuries, the treatment would usually be immobilization in a soft collar for a short time for comfort only. This by itself is a stable injury. (Reproduced with permission from Tay B, Eismont J. Injuries of the upper cervical spine. In: Garfin SR, Eismont FJ, Gordon R. Bell GR, Fischgrund JS, Bono CM, eds. Rothman-Simeone and Herkowitz's The Spine, Vol 2. Elsevier; 2017: 1285-1309.)

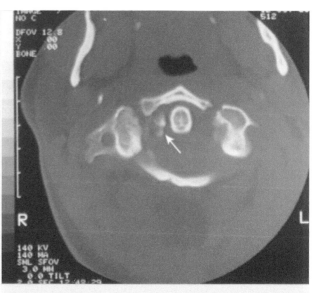

Fig. 8.2 This axial CT scan demonstrates a Jefferson fracture with splaying of the lateral masses of C1. The injury has caused an avulsion of the bony origin of the transverse ligament from the right lateral mass of C1 (*arrow*). (Reproduced with permission from Tay B, Eismont J. Injuries of the upper cervical spine. In: Garfin SR, Eismont FJ, Gordon R. Bell GR, Fischgrund JS, Bono CM, eds. Rothman-Simeone and Herkowitz's The Spine, Vol 2. Elsevier; 2017: 1285-1309.)

scans to assess bony healing and callus formation. The final test would then be cervical flexion and extension X-rays out of the orthosis (▶ Fig. 8.3). If there is no C1–C2 translation, then the patient would be changed to a soft collar for 1 month and then allowed to resume normal low-impact activities. On the other hand, if it remains unstable with C1–C2 translation after 2 to 3 months of immobilization, then surgery would be proposed and would be either a C1–C2 or an occiput–C2 fusion. The levels of the fusion would depend on the local bony anatomy, the degree of malalignment of the occipitocervical joint, and the location and patency of the vertebral arteries. It should be emphasized that drilling, tapping, and screw insertion into the atlas lateral masses can be extremely challenging and may not be possible if the atlas lateral masses are completely loose and independently mobile. In Landells series of 13 patients with type II atlas fractures, all were treated conservatively with a rigid orthosis and only one required C1–C2 fusion 1 year later after initial bracing because of lateral C1–C2 instability.

3. Type III: Fractures of a unilateral mass of the atlas are classified as type III. These may be subclassified as displaced and nondisplaced for treatment purposes. Lateral mass fractures with greater than 5 mm of displacement should be immobilized using a rigid cervical collar or rarely using a rigid occipito-cervical-thoracic brace. Minimal or nondisplaced injuries should be treated definitively with rigid cervical collar immobilization for 6 weeks.[21] In Landells series of 35 patients with atlas fractures, there were 16 type I, 13 type II, and 6 type III fractures. Of the 23 patients with more than 1-year follow-up, 57% reported significant symptoms including neck pain, scalp dysesthesias, and/or neck stiffness. Only one patient was treated surgically for late instability.[21]

8.7 Isolated Transverse Ligament Injuries

Transverse ligament injury is subdivided by Dickman et al into intrasubstance tears (type I) and bony avulsion injuries (type II).[27] The transverse ligament is composed primarily of collagen fibers making it fairly inelastic and susceptible to injury.[28] If instability is suspected, but diagnostic findings remain inconclusive, an MRI should be done to evaluate transverse ligament integrity.[13] A complete disruption of the transverse ligament will always cause atlantoaxial instability and necessitate surgical C1–C2 fusion since the ligament itself is not amenable to primary healing or to direct repair (▶ Fig. 8.5).

While an ADI greater than 3.5 mm in adults and 5 mm in children on lateral radiographs indicates C1–C2 instability, the actual bony avulsion fragment seen in type II transverse ligament injuries can only be detected with CT imaging. Management of bony avulsion injuries from C1 lateral masses requires rigid external cervical immobilization. Seventy-four percent of patients with type II injuries treated in this manner had successful patient outcomes in the series by Dickman and Sonntag.[27] If instability persists despite conservative treatment, then a posterior C1–C2 fusion is the recommended treatment.

8.8 Lateral Atlanto-Axial Subluxation

Significant lateral subluxation of the spine at C1-2 is uncommon and is only seen when the odontoid is absent, deficient, or fractured. The treatment for those patients with an odontoid

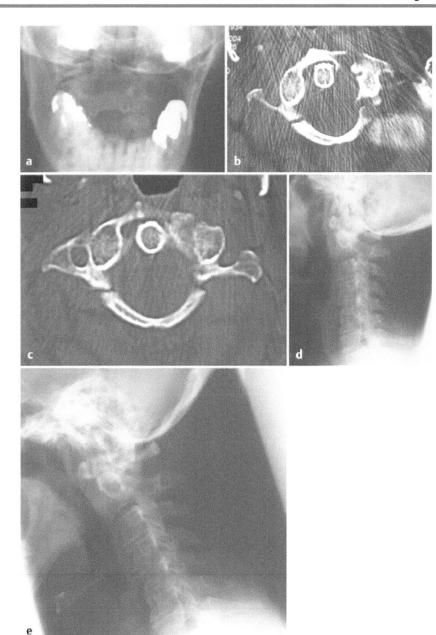

Fig. 8.3 This patient suffered a displaced Jefferson fracture and was treated in a halo vest without reduction. (**a**) The open-mouth view of C1–C2 shows a combined 10 mm overhang. (**b**) The CT scan shows an 8 mm lateral displacement of the C1 left lateral mass. (**c**) The final follow-up CT scan shows no further lateral displacement with interval callus formation. (**d, e**) Flexion and extension plain films demonstrate no radiographic evidence of instability at the occipitocervical junction or at C1–C2. (Reproduced with permission from Tay B, Eismont J. Injuries of the upper cervical spine. In: Garfin SR, Eismont FJ, Gordon R. Bell GR, Fischgrund JS, Bono CM, eds. Rothman-Simeone and Herkowitz's The Spine, Vol 2. Elsevier; 2017: 1285-1309.)

fracture will follow the guidelines of treatment given in Chapter 7. For those with os odontoideum or other odontoid deficiencies, it is possible for patients to develop a post traumatic lateral subluxation. In these cases, the alar ligaments are absent or deficient and the C1-2 joint capsules and the tectorial membrane are the only stabilizing structures. If the lateral subluxation is significant, then a posterior C1-2 fusion is indicated (Fig. 8.5). The authors are not aware of an exact number of millimeters of lateral subluxation of C1 on C2 before dangerous instability occurs. It would seem that five millimeters would probably be enough to demonstrate joint capsule instability but that is only the authors' estimate.

8.9 Surgical Stabilization

Fusions using wires with bone grafts have been used in the past but require prolonged immobilization and are the weakest of the available biomechanical constructs. Currently C1 lateral mass screws combined with C2 pedicle or translaminar screws and C1–C2 connecting rods are used to provide excellent fixation and C1–C2 fusion.[29,30,31] All 37 patients in Harm's original report had a solid C1–C2 fusion. C1–C2 transarticular screw fixation is another accepted treatment option if the vertebral artery anatomy is amenable to safe placement of the screws.[32] It is critical with C1–C2 transarticular screws that the medial and superior borders of the C2 pedicle be respected in order to avoid vertebral artery injury. A study by Paramore et al reviewed cervical CT scans with reconstruction views of 94 patients and found a high-riding transverse foramen on at least one side of the C2 vertebra that would prohibit placement of transarticular screws in 17 patients. In another five patients, screw placement was risky leaving a total of 23% of patients at risk for vertebral artery injury.[33] If transarticular C1–C2 screws are being considered, it is imperative that the CT reconstructed views of C1 and C2 be carefully reviewed in

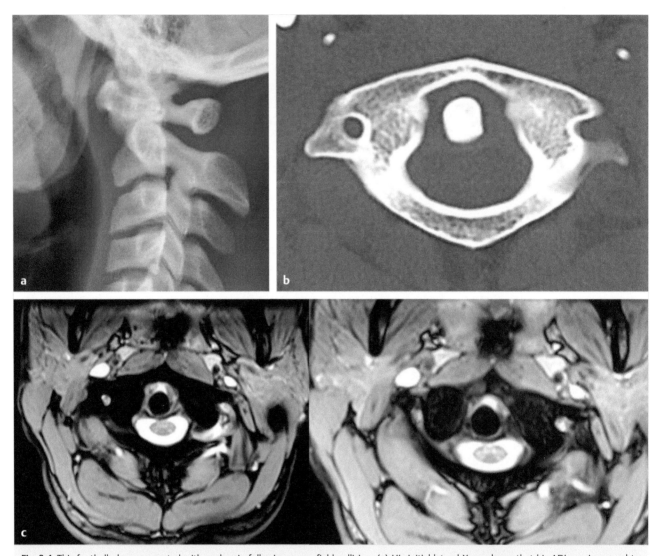

Fig. 8.4 This football player presented with neck pain following an on-field collision. (**a**) His initial lateral X-ray shows that his ADI was increased to 4.5 mm. (**b**) His CT scan at C1 also shows an increased ADI. There is no avulsion fracture from the C1 lateral mass. (**c**) His T-2 axial MRI images show that his transverse ligament is continuous but may have a smaller thickness directly behind the odontoid. (*continued*)

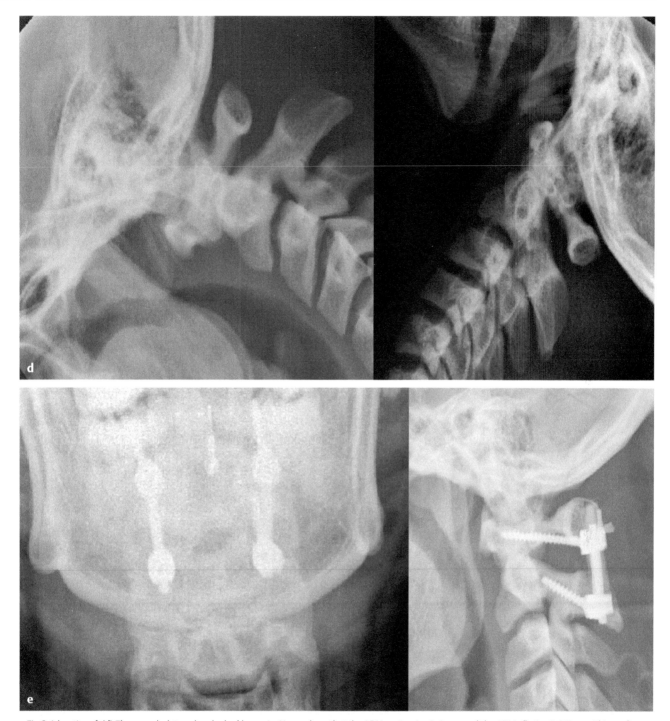

Fig 8.4 (*continued*) (**d**) Three weeks later when he had less pain, X-rays show that the ADI in extension is 1 mm and the ADI in flexion is 9.5 mm. This confirms that there is obviously an incompetent transverse ligament. (**e**) He was treated with a posterior C1–C2 fusion. With a one level sub-axial anterior fusion, a patient could be cleared for a return to football. A patient with a one level fusion at C1–C2, however, would not be allowed to return to football.

order to identify those patients who should not be treated using C1–C2 transarticular screws. Grob's original report of 161 patients showed a solid fusion in all but 1 patient. A survey of the AANS/CNS, however, showed that of 1,318 patients with C1–C2 transarticular screws, 31 patients had a known vertebral artery injury (2.4%) and 23 patients had a suspected vertebral artery injury (1.7%).[34] Anterior C1–C2 screw placement is also described but does not allow for adequate bone grafting and may lead to difficulties with respect to airway

obstruction and dysphagia.[35] Occipitocervical fusion may be considered for atlantoaxial stabilization when there is an aberrant course of the vertebral artery, the anatomy of the posterior elements is not suitable for fixation, or the ability to reduce the atlantoaxial joint is in question.[36]

With a C1–C2 fusion, there will be a loss of 50% of the normal cervical rotation. With an O–C2 fusion there will be the same 50% loss of rotation but, in addition, there will be a 50% loss of cervical flexion-extension.

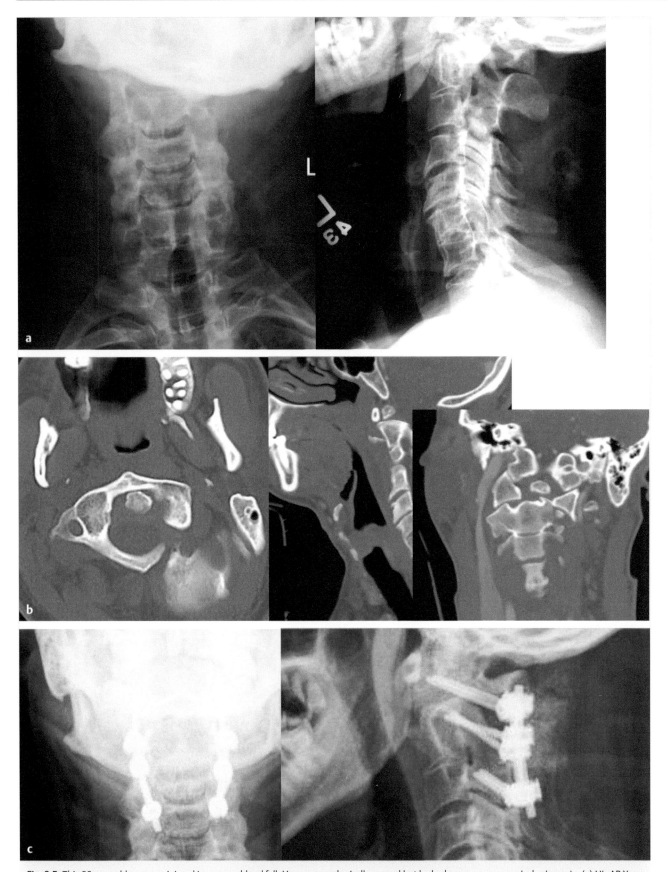

Fig. 8.5 This 66-year-old man was injured in a ground-level fall. He was neurologically normal but he had severe upper cervical spine pain. **(a)** His AP X-ray shows a 20° scoliosis deformity between his skull and C3. His lateral X-ray shows a chronic C2–C3 fusion and increased anterior soft tissue swelling. **(b)** His sagittal CT scan confirms an os-odontoideum and the coronal CT scan shows the 1 cm left lateral subluxation of C1 on C2. It also confirms that the 20° of head tilt all occurs at the C1–C2 level. The axial CT shows that the C1 ring is intact. **(c)** Postoperative X-rays show restoration of normal C1–C2 alignment. The arthrodesis utilized C1 and C3 lateral mass screws and C2 pars screws.

References

[1] Spivak JM, Weiss MA, Cotler JM, Call M. Cervical spine injuries in patients 65 and older. Spine. 1994; 19(20):2302–2306

[2] Sherk HH, Nicholson JT, Chung SM. Fractures of the odontoid process in young children. J Bone Joint Surg Am. 1978; 60(7):921–924

[3] Birney TJ, Hanley EN, Jr. Traumatic cervical spine injuries in childhood and adolescence. Spine. 1989; 14(12):1277–1282

[4] Givens TG, Polley KA, Smith GF, Hardin WD, Jr. Pediatric cervical spine injury: a three-year experience. J Trauma. 1996; 41(2):310–314

[5] Kiwerski JE. Injuries to the spinal cord in elderly patients. Injury. 1992; 23(6):397–400

[6] Weingarden SI, Graham PM. Falls resulting in spinal cord injury: patterns and outcomes in an older population. Paraplegia. 1989; 27(6):423–427

[7] DeVivo MJ, Kartus PL, Rutt RD, Stover SL, Fine PR. The influence of age at time of spinal cord injury on rehabilitation outcome. Arch Neurol. 1990; 47(6):687–691

[8] Werne S. Studies in spontaneous atlas dislocation. Acta Orthop Scand Suppl. 1957; 23 Suppl 23:1–150

[9] Vaccaro AR, Klein GR, Flanders AE, Albert TJ, Balderston RA, Cotler JM. Long-term evaluation of vertebral artery injuries following cervical spine trauma using magnetic resonance angiography. Spine. 1998; 23(7):789–794, discussion 795

[10] McGrory BJ, Klassen RA, Chao EY, Staeheli JW, Weaver AL. Acute fractures and dislocations of the cervical spine in children and adolescents. J Bone Joint Surg Am. 1993; 75(7):988–995

[11] Heller JG, Viroslav S, Hudson T. Jefferson fractures: the role of magnification artifact in assessing transverse ligament integrity. J Spinal Disord. 1993; 6(5):392–396

[12] Spence KF, Jr, Decker S, Sell KW. Bursting atlantal fracture associated with rupture of the transverse ligament. J Bone Joint Surg Am. 1970; 52(3):543–549

[13] Dickman CA, Mamourian A, Sonntag VKH, Drayer BP. Magnetic resonance imaging of the transverse atlantal ligament for the evaluation of atlantoaxial instability. J Neurosurg. 1991; 75(2):221–227

[14] McCulloch PT, France J, Jones DL, et al. Helical computed tomography alone compared with plain radiographs with adjunct computed tomography to evaluate the cervical spine after high-energy trauma. J Bone Joint Surg Am. 2005; 87(11):2388–2394

[15] Munera F, Rivas LA, Nunez DB, Jr, Quencer RM. Imaging evaluation of adult spinal injuries: emphasis on multidetector CT in cervical spine trauma. Radiology. 2012; 263(3):645–660

[16] Katzberg RW, Benedetti PF, Drake CM, et al. Acute cervical spine injuries: prospective MR imaging assessment at a level 1 trauma center. Radiology. 1999; 213(1):203–212

[17] Klein GR, Vaccaro AR, Albert TJ, et al. Efficacy of magnetic resonance imaging in the evaluation of posterior cervical spine fractures. Spine. 1999; 24(8):771–774

[18] Muchow RD, Resnick DK, Abdel MP, Munoz A, Anderson PA. Magnetic resonance imaging (MRI) in the clearance of the cervical spine in blunt trauma: a meta-analysis. J Trauma. 2008; 64(1):179–189

[19] Connolly B, Turner C, DeVine J, Gerlinger T. Jefferson fracture resulting in Collet-Sicard syndrome. Spine. 2000; 25(3):395–398

[20] Levine AM, Edwards CC. Fractures of the atlas. J Bone Joint Surg Am. 1991; 73(5):680–691

[21] Landells CD, Van Peteghem PK. Fractures of the atlas: classification, treatment and morbidity. Spine. 1988; 13(5):450–452

[22] Levine AM, Edwards CC. Treatment of injuries in the C1-C2 complex. Orthop Clin North Am. 1986; 17(1):31–44

[23] Fowler JL, Sandhu A, Fraser RD. A review of fractures of the atlas vertebra. J Spinal Disord. 1990; 3(1):19–24

[24] Hadley MN, Dickman CA, Browner CM, Sonntag VK. Acute traumatic atlas fractures: management and long term outcome. Neurosurgery. 1988; 23(1):31–35

[25] McGuire RA, Jr, Harkey HL. Primary treatment of unstable Jefferson's fractures. J Spinal Disord. 1995; 8(3):233–236

[26] Lee TT, Green BA, Petrin DR. Treatment of stable burst fracture of the atlas (Jefferson fracture) with rigid cervical collar. Spine. 1998; 23(18):1963–1967

[27] Dickman CA, Sonntag VK. Injuries involving the transverse atlantal ligament: classification and treatment guidelines based upon experience with 39 injuries. Neurosurgery. 1997; 40(4):886–887

[28] Dvorak J, Schneider E, Saldinger P, Rahn B. Biomechanics of the craniocervical region: the alar and transverse ligaments. J Orthop Res. 1988; 6(3):452–461

[29] Fiore AJ, Haid RW, Rodts GE, et al. Atlantal lateral mass screws for posterior spinal reconstruction: technical note and case series. Neurosurg Focus. 2002; 12(1):E5

[30] Harms J, Melcher RP. Posterior C1-C2 fusion with polyaxial screw and rod fixation. Spine. 2001; 26(22):2467–2471

[31] Aryan HE, Newman CB, Nottmeier EW, Acosta FL, Jr, Wang VY, Ames CP. Stabilization of the atlantoaxial complex via C-1 lateral mass and C-2 pedicle screw fixation in a multicenter clinical experience in 102 patients: modification of the Harms and Goel techniques. J Neurosurg Spine. 2008; 8(3):222–229

[32] Grob D, Jeanneret B, Aebi M, Markwalder TM. Atlanto-axial fusion with trans-articular screw fixation. J Bone Joint Surg Br. 1991; 73(6):972–976

[33] Paramore CG, Dickman CA, Sonntag VK. The anatomical suitability of the C1–2 complex for transarticular screw fixation. J Neurosurg. 1996; 85(2):221–224

[34] Wright NM, Lauryssen C, American Association of Neurological Surgeons/ Congress of Neurological Surgeons. Vertebral artery injury in C1–2 transarticular screw fixation: results of a survey of the AANS/CNS section on disorders of the spine and peripheral nerves. J Neurosurg. 1998; 88(4):634–640

[35] Reindl R, Sen M, Aebi M. Anterior instrumentation for traumatic C1-C2 instability. Spine. 2003; 28(17):E329–E333

[36] Wang S, Wang C, Liu Y, Yan M, Zhou H. Anomalous vertebral artery in craniovertebral junction with occipitalization of the atlas. Spine. 2009; 34(26):2838–2842

9 Traumatic Atlantoaxial Rotatory Fixation

Darnell T. Josiah and Daniel K. Resnick

Abstract

Traumatic atlantoaxial rotatory fixation is a rare entity that is seen in children after minor trauma with inherent ligamentous laxity, whereas the principal cause in adults is high-energy trauma. In this chapter, we review the etiologies along with the injury patterns and treatment options available in caring for these patients.

Keywords: atlantoaxial rotatory subluxation, classification, torticollis, atlantoaxial subluxation

9.1 Introduction

Rotatory deformities of the atlantoaxial joint are relatively rare in adults. Persistent subluxation causing torticollis was termed rotatory fixation of the atlantoaxial joint by Wortzman and Dewar in 1968. The condition was later referred to as atlantoaxial rotatory fixation (AARF) by Fielding and Hawkins in 1977, as fixation of the atlas on the axis may occur with subluxation.[1] This condition has been also previously termed rotatory dislocation, rotatory subluxation, rotatory displacement, and rotatory fixation. Pediatric patients with AARF typically present with torticollis in a "cock-robin" posture. Infections followed by trauma are the leading cause of AARF.[2,3,4] The differential diagnosis of nontraumatic AARF includes congenital anomalies, metastatic tumors, ankylosing spondylitis, general ligamentous laxity (which can result from Down syndrome, Morquio syndrome, Marfan syndrome, and rheumatoid arthritis), and eosinophilic granulomas.[2] Grisel syndrome typically occurs in children after a serious head and neck infection, and causes subluxation of the atlantoaxial joint due to inflammatory ligamentous laxity.[3,5] Traumatic AARF, while predominantly a pediatric disorder, does occur in the adult population and should be included in the differential for patients presenting with torticollis even after minor trauma. Two classification systems have been described: The White and Panjabi system, and the more frequently used Fielding and Hawkins classification system.[1,3] This chapter discusses traumatic AARF.

9.2 The Atlantoaxial Joint

The atlantoaxial joint is specialized, highly complex, and moves approximately 600 times per hour.[6] The joint contributes to nearly 50% of axial neck rotation. The normal physiological range of motion of the atlas on the axis is 25 to 53 degrees to either side.[4,7]

9.2.1 Functional Anatomy

The transverse ligament (located behind the odontoid process) and the facet joint capsule prevent excessive anterior translation of C1 on C2. The paired alar ligaments, which connect the posterolateral apex of the odontoid to the lateral aspect of the foramen magnum, bilaterally limit anterior shifting and exces-

sive rotation of C1 on C2 to approximately 50 degrees. The alar ligaments also act as secondary stabilizers; cadaveric studies have shown that if the transverse ligament is cut, anterior subluxation past 4 to 5 mm is prevented by these structures.[1,4,7] Rotation > 56 degrees or a right to left difference of > 8 degree is suggestive of hypermobility. Rotational hypomobility is indicated if motion is < 28°.[4,8] The spinal canal, which is widest at C1–C2, narrows during physiological rotation of the atlas on the axis due to the ipsilateral lateral mass moving posteriorly. During physiological rotation to the right, the right vertebral artery traveling in the transverse foramina is stretched while the left vertebral artery is kinked. The corollary occurs when turning the head to the left.[9]

9.3 Classification of Atlantoaxial Rotatory Fixation

Two classification systems, largely based on imaging findings, have been described to determine the direction of atlas displacement on the axis. Fielding, in 1977, divided AARF into four categories of instability. These include the following:

- Type 1: Rotatory fixation with less than 3 mm anterior displacement of the atlas. There is translation of the facets without any increase in the atlantodental interval. Rotation occurs within the normal physiological range.
- Type 2: Rotatory fixation with 3 to 5 mm anterior displacement of the atlas. One of the articular masses acts as a pivot and there is deficiency of the transverse ligament. This is the second most common type.
- Type 3: Rotatory fixation with greater than 5 mm anterior displacement of the atlas. There is deficiency of the transverse and alar ligaments.
- Type 4: Rotatory fixation with posterior displacement of the atlas. This is the rarest form and occurs with a deficiency of the odontoid process.[1] Fielding reported on a series of 17 patients and assessments were based on plain radiographs before computed tomography (CT) was available. Five of these patients ultimately required cervical fusion despite cervical traction.[1]

9.4 Diagnosis

Clinically, these patients have painful torticollis with lateral neck flexion and contralateral rotation. Physical exam and a high index of suspicion are the key along with appropriate imaging for early diagnosis. CT imaging is essential for initial evaluation; axial CT scans along with sagittal and coronal cuts of the upper cervical spine aid in identifying the rotated position of the atlas on the axis (▶ Fig. 9.1a, b).[4] Injury in adults is most commonly related to high-energy trauma such as car crashes, falls, or sports accidents.[10] These patients often present with articular cartilage damage and facet joint fractures; extent of neurological injury depends on the integrity of the transverse ligament, the anterior or posterior displacement of C1 on C2, and the degree of encroachment of the spinal canal.[3,11]

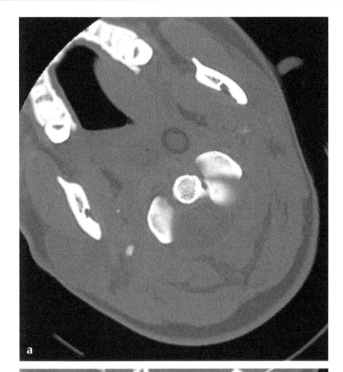

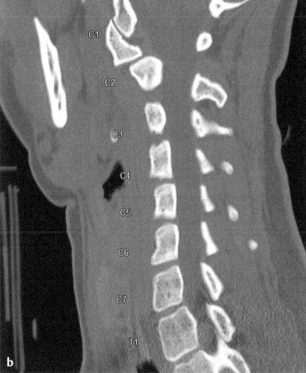

Fig. 9.1 (a) Axial computed tomography (CT) scan of the cervical spine showing the rotation of C1 to the right relative to C2. **(b)** Sagittal CT scan of the cervical spine showing the translation of C1 right lateral mass relative to C2.

9.5 Management

There are no predefined treatment protocols for the management of traumatic AARF; treatment typically begins with immobilization with the goal of reducing the deformity, controlling pain, limiting neurological injury, and restoring stability. Conservative treatment begins with immobilization via application of cervical traction with very low weights progressing to 30 or 35 lb in adults. The nature of the deformity often precludes reduction with simple longitudinal traction and a rotatory traction component may be necessary. In patients who have gross instability, closed reduction under general anesthesia should be performed with extreme caution due to the possibility of neurological injury.[3,11] Surgical treatment of these injuries remains controversial and various techniques of open reduction and internal fixation have been described. Atlantoaxial arthrodesis should be considered if the reduction is unstable, if the patient has sustained neurological injury, or if transverse ligament disruption with translation greater than 5 mm is observed. C1–C2 wiring or posterior fixation with hooks has a higher nonunion risk than screw fixation.[3,7,12]

9.6 Conclusion

Atlantoaxial rotatory injuries generally require immediate immobilization that can be either external or internal. Reduction with skeletal traction should be utilized before definitive treatment. Bilateral anterior translation and displacement greater that 3 mm, with the presence of neurological symptoms, should be considered unstable. A C1–C2 fusion with arthrodesis should be considered in these cases. Cases involving bilateral posterior translations with associated odontoid fractures should be reduced and then surgical fixation should be carried out. Unilateral anterior or posterior rotations/translations can be treated with closed reduction and external immobilization with a collar or halo if the transverse ligament is intact.[3,10,12]

References

[1] Fielding JW, Hawkins RJ. Atlanto-axial rotatory fixation. (Fixed rotatory subluxation of the atlanto-axial joint). J Bone Joint Surg Am. 1977; 59(1):37–44

[2] Jeon SW, Jeong JH, Moon SM, Choi SK. Atlantoaxial rotatory fixation in adults patient. J Korean Neurosurg Soc. 2009; 45(4):246–248

[3] Moore KR, Frank EH. Traumatic atlantoaxial rotatory subluxation and dislocation. Spine. 1995; 20(17):1928–1930

[4] Roche CJ, O'Malley M, Dorgan JC, Carty HM. A pictorial review of atlanto-axial rotatory fixation: key points for the radiologist. Clin Radiol. 2001; 56(12):947–958

[5] Guleryuz A, Bagdatoglu C, Duce MN, Talas DU, Celikbas H, Köksel T. Grisel's syndrome. J Clin Neurosci. 2002; 9(1):81–84

[6] Bland JH. Rheumatoid subluxation of the cervical spine. J Rheumatol. 1990; 17(2):134–137

[7] Venkatesan M, Bhatt R, Newey ML. Traumatic atlantoaxial rotatory subluxation (TAARS) in adults: a report of two cases and literature review. Injury. 2012; 43(7):1212–1215

[8] Pang D. Atlantoaxial rotatory fixation. Neurosurgery. 2010; 66(3) Suppl: 161–183

[9] White AA, III, Panjabi MM. The basic kinematics of the human spine. A review of past and current knowledge. Spine. 1978; 3(1):12–20

[10] Crook TB, Eynon CA. Traumatic atlantoaxial rotatory subluxation. Emerg Med J. 2005; 22(9):671–672

[11] García-Pallero MA, Torres CV, Delgado-Fernández J, Sola RG. Traumatic atlantoaxial rotatory fixation in an adult patient. Eur Spine J. 2017. DOI: 10.1007/s 00586-016-4916-3

[12] Peyriere H, Graillon T, Pesenti S, Tropiano P, Blondel B, Fuentes S. Surgical management of post-traumatic atlantoaxial rotatory fixation due to C2 facet fracture: 5 clinical cases. Orthop Traumatol Surg Res. 2017; 103(1):67–70

10 Subaxial Cervical Trauma in the Adult Patient

Fadi B. Sweiss, Michaela Lee, and Michael K. Rosner

Abstract

This chapter on subaxial cervical trauma in the adult patients will address the principles of understanding such injuries as well as focus on the efficient diagnosis and management. Subaxial cervical trauma is common and is defined as an injury that occurs from C3 to C7. Failure of identifying subaxial cervical trauma on initial evaluation may result in delayed treatment and devastating spinal cord injury. Such injuries are commonly seen in practice and it is important to understand the epidemiology, clinical and diagnostic features, and treatment options required to provide optimal care.

Keywords: subaxial cervical spine trauma, epidemiology, classification, diagnosis, treatment

10.1 Epidemiology

Subaxial cervical spine trauma accounts for 2 to 3% of injuries sustained by blunt trauma,[1,2] and is found in 21% of patients with traumatic spinal injury.[3] In North America, approximately 150,000 people per year suffer from cervical spine injuries. Of those, around 11,000 also suffer from spinal cord injuries.[2] Approximately 75% of all blunt cervical spine injuries occur in the subaxial cervical spine[4] with 50% of the injuries located between the levels C5 and C7.[5] Several studies have found a bimodal distribution of injuries with an increased risk of injury in young males (ages 15 to 45 years) as well as in older males and/or females (ages 65 to 85 years). Elderly females are four times more likely to suffer spinal trauma in comparison to their male counterparts.[3] Motor vehicle accidents account for a large percentage of cervical spine injuries and tend to occur in younger individuals whereas older individuals tend to have injuries that result largely from ground-level falls.[3]

10.2 Initial Management

The importance of recognizing potential subaxial cervical spine trauma cannot be overlooked. A standardized clinical and radiographic evaluation is paramount to prevent worsening of such injuries and the devastating sequelae that can result due to misdiagnosis. Following stabilization, as guided by the Advanced Trauma Life Support algorithm, patients with concern for cervical spine injury should be placed in a rigid cervical collar. Collars should be sized and fitted appropriately to ensure immobilization. All patients should be log rolled with cervical spine precautions during the secondary survey to prevent further injury. Outward signs of trauma to the head, neck, and upper torso can hint to the mechanism of injury during the traumatic event.

In addition, inspection of cervical posture for malalignment, including angular or rotational, can hint to dislocation or subluxation.[5] After completion of the primary and secondary survey, a detailed history can be of aid to determine risk factors as well as energy patterns for those who sustain subaxial cervical spine trauma. History of ankylosing spondylitis, diffuse idiopathic skeletal hyperostosis (DISH), or connective tissue disorders that are associated with ligamentous hyperlaxity should be identified as it increases the risk of subaxial cervical spine trauma.[5] A thorough physical exam should be performed on all patients with suspected subaxial cervical spine injuries including palpation of the entire spine with focus on tenderness and evaluation for any "step-offs" that could be present. Assessment and evaluation of each muscle group and sensory distributions can help identify levels of potential injury. Continuing to perform subsequent and frequent neurological exams is necessary, especially when spinal cord injury is evident because it allows for determination of injury progression versus symptom improvement.

10.2.1 Diagnostic Imaging

Subaxial cervical spine injuries are often misdiagnosed. Thus, understanding the various types of imaging modalities that can be utilized to diagnose such injuries is important. This can significantly reduce the number of unnecessary diagnostic images obtained that demonstrate negative findings. Obtaining the correct diagnostic imaging will expedite diagnosis and proper care of the injured patient.

Multiplanar computed tomography (CT) scans of the cervical spine have become the imaging modality of choice in the initial work-up of trauma patients. They have a sensitivity and specificity of 99 and 100%, respectively. In comparison, plain radiographs of the cervical spine have a sensitivity ranging from 43 to 70%.[6,7] CT scans are rapidly accessible and provide sufficient information in a timely fashion, which is necessary for accurately diagnosing severe injuries that require emergent intervention. Although ligamentous injuries cannot be fully assessed by CT scans, recent studies have suggested a CT scan with sagittal and coronal reconstruction is sufficient for diagnosis and further imaging is not warranted.[5]

The role of magnetic resonance imaging (MRI) has been controversial because despite its high sensitivity, it has a low specificity, which can lead to false positive results.[5] Nonetheless, MRI provides detailed information regarding the discoligamentous complex (DLC) as well as subaxial instablility.[5] The role of MRI was found to be important in older patients more than 60 years of age, and in patients that are obtunded, have cervical spondylosis, polytrauma, and patients with neurological deficits. These were noted to be predisposing factors for further injuries that were missed on CT scan but identified on MRI.[8] Kaiser et al described that with the resolution of CT scans increasing, the rate of missed clinically significant injuries remains at 6%.[9] It is impossible to predict patients who have occult injuries when CT scan of cervical spine is negative, even when a minor mechanism of injury may be responsible. The authors concluded that all blunt trauma patients with altered mental status should continue to undergo MRI for adequate cervical spine clearance even with a negative CT scan.[9] In contrast, Khanna et al concluded that the use of MRI for cervical spine clearance adds little information with the presence of a negative CT scan and a normal neurological examination.[10]

The authors did state that MRI may have a role on a delayed basis in patients with persistent neck pain.[10]

10.2.2 Cervical Traction

Prompt reduction with cervical traction is of utmost importance for patients with cervical dislocation. Early reduction results in decompression of the spinal canal in patients with neurological impairments and helps to obtain alignment prior to surgery.[11] Traction is not warranted for the management of extension-distraction injuries as this may lead to worsening deformity and risk for neurological compromise.[12] With traction, realignment of up to 70% of cervical dislocations can be achieved.[13] A retrospective review of 53 patients with cervical facet dislocations showed that closed reduction was achieved in 90% of patients by using a combination of traction, positioning, and occasional manipulation. Of this group, 68% had significant neurological improvement.[14]

Cervical traction can be safely done after admission to the intensive care unit to limit transport once completed. Patients should be given adequate pain control and light sedation to tolerate the procedure while maintaining responsiveness to participate in neurological exams during manipulation. Gardner–Wells tongs may be applied, and traction can be performed in the flexion, extension, or neutral positions depending on placement in relationship to the pinna.[11] Approximately 5 pounds of weight should be added per level of injury. Any manipulation requires subsequent close clinical and radiological observation to avoid overdistraction and further neurological injuries. In the setting of unilateral locked facets, the surgeon can reduce the injury by flexing and rotating the cervical spine. The manipulation can only be done in patients with a reliable neurological exam.[15] Once reduced, cervical extension and lighter traction should be maintained to prevent loss of reduction.

The surgeon should avoid traction in patients who are obtunded, inebriated, sedated/intubated, or unable to comply with a neurological exam.[15] In these situations, intraoperative or open reduction may be necessary. Contraindications include rostral injuries, such as atlantoaxial or occipital cervical dislocations.[16] MRI prior to closed reduction can be used to identify traumatic cervical disc herniation, but ultimately delays spinal decompression. Early reductions have the potential to improve neurological function and should always be attempted in a timely fashion.[15]

10.3 Classification

A myriad of classification systems has been used to aid in the decision-making process for subaxial cervical trauma. Earlier classification systems relied on plain radiographic imaging as well as mechanisms of injury. These early classification systems did not, however, factor in the patient or the patient's neurological status.

10.3.1 Classification Systems

One of the first universally accepted classification systems for indirect, lower cervical spine fractures and dislocations was described by Allen et al in 1982.[17] The Allen–Ferguson system focused on the mechanism of injury which could be extrapolated from plain radiographic images. The system was generated from a retrospective analysis of 165 patients with closed, indirect fractures and dislocations of the lower cervical spine. Injuries were classified into six categories which included flexion-compression, vertical compression, flexion-distraction, extension-compression, extension-distraction, and lateral flexion. Each of these categories were further divided into subcategories, which correlated to the severity of injury. This classification system was modified by Harris et al in 1986 and focused on rotational rather than distractive forces.[18] The categories in the Harris system included flexion, flexion-rotation, hyperextension-rotation, vertical compression, extension, and lateral flexion.

The AO Classification System

In 1994, Magerl et al described a classification system for thoracolumbar spine injuries, which was commonly applied to cervical spine injuries and primarily relied on pathomorphological criteria and plain radiographic imaging.[19] Classification criteria included the main mechanism of injury and pathomorphological uniformity as well as consideration of prognostic aspects regarding healing potential. The AO system classified injuries as type A (axial force resulting in vertebral body compression), type B (anterior and posterior element injuries with distraction), and type C (anterior and posterior element injuries with rotation; ▶ Table 10.1).[19] The AO subaxial cervical spine injury classification system did provide adequate reliability and was thought to be a valuable tool for communication, patient care, and research purposes.[20]

Table 10.1 The AO Classification System[19]

Type	A Compression			B Distraction			C Rotational		
Group	A1 Impaction fractures	A2 Split fractures	A3 Burst fractures	B1 Posterior ligamentous	B2 Posterior osseous	B3 Anterior disc disruption	C1 Type A with rotation	C2 Type B with rotation	C3 Rotational burst
Subgroup	A1.1 End plate impaction	A2.1 Sagittal split	A3.1 Incomplete burst	B1.1 With disc rupture	B2.1 Transverse bicolumn	B3.1 Hyperextension subluxation	C1.1 Rotational wedge fracture	C2.1 B1 lesion w/ rotation	C3.1 Slice fracture
	A1.2 Wedge impaction	A2.2 Coronal split	A3.2 Burst split	B1.2 With type A fracture	B2.2 With disc rupture	B3.2 Hyperextension spondylosis	C1.2 Rotational split fracture	C2.2 B1 lesion w/ rotation	C3.2 Oblique fracture
	A1.3 Vertebral body collapse	A2.3 Pincer fracture	A3.3 Complete burst		B2.3 With type A fracture	B3.3 Posterior dislocation	C1.3 Rotational burst fracture	C2.3 B3 lesion w/ rotation	

Source: Magerl et al.[19]

Subaxial Injury Classification System

The Subaxial Injury Classification (SLIC) System and injury severity score was developed based on weaknesses of previous classification systems.[21] As discussed, previous systems were developed based solely on the force vectors extrapolated from the injury patterns seen on plain radiographic films. Vaccaro et al describes the importance of incorporating both neurological status and emphasis on the stability of different injuries.[21] It allows the physician to account for three major characteristics to assist in decision-making, which include injury morphology, integrity of the DLC, and the neurological status of the patient.[22] These three factors are evaluated independently and the summation provides a final score which can assist in management. SLIC is one of the most widely used systems today and is summarized in ▶ Table 10.2.[21]

Many believe that the SLIC system can be integrated with daily practice and can be easily applied while remaining comprehensive. Studies have also shown that it is reproducible among surgeons.[23] A retrospective analysis of patients previously treated for subaxial cervical spine trauma determined that when the SLIC system was applied, 90% of those patients matched the conservative or surgical approaches that were proposed.[24] However, larger and higher quality evidence that can validate the SLIC system are lacking.

Table 10.2 The SLIC system[21]

	Points
Injury morphology	
• No abnormality	0
• Compression	1
• Burst	+ 1
• Distraction	2
• Translation	3
Integrity of the DLC	
• Intact	0
• Indeterminate	1
• Disrupted	2
Neurologic status	
• Intact	0
• Nerve root injury	1
• Complete	2
• Incomplete	3
• Persistent cord compression	+ 1

Score	Treatment
≥ 5	Operative
4	Operative vs. nonoperative
≤ 3	Nonoperative

Abbreviation: DLC, discoligamentous complex.
Source: Vaccaro et al.[21]

10.4 Nonsurgical Management

In the setting of subaxial cervical spine injuries, nonsurgical management with external immobilization can be considered for injuries that are deemed stable. There is no consensus regarding the types of injuries stable enough for nonoperative treatment. However, the stability of the injury pattern, neurological status of the patient, and the patient's comorbidities are all factors that should be considered.[5] If using the SLIC system, a score of 3 or less can be considered stable and treated with cervical orthoses. Such management can also be done in patients with a SLIC score of 4. However, the decision for nonoperative versus operative treatment may be based on the surgeon's experience and patient's comorbidities.[5]

Nonoperative treatment should be restricted to only bony injuries and should not be considered for patients with DLC injuries.[25] Although cervical orthosis is not required in the stable injury, it does emphasize the importance of activity restrictions and provides comfort.[5,15] Cervical orthosis can provide adequate stability in fractures without ligamentous injuries. This varies when it comes to fractures of the cervical facet that are less predictable in terms of instability. In a retrospective series of 68 patients with cervical facet fracture-dislocation injuries, external immobilization could provide stability in injuries with < 1 mm of displacement.[26] Typically, external immobilization for stable fractures is required for at least 6 to 12 weeks with close interval follow-up. Prior to cervical spine clearance, the physician should obtain dynamic plain cervical spine radiographs to rule out evidence of instability. If no abnormalities are present, immobilization can be discontinued.

In patients with ligamentous injuries, the physician should be extremely cautious when foregoing surgical management for external immobilization. A review of 64 patients with subaxial cervical spine injuries strongly correlated the presence of ligamentous injury with or without severe vertebral body injury to failure of nonoperative management. When these injuries were not present, the authors were able to conclude that successful treatment with bracing was achieved.[27] Even after immobilization, pain can persist and instability can continue. Further imaging should be done at that time to determine the burden of injury and evaluate for possible surgical treatment (▶ Fig. 10.1).

10.5 Surgical Management

10.5.1 Timing of Surgery

Unstable injuries and fractures that have failed conservative management, or patients with the potential for neurological compromise should be treated surgically. The benefits of early decompression have been well described in the literature. The Surgical Timing in Acute Spinal Cord Injury Study (STASCIS) concluded that decompression prior to 24 hours after cervical spinal cord injury can be performed safely and was associated with improved neurological outcome.[28] Nearly 20% of patients had improvement of ≥ 2 in the ASIA impairment score in comparison to surgery occurring after 24 hours (late surgery group,

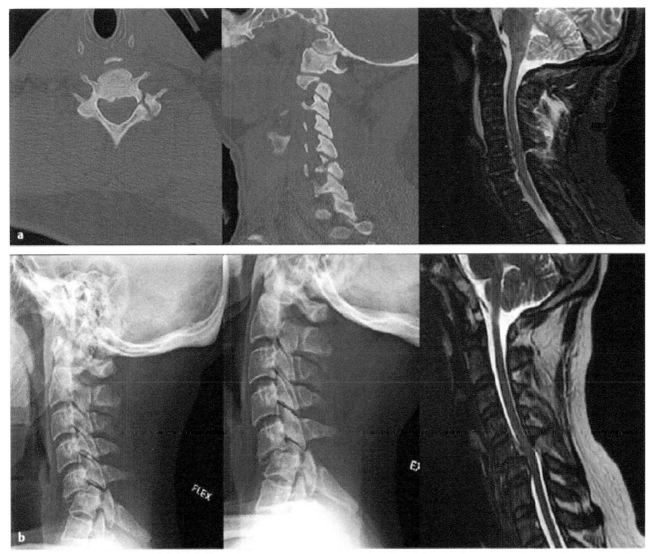

Fig. 10.1 (a) Axial computed tomography (CT) scan of the cervical spine showing a left C6 facet fracture extending into the pedicle. Sagittal view also shows extent of fracture without dislocation/distraction or sagittal imbalance. Magnetic resonance imaging (MRI) of the cervical spine stir sequence shows significant posterior ligamentous injury extending from C2 to C7. Decision was made to manage patient nonoperatively with cervical orthosis. (b) Anteroposterior and lateral plain radiographs of the cervical spine completed at 6 weeks follow-up for clearance of cervical orthosis. Images were significant for a left C5–C6 unilateral jumped facet with anterolisthesis of C5 on C6. MRI of the C spine with stenosis and posterior displacement of the spinal cord at the level of injury. (*continued*)

9%), with no differences regarding adverse outcomes.[28] Therefore, surgical decompression and stabilization should be completed once the patient is hemodynamically stable and is deemed safe for surgery.

10.5.2 Approach to Surgery

Surgical management of subaxial cervical spine trauma depends on instability and the presence of neurological deficits. Instrumentation and fusion, in comparison to external immobilization, provides immediate stability while maintaining alignment and promoting bony fusion.[25] It is critical for the surgeon to determine the best surgical approach to address cervical decompression, alignment, and stabilization. Therefore, it is important for the surgeon to evaluate preoperative images to understand the extent of injury sustained from subaxial cervical spine trauma. Surgery can be performed through an anterior, posterior, or combined approach. Factors including cause of compression, primary site of compression, number of levels involved, alignment of the cervical spine, and medical comorbidities can guide the surgical approach best suited for the patient.[29] In 2007, the Spine Trauma Study Group developed an evidence-based algorithm to help determine the best surgical approach for subaxial cervical spine trauma.[30] The algorithm was developed using the SLIC system and addressed the indication for surgery. However, emphasis should be placed on treatment individualized to the patient according to the characteristics of the injury as well as the surgeon's preference and experience.[15]

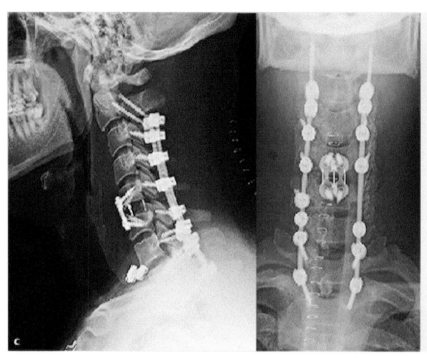

Fig 10.1 (*continued*) (**c**) Intraoperative reduction using manipulation after failed reduction. Patient at high risk for kyphosis based on preoperative imaging prompting reinforcement of C5–C6 stand-alone interbody fixation with plate. This was followed by a C2–T2 posterior instrumentation and fusion.

Anterior versus Posterior Approaches

Traumatic subaxial cervical spine trauma can be treated with anterior or posterior approaches depending on the pattern of injury. Advantages to the anterior approach include safe and straightforward positioning, minor surgical trauma, and direct anterior decompression of the neural elements (removal of ventral compressive structures such as disc and bone).[11] Anterior approaches include anterior cervical discectomy, or corpectomy, and fusion that remains the procedure of choice for compression/burst fractures with ventral compression and without significant disruption of posterior elements (▶ Fig. 10.2). Anterior approaches are associated with fewer complications and a higher fusion rate in comparison to posterior approaches. However, there is a higher rate of postoperative swallowing difficulties and hoarseness secondary to edema from manipulation or traction of soft tissues and the esophagus. There is potential risk of injury to the recurrent laryngeal nerve as well. In 2017, a multicenter retrospective study found that the risk for symptomatic recurrent laryngeal nerve palsy following cervical spine surgery ranged from 0.6 to 2.9%.[31] Although rare, the authors found that 16% of patients may experience partial resolution with residual effects while 74% of cases resolved completely.[31]

In contrast, posterior approaches are based on posterior decompression and rigid fixation techniques and should be reserved for unstable injuries without significant ventral compression. These include lateral mass or pedicle fixation with or without laminectomies. Posterior approaches are good alternatives for distraction and rotational/transitional injuries as reduction forces can be used to improve overall alignment intraoperatively.[15] Postoperative pain is significantly greater with posterior approaches given the extensive tissue disruption needed for proper exposure. Nonetheless, no significant differences in neurological recovery or patient-reported outcome measures are noted when anterior and posterior approaches are compared.[32,33] Therefore, both anterior and posterior

approaches are options for decompression and fusion. It is the pathology associated with the injury that will help guide the surgeon to utilizing the most appropriate approach.

In a randomized cohort, 52 patients were evaluated to compare anterior versus posterior stabilization and fusion. There was no significant difference in neurological recovery or fusion rates depending on the approach that was undertaken.[32] This was also confirmed by Kwon et al in 42 patients with unilateral facet injuries. The authors concluded that there was a lower rate of wound complications and less postoperative pain with anterior approaches. However, they did report a higher rate of fusion with anterior approaches.[33] In a retrospective review of 99 patients with subaxial cervical spine injuries treated with instrumented anterior or posterior stabilization, no significant difference was noted in complication rates between the two groups.[34] Toh et al evaluated 31 patients with burst or flexion distraction injuries in the subaxial cervical spine treated with anterior, posterior, or combined approaches. The authors found that anterior decompression and fusion restored spinal canal diameter and improved neurological function in 9 of 24 patients. There was no significant improvement in patients who were treated posteriorly alone.[35] Duggal et al conducted a study using cadavers to re-create unilateral facet dislocation. This was followed by sequential instrumentation with screws and plates to evaluate biomechanical differences between anterior and posterior approaches. The authors found that lateral mass plating was more effective in limiting motion than anterior plating.[36]

Combined Approach

The role of combined approaches in subaxial cervical spine trauma has been increasing. The approach provides the strongest fixation and significantly limits motion.[37] Combined anterior and posterior approaches should be considered when there are components of significant discoligamentous injuries in the

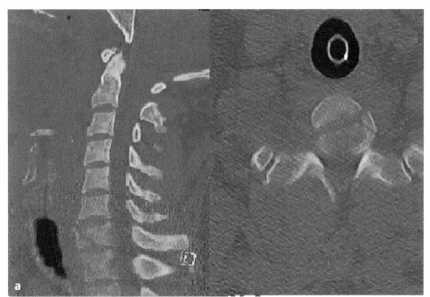

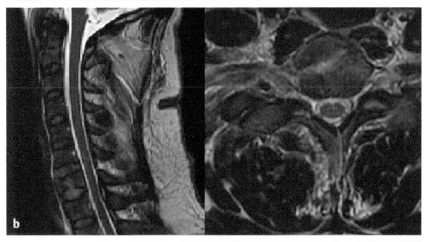

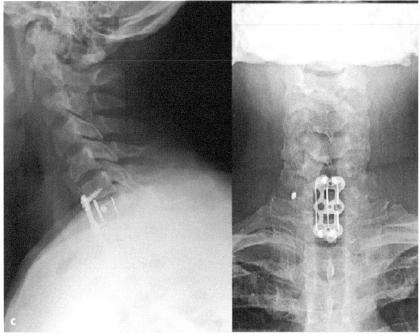

Fig. 10.2 (**a**) Computed tomography (CT) scan of the cervical spine, sagittal and axial images, significant for C7 burst fracture with slight retropulsion into the cervical canal. (**b**) Magnetic resonance imaging (MRI) of the C spine with congenital canal narrowing without significant retropulsion or cervical stenosis. (**c**) Anteroposterior and lateral plain radiographs of the cervical spine following C7 corpectomy and C6–T1 anterior fusion with plate.

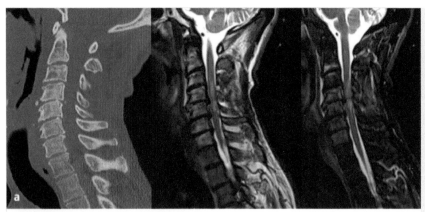

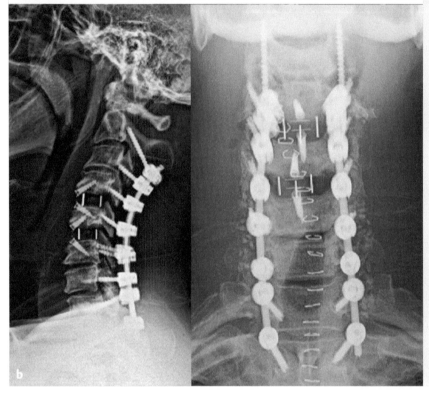

Fig. 10.3 (a) Computed tomography (CT) scan of the cervical spine showing multilevel degenerative disease with an acute displaced avulsion fracture of C4 anterior osteophyte with associated paravertebral swelling. Magnetic resonance imaging (MRI) of the C spine was significant for disruption of the anterior longitudinal ligament and cervical stenosis with cord signal abnormalities extending from C3 to C6. Also significant for posterior ligamentous injuries extending from C2 to T3. (b) Anteroposterior and lateral plain films of the cervical spine following C4–C5, C5–C6 anterior cervical discectomy and fusion; C3–C7 laminectomies; and C2–T2 posterior instrumentation and fusion.

setting of extensive posterior ligamentous injury (▶ Fig. 10.3). The combined approach allows for adequate discectomy, reduction, anterior column reconstruction with grafting, reconstitution of the posterior tension band with stabilization and fusion, and restoration of sagittal alignment.[15] Poor bone quality, such as in those with severe osteoporosis, DISH, ankylosing spondylitis, or other chronic conditions, increase the likelihood of an unstable injury pattern and a high rate of neurological injury with or without progressive decline[15] (▶ Fig. 10.4). The anterior stage should include all levels in which ventral injury is apparent and can be done with anterior cervical discectomy and fusion (ACDF) or corpectomy. The posterior stage should extend to all levels where posterior ligamentous injury is apparent. Laminectomies should also be completed for further decompression. For compression/burst fracture with posterior ligamentous injury, the anterior approach can be completed followed by posterior decompression and fusion ("front/back"). When unable to reduce facet dislocation with traction or manipulation, reduction should initially be done posteriorly ("back/

front/back"). Based on surgeon experience and patient's medical stability, the combined approached can be carried out in multiple ways in the same or multiple settings.

10.6 Postoperative Management

After surgical correction for subaxial cervical spine injuries, close observation should continue in the perioperative period. Patients should remain on prophylactic antibiotics for 24 hours. Frequent neurological exams should be completed, and the surgeon should be notified immediately of any subtle neurological changes or sudden increase in drain output. After anterior approaches, paravertebral swelling can lead to difficulty in swallowing and patients should be evaluated for aspiration risk. Lateral plain films of the cervical spine can help evaluate worsening or improvement of paravertebral swelling which can be done daily until resolved. Moreover, rapidly expanding hematomas can immediately progress to airway compromise. Emergent airway protection and hematoma evacuation at the

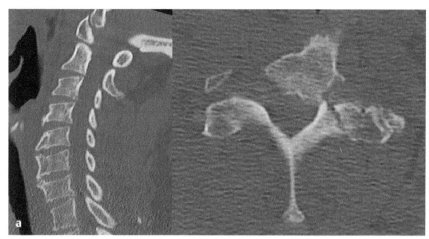

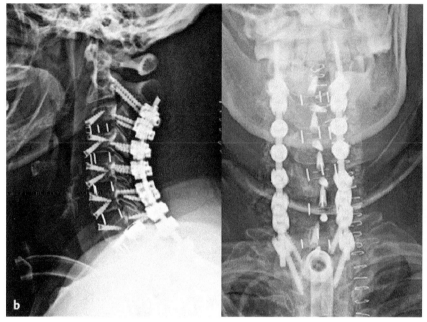

Fig. 10.4 (a) Computed tomography (CT) scan of the C spine, sagittal and axial images, significant for left C7 facet fracture with acute fractures of anterior osteophytes widening of the disc spaces at C3–C4, C4–C5, C5–C6, C6–C7, and C7–T1 in the setting of diffuse idiopathic skeletal hyperostosis. Concern for extension/distraction injury with severe subaxial cervical spine instability. Patient taken emergently to the operating room. (b) anteroposterior and lateral plain radiographs of the cervical spine following C3–C4, C4–C5, C5–C6, C6–C7, C7–T1 anterior cervical discectomy and fusion; C3–C7 laminectomies; and C2–T2 posterior instrumentation and fusion.

bedside or in the operating room should be done without delay. Following posterior approaches, pain should be adequately controlled, and patients should be observed for C5 palsy. Any subtle or progressive neurological changes may prompt evaluation with CT scan of the cervical spine to rule out an epidural hematoma with compression of the spinal cord. If present, the patient should be taken emergently for evacuation to preserve neurological function.

With an uneventful postoperative course, anteroposterior and lateral plain films should be obtained as a baseline for future comparisons and to evaluate for proper placement of instrumentation. Subcutaneous heparin or low-molecular-weight heparin, sequential compression devices, and early ambulation should be initiated to help in the prevention of deep vein thrombosis (DVT). The need for cervical orthosis after surgery should be determined by the surgeon. Although now stabilized, cervical collars can emphasize the importance of activity restrictions to the patient and care providers while providing comfort. In the setting of limited mobility, patients should be turned frequently to prevent decubitus ulcers. It is important to practice proper positioning and turning techniques to prevent stress on the patients construct and subsequent failure. Ultimately, the patient should be transitioned to a rehabilitation unit where intense physical and occupational therapy can begin.

References

[1] Hoffman JR, Mower WR, Wolfson AB, Todd KH, Zucker MI, National Emergency X-Radiography Utilization Study Group. Validity of a set of clinical criteria to rule out injury to the cervical spine in patients with blunt trauma. N Engl J Med. 2000; 343(2):94–99

[2] Lowery DW, Wald MM, Browne BJ, Tigges S, Hoffman JR, Mower WR, NEXUS Group. Epidemiology of cervical spine injury victims. Ann Emerg Med. 2001; 38(1):12–16

[3] Tee JW, Chan CH, Fitzgerald MC, Liew SM, Rosenfeld JV. Epidemiological trends of spine trauma: an Australian level 1 trauma centre study. Global Spine J. 2013; 3(2):75–84

[4] Goldberg W, Mueller C, Panacek E, Tigges S, Hoffman JR, Mower WR, NEXUS Group. Distribution and patterns of blunt traumatic cervical spine injury. Ann Emerg Med. 2001; 38(1):17–21

[5] Feuchtbaum E, Buchowski J, Zebala L. Subaxial cervical spine trauma. Curr Rev Musculoskelet Med. 2016; 9(4):496–504

[6] Antevil JL, Sise MJ, Sack DI, Kidder B, Hopper A, Brown CV. Spiral computed tomography for the initial evaluation of spine trauma: a new standard of care? J Trauma. 2006; 61(2):382–387

[7] Nuñez DB, Jr, Ahmad AA, Coin CG, et al. Clearing the cervical spine in multiple trauma victims: a time-effective protocol using helical computed tomography. Emerg Radiol. 1994; 1(6):273–278

[8] Pourtaheri S, Emami A, Sinha K, et al. The role of magnetic resonance imaging in acute cervical spine fractures. Spine J. 2014; 14(11):2546–2553

[9] Kaiser ML, Whealon MD, Barrios C, Kong AP, Lekawa ME, Dolich MO. The current role of magnetic resonance imaging for diagnosing cervical spine injury in blunt trauma patients with negative computed tomography scan. Am Surg. 2012; 78(10):1156–1160

[10] Khanna P, Chau C, Dublin A, Kim K, Wisner D. The value of cervical magnetic resonance imaging in the evaluation of the obtunded or comatose patient with cervical trauma, no other abnormal neurological findings, and a normal cervical computed tomography. J Trauma Acute Care Surg. 2012; 72(3): 699–702

[11] Aebi M. Surgical treatment of upper, middle and lower cervical injuries and non-unions by anterior procedures. Eur Spine J. 2010; 19(1) Suppl 1:S33–S39

[12] Ludwig SC, Karp JE. Flexion and cervical distraction injuries characterized by the SLIC system. In: Vaccaro AR, Fehlings MG, Dvorak MF, eds. Spine and Spinal Cord Trauma. New York, NY: Thieme; 2011. 284–294

[13] Hadley MN. Guidelines for management of acute cervical injuries. Neurosurgery. 2002; 50(3) Suppl:S1

[14] Star AM, Jones AA, Cotler JM, Balderston RA, Sinha R. Immediate closed reduction of cervical spine dislocations using traction. Spine. 1990; 15(10):1068–1072

[15] Joaquim AF, Patel AA. Subaxial cervical spine trauma: evaluation and surgical decision-making. Global Spine J. 2014; 4(1):63–70

[16] Farmer J, Vaccaro A, Albert TJ, Malone S, Balderston RA, Cotler JM. Neurologic deterioration after cervical spinal cord injury. J Spinal Disord. 1998; 11(3):192–196

[17] Allen BL, Jr, Ferguson RL, Lehmann TR, O'Brien RP. A mechanistic classification of closed, indirect fractures and dislocations of the lower cervical spine. Spine. 1982; 7(1):1–27

[18] Harris JH, Jr, Edeiken-Monroe B, Kopaniky DR. A practical classification of acute cervical spine injuries. Orthop Clin North Am. 1986; 17(1):15–30

[19] Magerl F, Aebi M, Gertzbein SD, Harms J, Nazarian S. A comprehensive classification of thoracic and lumbar injuries. Eur Spine J. 1994; 3(4):184–201

[20] Vaccaro AR, Koerner JD, Radcliff KE, et al. AOSpine subaxial cervical spine injury classification system. Eur Spine J. 2016; 25(7):2173–2184

[21] Vaccaro AR, Hulbert RJ, Patel AA, et al. Spine Trauma Study Group. The subaxial cervical spine injury classification system: a novel approach to recognize the importance of morphology, neurology, and integrity of the disco-ligamentous complex. Spine. 2007; 32(21):2365–2374

[22] Zahir U, Ludwig SC, Daily AT, Vaccaro AR. The subaxial cervical spine injury classification scale (SLIC). In: Vaccaro AR, Fehlings MG, Dvorak MF. Spine and Spinal Cord Trauma. New York, NY: Thieme; 2011:265–274

[23] Joaquim AF, Lawrence B, Daubs M, Brodke D, Patel AA. Evaluation of the subaxial injury classification system. J Craniovertebr Junction Spine. 2011; 2(2):67–72

[24] Lee WJ, Yoon SH, Kim YJ, Kim JY, Park HC, Park CO. Interobserver and intraobserver reliability of sub-axial injury classification and severity scale between radiologist, resident and spine surgeon. J Korean Neurosurg Soc. 2012; 52(3):200–203

[25] Ludwig SC, Karp JE. Flexion and cervical distraction injuries characterized by the SLIC system. In: Vaccaro AR, Fehlings MG, Dvorak MF, eds. Spine and Spinal Cord Trauma. New York, NY: Thieme; 2011:284–294

[26] Hadley MN, Fitzpatrick BC, Sonntag VK, Browner CM. Facet fracture-dislocation injuries of the cervical spine. Neurosurgery. 1992; 30(5):661–666

[27] Lemons VR, Wagner FC, Jr. Stabilization of subaxial cervical spinal injuries. Surg Neurol. 1993; 39(6):511–518

[28] Fehlings MG, Vaccaro A, Wilson JR, et al. Early versus delayed decompression for traumatic cervical spinal cord injury: results of the Surgical Timing in Acute Spinal Cord Injury Study (STASCIS). PLoS One. 2012; 7(2):e32037

[29] Fehlings MG, Barry S, Kopjar B, et al. Anterior versus posterior surgical approaches to treat cervical spondylotic myelopathy: outcomes of the prospective multicenter AOSpine North America CSM study in 264 patients. Spine. 2013; 38(26):2247–2252

[30] Dvorak MF, Fisher CG, Fehlings MG, et al. The surgical approach to subaxial cervical spine injuries: an evidence-based algorithm based on the SLIC classification system. Spine. 2007; 32(23):2620–2629

[31] Gokaslan ZL, Bydon M, De la Garza-Ramos R, et al. Recurrent laryngeal nerve palsy after cervical spine surgery: a multicenter AOSpine clinical research network study. Global Spine J. 2017; 7(1) Suppl:53S–57S

[32] Brodke DS, Anderson PA, Newell DW, Grady MS, Chapman JR. Comparison of anterior and posterior approaches in cervical spinal cord injuries. J Spinal Disord Tech. 2003; 16(3):229–235

[33] Kwon BK, Fisher CG, Boyd MC, et al. A prospective randomized controlled trial of anterior compared with posterior stabilization for unilateral facet injuries of the cervical spine. J Neurosurg Spine. 2007; 7(1):1–12

[34] Lambiris E, Kasimatis GB, Tyllianakis M, Zouboulis P, Panagiotopoulos E. Treatment of unstable lower cervical spine injuries by anterior instrumented fusion alone. J Spinal Disord Tech. 2008; 21(7):500–507

[35] Toh E, Nomura T, Watanabe M, Mochida J. Surgical treatment for injuries of the middle and lower cervical spine. Int Orthop. 2006; 30(1):54–58

[36] Duggal N, Chamberlain RH, Park SC, Sonntag VK, Dickman CA, Crawford NR. Unilateral cervical facet dislocation: biomechanics of fixation. Spine. 2005; 30(7):E164–E168

[37] An HS. Cervical spine trauma. Spine. 1998; 23(24):2713–2729

11 Subaxial Cervical Spine Trauma in the Pediatric Patient

Catherine A. Mazzola and Nicole Silva

Abstract

Pediatric subaxial cervical injury (PSCI) is very different from its adult counterpart. The immature spine has unique biomechanics. The identification of cervical spine injury in children is important; however, too often unnecessary computed tomography (CT) imaging studies are obtained that expose children to dangerous radiation. Knowledge of the embryology and anatomical development of the cervical spine is crucial. Understanding the pediatric neurological examination, identifying risk factors for cervical spine injury, and knowing the appropriate imaging studies to order are imperative in caring for the pediatric trauma patient. Once PSCI is identified, making the appropriate recommendations for treatment is essential. Options for treatment vary depending on the type and severity of injury and the age of the child. Postoperative and postinjury rehabilitation for pediatric patients are important steps in restoring function and allowing for optimal recovery. The goal is always to maintain independence, spinal stability and range of motion, strengthen the spine, and if possible, to avoid future injury, long-term disability, or complications.

Keywords: cervical, child, children, injury, instability, pediatric, spinal, spine, subaxial, trauma

11.1 Introduction

Due to the incomplete maturation of the child's spine, pediatric subaxial cervical injury (PSCI) in children is somewhat different than its adult counterpart. The anatomical and developmental characteristics of the pediatric spine impact the clinical presentation, imaging characteristics, patterns of injury, and treatment.[1] In the pediatric population, subaxial spinal injuries are mostly due to motor vehicle accidents, pedestrian struck by motor vehicles, and sports-related injuries.[1,2] Although there have been major efforts to prevent these injuries, in the development of better car seat technology, safety belts, helmets, and education programs, injuries still occur. In the ambulatory field, immobilization and stabilization of the cervical spine are paramount after airway, breathing, and circulation issues have been addressed. Transportation to a trauma center and appropriate imaging, followed by a detailed neurological examination take precedence. Identification and treatment of subaxial treatment should follow best clinical practice guidelines.

11.2 Embryology, Anatomy, and Development

The upper cervical spine consists of the C1 atlas which is formed by three ossification centers and the C2 axis with five primary and two secondary ossification centers.[1,3] Development of the lower vertebral bodies begins with three primary ossification centers, with one in the body and two laterally in the neural arches at each vertebral level, and secondary ossifications centers at the superior and inferior epiphyseal ring.[3] The morphometric and growth characteristics of the pediatric cervical spine have been described. In the midsagittal plane, 50% of cervical spinal growth occurs before the age of 9 years with spinal height continuing to increase in males, tapering off at the age of 17.[4] In females, 66.8% of the height development occurs before 9 years of age. Girls stop growing in height at an average age of 14 years.[4] In children, the head-to-body ratio is larger than it is in adults creating instability with a higher center of gravity and fulcrum of the neck.[1] This fulcrum of movement shifts as the child matures, moving from C2 to C3 as an infant, to C4–C5 at the age of 5 or 6 years, and C5–C6 during adolescence and adulthood[5] (▶ Table 11.1 and ▶ Table 11.2).

11.3 Biomechanics and Morphometrics of the Pediatric Subaxial Spine

The subaxial cervical spine includes the vertebral levels of C3 to C7 (▶ Fig. 11.1). The immature cervical vertebra has a small body attached to the lamina with short, narrow pedicles and spinal processes that are underdeveloped and bifid. The transverse processes of the C3 to C6 vertebral levels are small and short with foramen transversarium. Although initially more wedge shaped than adult vertebrae, the more mature C3 and C4 levels resemble a typical cerebral vertebral body in size and structure, but the C7 can be considered a transitional vertebra. It resembles the thoracic vertebral body in size with a large posterior spinal process, but with a configuration more similar to a cervical vertebra. In addition, the transverse process of C7 is larger and occasionally will not have a foramen transversarium.[4,6]

Table 11.1 Average cervical spine midsagittal growth measurements

	Female average C2–C7 (mm)	Male average C2–C7 (mm)
Cervical spine midsagittal measurements		
0–12 mo	69.11	70.68
2–5 yr	82.00	82.62
6 yr–adulthood	106.50	109.91

Data adapted from Johnson et al.[4]

Table 11.2 Average cervical spine vertebral body height and depth measurements

	Male					Female				
Cervical spine vertebral body height measurements (mm)	C3	C4	C5	C6	C7	C3	C4	C5	C6	C7
0–12 mo	5.54	5.51	5.56	5.85	6.43	5.55	5.51	5.62	5.77	6.46
2–5 yr	6.65	6.65	6.74	6.83	7.7	6.65	6.63	6.63	6.76	7.69
6 yr–adulthood	9.82	9.56	9.40	9.52	11.0	9.73	9.39	9.41	9.49	10.57
Cervical spine vertebral body depth measurements (mm)	C3	C4	C5	C6	C7	C3	C4	C5	C6	C7
0–12 mo	9.91	9.83	9.96	10.5	10.96	8.86	8.92	8.89	9.46	9.83
2–5 yr	10.79	10.57	10.16	11.19	11.65	10.25	10.10	9.74	10.75	11.08
6 yr–adulthood	14.09	13.82	13.82	14.45	14.74	12.9	12.59	12.65	13.25	13.49

Data adapted from Johnson et al.[4]

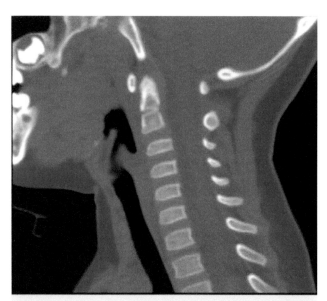

Fig. 11.1 Sagittal computed tomography (CT) of the subaxial cervical spine.

It is very important to consider the hypermobility and ligamentous laxity of the immature subaxial spine during development.[3] The articular processes will have a more axial position, with vertebral bodies that are wedged-shaped, contributing to increased movement of the spine.[5] This is especially noted in children under the age of 8 years.[5] The facet joints in the pediatric subaxial spine are more horizontally oriented allowing for easier subluxation.[6] The anterior longitudinal ligament (ALL) and posterior longitudinal ligament (PLL) are draped over the anterior and posterior vertebral body surfaces, respectively, from their attachment at C1 all the way to the sacrum.[5] Although the ALL and PLL provide stability to the subaxial spine, these ligaments are lax and underdeveloped in children increasing flexibility.[5] The uncovertebral joint does not develop completely until the age of 8 years.[5] Hypermobility and decreased resistance to injury are due to multiple factors that affect the immature pediatric spine.[5,6]

11.4 Epidemiology and Patterns of Injury

11.4.1 Demographics and Epidemiology

According to the Centers for Disease Control (CDC), motor vehicle accidents are the leading cause of death in children up to the age of 14 years.[7] Recent data analyses of all pediatric trauma admissions, from the Kids' Inpatient Database (KID), suggest that between 2000 and 2012, the prevalence of pediatric cervical spine injury (PCSI) was 2.07% and the mortality rate was 4.87%.[2] The most frequent cause of pediatric cervical spine trauma was motor vehicle accidents which accounts for about 57.51%.[2] Cervical spine injury in pediatric injuries are more common than thoracic and lumbar spinal injuries, accounting for about 60 to 80% of all spinal injuries.[8] The most common cause of pediatric spine injury, from most to least prevalent, are motor vehicle accidents including pedestrian struck by a motor vehicle, followed by falls, sports, diving accidents, firearms, and child abuse.[1,2,9] Motor-vehicle-related trauma is more common in younger children while older children are more likely to suffer from sports-related injuries.[10] While in infants, the upper part of the cervical spine is most commonly injured; in school-aged children, the lower level of the subaxial spine is more frequently injured because of caudal shift of the fulcrum of the movement of the spine in older childhood.[1,5,10] Finally, there are many connective tissue disorders such as Down syndrome, Marfan syndrome, and other disorders that predispose children to subaxial cervical spine injuries.[1]

11.4.2 Types and Patterns of Injury

Spinal Cord Injury/SCIWORA

Spinal cord injury (SCI) is more common in younger children due to increased ligamentous laxity.[3,5] Treatment of SCI in children is very similar to that of the adult SCI, with extent of recovery limited to degree of initial neurological impairment.[3] The diagnosis of SCI without radiological abnormality (SCIWORA) is less common with the advent of improved magnetic resonance imaging (MRI) techniques. When a child presents with a clinical deficit, there is usually an abnormality found on imaging. It is rare that a child presents with neurological findings without any evidence of spinal column or SCI.

Vascular Injury

Vascular injury should be suspected in PCSI, especially when neurological deficits or fracture through the foramen transversarium are present. The vertebral artery travels through the foramen transversarium of the cervical vertebrae.[6] Vascular injury in the cervical spine can cause brain stem or spinal cord infarct, hematoma, and/or hemorrhage.[5] Concomitant craniocervical arterial dissection (CCAD), is a life-threatening injury that may occur with any cervical trauma.[3] The gold standard diagnostic study for evaluation of vascular injury is the cervical angiogram. Magnetic resonance angiography (MRA) or computed tomography angiography (CTA) may be carried out to either rule out or intervene in evaluate vascular injury in PCSI. It is important to be cognizant of the very real risk of vascular injury in children with increased risk of cervical mobility, ligamentous laxity, and subluxation.[3] Vertebral artery dissection, disruption, and occlusion have been well described.

Ligamentous Injury and Subluxations (Without Fracture)

Children with immature spinal development are more prone to ligamentous injury.[10] Under the age of 12 years, normal physiological ranges of motion of the cervical vertebrae can be up to 4 mm from neutral in C2 to C4, and about 3 mm from neutral position in levels below C4 (when comparing neutral position to maximal flexion).[11] Subaxial pseudosubluxation, with minimal subluxation (typically C2–C3 or C3–C4), is common in children and is often noted on radiographic imaging between C2 to C4 as up to 4 mm of movement from neutral.[3] This should not be mistaken from a true subluxation for patients under the age of 8 years, which is a movement of greater than 4.5 mm between C2 and C3 or C3 and C4 or greater than 3.5 mm at any other lower level.[5] Another common way to measure ligamentous injury is measuring the degree of angulation between adjacent vertebra, which should be less than 7 degrees.[11] Children with X-ray evidence of true subluxation should be placed in a hard collar, and MRI should be obtained with and without intravenous contrast to assess integrity of cervical ligaments. If there is ligamentous injury or inflammation, stabilization (temporary in collar, or permanent, internal stabilization) may be needed.

Bilateral Facet Fractures/Dislocations

Facet dislocations are posterior column injuries and they represent the second most common injury pattern in PCSI.[11] Bilateral facet dislocation occurs when there is flexion-distraction or rotation-compression injury. Typically, plain radiographs are sufficient to rule out facet dislocation, but CT scan may be needed to rule out subtle fractures, and MRI may be necessary to evaluate ligamentous and/or SCI.[11] Children with bilateral facet fractures and dislocation are likely to present with neurological findings.

Unilateral Facet Fracture

Unilateral facet fractures are the most frequently missed cervical spine injury on plain X-rays and they vary with severity based on the stability of the patient's subaxial cervical spine.[11] CT imaging is better for the evaluation of unilateral facet fractures, but they may also be identified on MRI. They may occur with flexion, distraction when in rotation, and they lead to subluxation and monoradiculopathy that improves with traction. Most facet dislocations occur within the subaxial spine.

Single-Level Disc/Teardrop Injury

Cervical teardrop fractures are unique injuries that pose an unstable condition of possible neurological deficits due to posterior displacement of the fractured vertebra and impingement on the spinal cord.[12] This injury will cause widening of the interlaminar and interspinous spaces with kyphotic deformity seen on imaging.[12] It is a rare injury in children and usually results from traumatic flexion or extension.[13,14] Most of these injuries will require immobilization and stabilization.

Single-Level Burst Fracture

Burst fractures are anterior column injuries due to axial loading and compressive forces transmitted through the annulus fibrosus and onto the neighboring vertebral bodies.[11] These fractures typically occur with a forced forward flexion movement that impairs the posterior stabilization mechanism.[15] Single-level burst fractures may occur with or without neurological injury. Retropulsed bone fragments may need to be removed through an anterior approach, followed by anterior and possibly posterior stabilization.

Single-Level Compression Fracture

Compression fractures are very similar to burst fractures and can result in a significant instability of vertebral height loss and spinal cord stenosis.[15] Mild compression fractures typically occur without neurological sequelae, but severe compression fractures may be associated with neurological deficits. Rigid cervical orthosis may be utilized. Patients should be carefully followed to rule out progressive kyphosis and instability.

Single-Level Vertebral Fractures (Other Types)

Fractures are the most common type of injury in subaxial cervical spine and risk of fracture increases with age of the child.[2] Single-level vertebral fractures are most commonly the result of sports-related injuries in older children, and the patterns of fracture are similar to those seen in adult cervical fractures.[16]

Transverse process fractures

Although rare, transverse process fractures may cause painful radiculopathies. They are not unstable and do not require bracing. Transverse process fractures result from an extreme rotation or lateral bending movement.

Spinous process fractures

Also known as a "clay shoveler fracture," this type of fracture occurs when the end of the spinous process is broken off by a physical force or when paraspinal muscles pull so hard on the spinous process, that it breaks off part of the spinous process. Spinous process fractures may result from severe flexion or extension or a direct blow to the neck. Spinous process fractures may be indicative of ligamentous injury, so rigid orthoses should be utilized until MRI can be done. Immobilization and stabilization for a few weeks in a hard collar may be adequate treatment.

Multilevel Burst and Other Fractures

Complicated burst and other fractures are the result of high-energy trauma and must be treated with the extreme caution. These children typically present with neurological deficits. Cervical immobilization and stabilization are crucial in the treatment of these injuries. Spinal cord decompression and cervical spine fusion through an anterior, posterior, or combined approach may be indicated.

11.5 Prehospital Management

Management of the ABCs (airway, breathing, and circulation) followed by immobilization and stabilization of the spine are the most important considerations for children with spinal injuries. Immobilization of the cervical spine in a size-appropriate manner is essential. Over the age of 8 years, backboard and cervical collar immobilization should be used. However, it is recommended that a standard backboard should be modified for patients under the age of 8 years due to their large head-to-body ratios, which causes flexion of the cervical spine in the supine position.[11] The patient's torso may be elevated in order to maintain a neutral cervical alignment.[11] Children under the age of 8 years should be immobilized by building up the torso on a regular backboard.[11] Infants cannot be placed in a cervical collar and should be stabilized with sandbags or foam head blocks, which are secured at both sides of the head and taped to a modified backboard.[10,11]

11.6 Clinical Examination

Clinical examination of the pediatric trauma patient is challenging due to many reasons. It is extremely important to get a thorough history of the patient's injury. Mechanism of injury often indicates the severity of trauma expected. When the history does not correlate with the physical or radiological findings, the clinical history may be suspect or child abuse may be considered. A complete physical examination is important. Evidence of any obvious lacerations, abrasions, and/or ecchymoses are important to document. Battle sign, or ecchymosis around the mastoid bones, bruising around the neck, or cervical hematomas are ominous signs. Cervical collar and backboard immobilization should be utilized until a patient with a suspected injury is cleared by X-ray imaging. It is crucial to perform an age-appropriate, comprehensive neurological exam as deficits

correlate well with PCSI.[3] Presenting symptoms may be neck pain and rigidity, altered mental status, focal neural deficits, torticollis, numbness, radicular pain, or weakness.[1,10]

Although there are no comprehensive pediatric screening guidelines, there are several adult guidelines that are commonly used in both the United States and Canada by medical professionals. It is difficult to get a traumatized child to cooperate and complete a full neurological examination, especially when the child is upset, anxious, and afraid.[10] The National Emergency X-Radiography Utilization Study (NEXUS) identifies five criteria which stratify patients based on the likelihood of having sustained injury to the spinal cord including

1. No midline cervical tenderness.
2. No focal neural deficits.
3. Normal alertness.
4. No intoxication.
5. No painful distracting injury.[10,17]

Children who meet all five criteria are unlikely to have PSCI.[10,15]

In comparison, the Canadian "C-Spine Rule" recommends that clinicians ask following three questions:

1. Is there any high-risk factor present that mandates radiographic assessment (i.e., a dangerous mechanism of injury)?
2. Is there any low-risk factor present that allows for the safe assessment of range of motion (i.e., is the patient able to ambulate independently)?
3. Is the patient able to actively rotate his or her neck 45 degrees to the left and right?

A negative answer to the first question and/or affirmative answers to the last two questions rules out the possibility of cervical spine injury in adult patients with a high specificity.[10,18]

The National Institute for Health and Care Excellence (NICE) Guidelines have identified three high-risk inclusion criteria:

1. Age 65 years or older.
2. Dangerous mechanisms of injury (fall from a height of greater than 1 m or five steps, axial load to the head, rollover motor vehicle accident, ejection from a motor vehicle, accident involving motorized recreational vehicles, bicycle collisions, horse riding accidents).
3. Paresthesia in the upper or lower limbs.[19]

In pediatric trauma patients, evaluation of clinical and neurological status is difficult. Adult guidelines are not applied to pediatric patients with SCI and thus, we recommend using a combination of these guidelines with special attention to the maturing spine of the child.[20] For children under the age of 2 years, we recommend a high index of suspicion for occult PSCI.[20] In summary, PCSI should be considered if any of the following criteria are met[10]:

1. After a fall from 10 feet or greater (or body height if < 8 years).
2. Motor vehicle accident (MVA).
3. Glasgow Coma Scale (GCS) < 14.
4. Neurological deficit.
5. Significant head, face, or neck trauma.
6. Neck pain or torticollis.
7. Distraction injury or intoxication.[10]

PSCI algorithms are being continuously developed for attainment of the best possible outcomes in these cases.[20]

11.7 Diagnostic Imaging and Indications

There is significant controversy in the literature regarding the proper use of imaging in pediatric patients with subaxial injuries. Exposure to radiation is a concern in younger patients. Imaging of PSCIs should be conducted in unison with clinical and neurological findings.

11.7.1 X-ray Imaging of the Subaxial Cervical Spine in Children

Plain radiographs are often obtained shortly after initial assessment, if PSCI is suspected.[8,10] X-rays are useful for the rapid, early detection of severe injuries such as cervical spine fractures and subluxations (▶ Fig. 11.2 and ▶ Fig. 11.3). In an intact and cooperative child, negative clinical and neurological examinations combined with negative cervical spine imaging studies rule out cervical spine injuries.[21] X-ray imaging may help identify subtle injuries that mandate MRI in PSCI.[22] It is recommended that children who do not meet NEXUS criteria should receive anteroposterior and lateral cervical spine X-rays.[5,23] However, recent studies have questioned the utility of flexion, extension, and oblique views unless there is postinjury spinal tenderness persistent in a neurologically intact pediatric patient.[8,10]

11.7.2 Computed Tomography

CT imaging is associated with some radiation risk to the pediatric patient. The thyroid gland is especially sensitive to radiation exposure. Parents are increasingly aware of radiation risks and are interested in avoiding excessive radiation exposure when

possible in the context of PSCI.[5,10] CT imaging is associated with radiation doses that are 90 to 200 times more than that associated with a plain radiograph.[21] Most clinically significant findings on a CT would also be seen in X-rays, making diagnostic CT imaging generally unnecessary in the pediatric population.[10] A recent study showed that CT of the cervical spine after plain cervical spine radiographs only minimally improved diagnostic accuracy.[21] As children under 8 years of age are more prone to ligamentous injury, CT imaging is usually followed by MRI anyway.[5,10,24] However, an alternative to CT imaging of the cervical spine includes a limited or focused CT which exposes patients to far less radiation exposure. Limited CT scans can better define fracture and/or pathologies detected on X-ray imaging and may also help in operative planning.[10] The authors strongly recommend avoiding unnecessary imaging and needless radiation exposure.[22] We have found that clinical examinations and cervical spine X-rays in conjunction with MRI are usually sufficient to rule out PSCI.

11.7.3 Magnetic Resonance Imaging

The authors recommend MRI for pediatric patients with neurological deficits for the evaluation of soft-tissue injuries (including the intervertebral discs, ligaments, and spinal cord).[8] MRI is imperative for the diagnosis of subaxial ligamentous injury and other soft-tissue injuries such as spinal cord contusions, herniated discs, and/or nerve root compression.[5,10] MRI has a high specificity and sensitivity for detecting subaxial injuries in pediatric patients.[10,24] For intubated and obtunded children, MRI is the best option in the first 24 to 48 hours in order to rule out severe SCI.[10] If a patient remains unconscious or is not cooperative then intubation for airway protection, with or without sedation, may be necessary in order to obtain imaging.

11.7.4 Imaging of Vascular Injury

Most vascular injuries can be visualized using MRI and/or MRA. MRI can detect epidural or subdural hematomas,

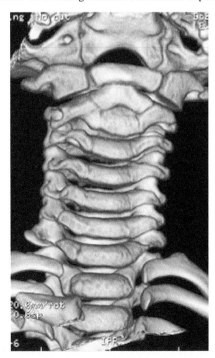

Fig. 11.2 Three-dimensional image of anterior view of the subaxial cervical spine.

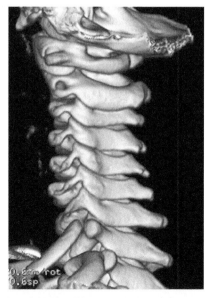

Fig. 11.3 Three-dimensional image of the lateral view of the subaxial cervical spine.

as well as spinal cord contusions, edema or intraparenchymal hemorrhage.[5,10] Arterial dissections are rare, life-threatening entities, which can be identified via MRA.[3] Dissections may be treated medically or surgically through either open or endovascular procedures, depending on pertinent clinical and radiological findings.

11.8 Management of Pediatric Subaxial Cervical Trauma

11.8.1 Nonoperative Management

No Stabilization/Soft Collars

If a child is neurologically intact and imaging studies are negative, and there is no pain, then treatment is not indicated and cervical immobilization can be removed. However, often the pediatric trauma patient presents with complaints of severe pain, without serious mechanism of injury and negative cervical spine X-rays. After MRI shows no injury, hard collar immobilization can be safely exchanged for a soft collar, although at times allowing a child to wear the cervical collar may decrease painful spasms, limit cervical movement. It may be removed when pain resolves.[5] Limiting range of motion may help reduce pain in a cervical sprain. Ligamentous sprain or subtle stretch injury heals well in pediatric patients with cervical immobilization.[23] There is some evidence that nonoperative management of these injuries may benefit from corticosteroids to reduce inflammation, yet use remains controversial and is not generally recommended in spinal injuries. Steroids may be associated with increased complications after PSCI and poor outcomes.[1,10] Utilization of antispasmodic agents or nonsteroidals may help with muscle spasm and pain.

Stabilization

Hard collars

Cervical sprains, certain ligamentous injuries, nondisplaced cervical fractures, and other PSCIs may be managed via application of a rigid or "hard" cervical orthosis.[5] It is important that the collar fits properly (in select cases, a customized sizing for small children may be necessary).[5] Immobilization is usually recommended for a period of 6 to 12 weeks for adequate healing of ligamentous or bony injury.[11] Some rigid orthoses may be easily removed by the children, so compliance with immobilization is an important consideration when treating PSCI.[11] Modifications may be made for rigid orthoses in these cases. When sending a child home with a rigid orthosis, it is important to instruct the parents on how to change the collar for bathing, and often it is helpful to provide a rigid foam collar for showering and bathing. The foam collars can be removed after bathing and the padded rigid orthosis may be replaced. Before discontinuing the orthosis, a full clinical examination (which assesses range of motion of the cervical spine) should be normal and MRI should show ligamentous integrity without residual edema and/or evidence of subluxation.

Halo stabilization

It can be used with care in infants older than 8 months of age. If there is cervical spine instability, options for immobilization include rigid orthoses and halo stabilization. Each of these is associated with its respective benefits and complications or concerns. While halo immobilization provides "custom fit" stabilization of the cervical spine, it may also cause complications. Placement of a child in a halo usually requires sedation or general anesthesia. Halo application may be accomplished in the emergency room, pediatric intensive care unit (PICU) or operating room (OR). Halo vests and head pieces come in various sizes, and it is best to measure the head circumference and thoracic circumference of the child when selecting or ordering a halo to be placed. Manufacturer's guidelines should be followed. Adequate immobilization can be obtained with four to eight pins with 2 pounds of torque for a 2-year-old child, increasing a pound per year up to the age of 6 years. In infants, ten pins should result in adequate fixation.[23] For children under the age of 2 years, pins should be finger tight, and not torqued, to avoid causing a skull fracture. If the pin head perforates the skull, dural laceration and cerebrospinal fluid leak or infection may occur. It is certainly good practice to be certain that the skin has been cleaned well and the pin head is covered with antibiotic ointment before placing the pins through the skin. Halo stabilization can have many complications in the pediatric patient and at times poorer outcomes than an internal fixation.[5,24] In patients under the age of 1 year, a custom rigid cervical orthosis may be preferred over a halo vest fixation.[5] Careful follow-up of children in halo vests is recommended; pin sites should be regularly checked for local cellulitis and infection. Halo rings and the rod connections should be regularly monitored for tightness. Occasionally, connections can become loose over time.

11.8.2 Operative Management

In about one-third of the children with PSCI, surgical intervention is necessary.[5] Surgeons must be extremely precise and cautious when using instruments in pediatric patients, as every case is unique and there is a paucity of pediatric-specific cervical instruments.[25] Especially in children under 6 years of age, it is difficult to adapt adult-sized cervical instruments to the developing cervical spine, with small vertebral body height-to-disc ratios and small, short pedicles.[25]

Despite spinal maturation in between ages 8 and 10 years, we encourage careful evaluation of each patient's anatomy when planning surgical intervention.[4] Since there is a substantial growth in the length of the spine after the age of 10 years in children, it is important to consider levels of instrumentation and location of instrumentation (▶ Table 11.1 and ▶ Table 11.2).[4] It may be beneficial to avoid pedicle screws in younger pediatric patients; in infants and very young children, sublaminar wiring may be safer.[26] In more challenging cases, hybrid or modified techniques can be implemented.[26] The challenge, of course, is to keep screws in the vertebral bone, whether using laminar or pedicle screws, or screws anchored in the vertebral body. Maintaining the integrity of the bone, allowing growth, and preserving maximal natural mobility, while stabilizing the level of injury, are all important factors to consider.

Anterior Decompression/Stabilization

The anterior cervical approach can be adapted for use in patients of any age and has been well described previously.[27]

The incision can be moved superiorly and inferiorly with visualization and exposure of at least three vertebral body segments and two disc spaces at a time.[27] Anterior stabilization is used in cases involving disc disruption in children greater than 5 years of age as well as unstable burst fractures.[5] Fusion can be achieved with either static or dynamic anterior cervical plates that fit the anatomical size of the child's developing spine.[25] Some have advocated using autograft from the iliac crest rather than using autograft for stabilization; however, iliac crest harvesting, itself, is associated with pain and complications. When needed, craniofacial plating systems may be used, but there are risks involved with using instruments "off-label."

Posterior Decompression/Stabilization

The posterior midline approach can be performed with access to the posterior and posterolateral portion of the spinal canal.[27] Posterior stabilization of the cervical spine may include pedicle screw fixation, lateral mass screw application, laminar screw application, sublaminar wiring techniques, and hybrid techniques as well. Hybrid techniques may be employed when the pedicle on one side is large enough for pedicle screw placement, but the contralateral side pedicle is too narrow. This salvage technique allows for bilateral posterior cervical fixation and immobilization.[26] The posterior cervical approach may be associated with postoperative muscle spasm; adequate pain management and muscle relaxants should be provided.[27]

Anterior and Posterior Decompression and Stabilization

In some cases, anterior and posterior decompression and stabilization are needed. Decompression of the spinal cord should be done as soon as the child is stabilized and it is safe to proceed with surgery. Decompression from the front or back is dictated by radiological findings. Stabilization should be accomplished if the child is stable. If there are bone fragments in the spinal cord and they are easily accessible, they should be removed, and the dura should be repaired and patched, if necessary. In the case of a dural tear, a lumbar drain may be considered following assessment of any concomitant head injuries. Once stabilization has been achieved, in some cases, anterior and posterior surgeries may be needed in order to ensure stabilization of the cervical spine. After application of anterior and posterior instrumentation, it is very important to continue to follow-up the patient until he or she stops growing.[27]

11.9 Rehabilitation of Children with Subaxial Spine Trauma

After PSCI, children often benefit from inpatient or outpatient rehabilitation. Physiatrists and therapists should be made aware of any restrictions. Mobilization of the child after trauma is important for pulmonary toilet. If it is safe to get the patient to ambulate, physical therapy should be initiated as soon as possible. For children with SCIs, rotation and log rolling, chest percussions, and incentive spirometry should be implemented when deemed safe. In addition, it may be important to monitor pulmonary volume, carbon dioxide retention, and oxygen satu-

ration. Even after internal fixation, many rehabilitation mechanisms can be utilized.[5] For children requiring external immobilization via rigid orthoses or halo fixation, it is important to assess the child's safety when navigating his or her environment. Children must be taught how to navigate stairs, curbs, and ramps safely.[5] Physiatry and physical therapy are strongly recommended to restore as much function and strength to the subaxial cervical spine as possible.

11.10 Clinical Outcomes

In general, poor outcomes are noted to be associated with young age, multiple comorbidities, and confirmed cervical cord injuries.[1] Although PSCI is generally more common in older children, injury sustained by a younger patient will have a higher mortality.[2] Surgical outcomes depend on the initial trauma and neurological deficits, as well as the type of instrumentation used for spinal stabilization. Infections associated with cervical spine surgery may occur in children and should be monitored at both short-term and long-term clinical follow-up. Outcomes are improved when ambulatory independence and neurological function can be maintained. Short-term outcomes are well monitored through the National Surgical Quality Improvement Program for children. Readmission for complications, death, and disability are now being prospectively tracked and followed. These data points will help us improve our outcomes as physicians and surgeons.

Long-term complications may occur due to stunted growth across fused spinal segments. There are ongoing studies looking at the effects of instrumentation on spinal growth and development.[28] In some patients with cervical fusion, a "crank-shaft" phenomenon may occur, in which restricted growth of the child's spine results in displacement of the spine, stress on adjacent levels, and subsequent cervical lordosis.[11] Hardware can also break and become displaced, leading to postoperative pain or spinal instability. It may be prudent to monitor bone health, density and vitamin D levels in children with PSCI to allow for optimal healing.

Finally, while children with PSCI may present with severe pain and muscle spasm, anxiety, depression, and/or fear should not be misinterpreted as "pain"; overprescribing of narcotics, opioids, and muscle relaxants should be avoided at all costs. Children and adolescents are especially at risk of developing tolerance and addiction to these medications. Alternative treatment modalities including heat and massage therapy, acupuncture, and administration of nonsteroidal medications may provide adequate muscle relaxation and pain reduction.

11.11 Conclusion

The anatomical, developmental, and incremental growth of the subaxial cervical spine in the pediatric patient creates a challenge for neurosurgical treatment. Even with major efforts to prevent traumatic injuries, children are still more vulnerable to cervical spine injuries than injuries of other segments of the spine. Thus, it is essential that any child sustaining a possible cervical spine injury be properly immobilized, transported to a trauma center, and worked up for a full clinical and radiographic examination. Although there is no established standard of care for subaxial cervical spine injuries in pediatric patients, we encourage universal efforts in the future toward the creation of a standard treatment paradigm.

References

[1] Leonard JR, Jaffe DM, Kuppermann N, Olsen CS, Leonard JC, Pediatric Emergency Care Applied Research Network (PECARN) Cervical Spine Study Group. Cervical spine injury patterns in children. Pediatrics. 2014; 133(5): e1179–e1188

[2] Shin JI, Lee NJ, Cho SK. Pediatric cervical spine and spinal cord injury: a national database study. Spine. 2016; 41(4):283–292

[3] Baumann F, Ernstberger T, Neumann C, et al. Pediatric cervical spine injuries: a rare but challenging entity. J Spinal Disord Tech. 2015; 28(7):E377–E384

[4] Johnson KT, Al-Holou WN, Anderson RC, et al. Morphometric analysis of the developing pediatric cervical spine. J Neurosurg Pediatr. 2016; 18(3): 377–389

[5] Madura CJ, Johnston JM , Jr. Classification and management of pediatric subaxial cervical spine injuries. Neurosurg Clin N Am. 2017; 28(1):91–102

[6] Dias MS, Brockmeyer DL. Anatomy, embryology, and normal development of the craniovertebral junction and cervical spine. In: Brockmeyer, DL, ed. Advanced Pediatric Craniocervical Surgery. New York, NY: Thieme; 2005:1–26

[7] U.S. Injury Statistics. 10 leading causes of nonfatal injury, United States. https://www.cdc.gov/injury/wisqars/facts.html.Published 2015. Accessed June 11, 2016

[8] Murphy RF, Davidson AR, Kelly DM, Warner WC , Jr, Sawyer JR. Subaxial cervical spine injuries in children and adolescents. J Pediatr Orthop. 2015; 35(2):136–139

[9] Babcock L, Olsen CS, Jaffe DM, Leonard JC, Cervical Spine Study Group for the Pediatric Emergency Care Applied Research Network. Cervical spine injuries in children associated with sports and recreational activities. Pediatr Emerg Care. 2016

[10] Arbuthnot MK, Mooney DP, Glenn IC. Head and cervical spine evaluation for the pediatric surgeon. Surg Clin North Am. 2017; 97(1):35–58

[11] Grabb PA, Hadley MN. Spinal column trauma in children. In: Albright L, Pollack I, Adelson D, eds. Spinal Column Trauma in Children. New York, NY: Thieme Medical Publishers, Inc.; 1999: 935–952

[12] Ware ML, Gupta N, Sun PP, Brockmeyer DL. Clinical biomechanics of the pediatric craniocervical junction and subaxial spine. In: Brockmeyer, DL. Advanced Pediatric Craniocervical Surgery. New York, NY: Thieme; 2006. 27–42

[13] Ware ML, Auguste KI, Gupta N, Sun PP, Brockmeyer DL. Traumatic injuries of the pediatric craniocervical junction. In: Brockmeyer, DL. Advanced Pediatric Craniocervical Surgery. New York, NY: Thieme; 2006. 55–74

[14] Xu G, Li W, Bao G, Sun Y, Wang L, Cui Z. Tear-drop fracture of the axis in a child with an 8-year follow-up: a case report. J Pediatr Orthop B. 2014; 23(3):299–305

[15] Signoret F, Jacquot FP, Feron JM. Reducing the cervical flexion tear-drop fracture with a posterior approach and plating technique: an original method. Eur Spine J. 1999; 8(2):110–116

[16] Feuchtbaum E, Buchowski J, Zebala L. Subaxial cervical spine trauma. Curr Rev Musculoskelet Med. 2016; 9(4):496–504

[17] Hoffman JR, Mower WR, Wolfson AB, Todd KH, Zucker MI, National Emergency X-Radiography Utilization Study Group. Validity of a set of clinical criteria to rule out injury to the cervical spine in patients with blunt trauma. N Engl J Med. 2000; 343(2):94–99

[18] Stiell IG, Wells GA, Vandemheen KL, et al. The Canadian C-spine rule for radiography in alert and stable trauma patients. JAMA. 2001; 286(15): 1841–1848

[19] National Institute for Health and Care Excellence (NICE). Spinal injury: assessment and initial management. NICE guideline; no. 41. London, UK

[20] Chung S, Mikrogianakis A, Wales PW, et al. Trauma association of Canada Pediatric Subcommittee National Pediatric Cervical Spine Evaluation Pathway: consensus guidelines. J Trauma. 2011; 70(4):873–884

[21] Somppi LK, Frenn KA, Kharbanda AB. Examination of pediatric radiation dose delivered after cervical spine trauma. Pediatr Emerg Care. 2017

[22] Moore JM, Hall J, Ditchfield M, Xenos C, Danks A. Utility of plain radiographs and MRI in cervical spine clearance in symptomatic non-obtunded pediatric patients without high-impact trauma. Childs Nerv Syst. 2017; 33(2):249–258

[23] Rosati SF, Maarouf R, Wolfe L, et al. Implementation of pediatric cervical spine clearance guidelines at a combined trauma center: twelve-month impact. J Trauma Acute Care Surg. 2015; 78(6):1117–1121

[24] Henry M, Riesenburger RI, Kryzanski J, Jea A, Hwang SW. A retrospective comparison of CT and MRI in detecting pediatric cervical spine injury. Childs Nerv Syst. 2013; 29(8):1333–1338

[25] Garber ST, Brockmeyer DL. Management of subaxial cervical instability in very young or small-for-age children using a static single-screw anterior cervical plate: indications, results, and long-term follow-up. J Neurosurg Spine. 2016; 24(6):892–896

[26] Quinn JC, Patel NV, Tyagi R. Hybrid lateral mass screw sublaminar wire construct: A salvage technique for posterior cervical fixation in pediatric spine surgery. J Clin Neurosci. 2016; 25:118–121

[27] Brockmeyer DL. Advanced surgery for the subaxial cervical spine in children. In: Brockmeyer DL, ed. Advanced Pediatric Craniocervical Surgery. New York, NY: Thieme; 2006:109–122

[28] Hwang SW, Gressot LV, Rangel-Castilla L, et al. Outcomes of instrumented fusion in the pediatric cervical spine. J Neurosurg Spine. 2012; 17(5): 397–409

12 Cervical Burst Fractures

Scott C. Wagner and Alan S. Hilibrand

Abstract

Subaxial cervical burst fractures occur relatively infrequently but are typically associated with a high rate of instability and neurological injury. Emergency evaluation, radiographic diagnosis, early classification, and appropriate surgical intervention—which may vary depending on the type of fracture and associated injuries—can yield overall good outcomes. This chapter will examine the evaluation, classification, and treatment options for subaxial cervical burst fractures. Patient characteristics and fracture patterns should be considered when determining the appropriate course of intervention; the treating surgeon's judgment is also paramount for successful management of these rare injuries.

Keywords: cervical burst fracture, Subaxial Injury Classification (SLIC), AOSpine Subaxial Cervical Spine Classification

12.1 Introduction

Subaxial cervical burst fractures are relatively uncommon injuries, with estimated incidence of 5 to 10% of all burst fractures.[1] Burst fractures were originally described in the early 1960s as injuries caused by herniation of the intervertebral disc through the endplate of the vertebral body.[2] Denis expanded upon this description, utilizing the three-column concept of spinal stability to define burst fractures as disruption of the anterior and middle columns, often with retropulsion of the middle column fragment into the spinal canal; though this description was specific for thoracolumbar fractures.[3] Historically, cervical burst fractures were also described as "teardrop" or "quadrangular" fractures,[4,5] and were believed to result from compressive forces along the vertical orientation of the cervical spine due to an axial load.[6] In their 2002 article describing treatment techniques, Fisher et al defined this fracture subtype as a "coronal split through the vertebral body, with dorsal displacement of the remaining vertebral body that leads to narrowing of the spinal canal."[5] The flexion movement cause by the axial force often disrupts the posterior ligamentous complex, resulting in significant instability at the injured level with a high risk of neurological compromise.[7]

Over the past decade, several classification systems have been described and validated, such as the Subaxial Injury Classification (SLIC) System and the AOSpine Subaxial Cervical Spine Injury Classification System. These have been developed in an attempt to standardize treatment protocols for spinal trauma.[8,9] Considered in the context of these classification schemes, cervical burst fractures can be systematically evaluated and potential treatment options can be considered based on current evidence. However, no universal treatment algorithm is available at present. Treatment options include conservative care with immobilization in patients without neurological deficits and no evidence of discoligamentous instability, an anterior corpectomy with strut grafting, a posterior cervical decompression and fusion, or a combination of these approaches for severely unstable injuries.[6,7]

12.2 Initial Evaluation

12.2.1 Clinical History and Physical Examination

Despite comprising only 3% of all blunt trauma, injury to the cervical spine is often among the most catastrophic injuries due to the frequency of associated spinal cord injury.[7,10] Upon initial presentation, any patient sustaining major trauma or suspected cervical spine injury should be managed according to Advanced Trauma Life Support (ATLS) principles, including protection of the airway and maintenance of circulation and breathing.[7] Inspection and palpation of the neck may reveal significant pain or gross deformity, and the cervical spine should immediately be protected in a hard collar (though these are typically placed in the field at the point-of-contact by first responders). With cervical immobilization in place, the patient should be log rolled to allow for inspection and palpation of the entire spinal column.[7] A thorough neurological examination, including sensory and motor evaluation, should be performed to identify any deficits, which can be used to determine the potential for spinal axis injury. After appropriate resuscitation has begun, the patient should undergo radiographic evaluation to screen for potential diagnoses on the basis of suspected type of injury.

12.2.2 Radiographic Evaluation

There is some controversy with regard to the use of plain films, including anteroposterior, lateral, open-mouth odontoid, and flexion-extension views of the cervical spine,[7] which is primarily related to differences in imaging capabilities across various institutions. Traditionally, plain radiographs were utilized to evaluate global alignment of the cervical spine, including areas of kyphosis or dislocation, as well as for changes in disc height or interspinous distance suggestive of flexion-distraction injuries.[7] However, some recent studies have suggested that the sensitivity of plain films to rule out cervical fractures or instability secondary to ligamentous injury ranges from 30 to 60%, and a paper by Sim et al[11] found that 95% of flexion-extension views were inadequate due to the inability to visualize T1 or poor patient effort.[12,13,14] Therefore, use of computed tomography (CT) imaging has become more common to provide rapid, high-quality screening for traumatic injuries, including the cervical spine. CT scans allow for much better evaluation of the occipitocervical and cervicothoracic junctions than traditional plain radiographs.[7] If a cervical burst fracture is identified on a CT scan, magnetic resonance imaging (MRI) has very high utility in evaluating associated discoligamentous and soft-tissue injuries. However, some recent literature has suggested that MRI may not be as reliable in identifying disruption of the posterior ligamentous complex (PLC), which has significant implications with regard to classification and treatment of these injuries.[15]

12.3 Classification

While an exhaustive review of published classification schemes for cervical trauma is beyond the scope of this chapter, the two most commonly utilized (and validated) systems include the SLIC and the AOSpine Subaxial Cervical Spine classification. These systems were created to consolidate fracture patterns, instability, and neurological status of the patient into a treatment algorithm that can be easily applied in most, if not all, cervical trauma scenarios. Cervical burst fractures can be adequately described utilizing these systems, and with other clinical factors, can be managed effectively.

12.3.1 Subaxial Injury Classification

With the Spine Trauma Study Group, Vaccaro et al[8] published the original SLIC system in 2007. The SLIC system is based on the specific presenting morphology of the fracture, the neurological status of the patient, and the integrity of the PLC as an indicator of posterior instability. Each factor is independently assigned a numerical value based on certain characteristics, and the values are then aggregated to yield a total score that can be used for directing treatment. For total scores < 4, conservative treatment is advocated; scores ≥ 5 suggest operative management; and an intermediate score of 4 indicates that the clinical judgment of the surgeon and the patient's comorbidities can dictate either conservative or surgical treatment. Fractures with burst morphology, which are defined in this system as a subtype of compression/flexion injuries, are assigned a numerical score of 2. The SLIC system is summarized in ▶ Table 12.1.

Table 12.1 The Subaxial Injury Classification (SLIC) System.[8] Total summative scores of less than 4 receive nonoperative treatment, while scores greater than or equal to 5 should undergo operative management. A score of 4 represents an indeterminate injury that should be left to the treating surgeon's judgment

Characteristic	Points
Morphology	
No abnormality	0
Compression	1
Burst	+ 1 = 2
Distraction (e.g., facet perch, hyperextension)	3
Rotation/translation	4
Discoligamentous complex (DLC)	
Intact	0
Indeterminate	3
Disrupted	4
Neurological status	
Intact	0
Root injury	1
Complete cord injury	2
Incomplete cord injury	3
Continuous cord compression	+ 1

12.3.2 AOSpine Subaxial Cervical Spine Classification

The AOSpine Knowledge Forum developed the AOSpine Cervical Spine Classification in an effort to improve upon the SLIC system which despite relatively high reliability was still plagued by inconsistencies between evaluators related to PLC integrity and morphology.[9] Like the SLIC system, the AOSpine Classification is based on fracture morphology and neurological status of the patient, but considers facet injuries rather than status of the PLC, and includes multiple case-specific modifiers such as critical disc herniation, metabolic bone disease, vertebral artery injury, and any suggestion of PLC disruption.[9] Fracture morphology is divided into three basic categories. Type A injuries are fractures that involve the vertebral body with an intact posterior tension band. Type B injuries involve failure of the anterior or posterior tension bands, but without associated translation of the spinal axis. Type C fractures demonstrate displacement of vertebral bodies in any direction. Several recent studies have shown adequate inter- and intraobserver reliability.[16,17] A scoring system for treatment guidance has not yet been developed. In this system, burst fractures are considered type A injuries, with subtypes described by status of the endplates: A3 fractures only involve one endplate, while A4 fractures involve both endplates and also include sagittal split fractures that involve the posterior wall.[9]

12.4 Treatment

The decision for conservative versus operative management of cervical burst fractures is dependent upon many clinical factors in addition to fracture pattern, and there is no universally accepted algorithm for these at present. As discussed, patients with a cervical burst fracture morphology and an overall SLIC score > 4 are treated surgically, while those with a score < 3 are managed conservatively. Nonsurgical management of a stable burst fracture involves a hard cervical orthosis, generally worn for 6 to 12 weeks until evidence of clinical and radiographic healing has been achieved.[6,7] Use of the orthosis is not mandatory, as these injuries are technically considered stable, but it may aid in providing support for soft tissue rest[6,7] and reduce postinjury subsidence of the fracture.

Unstable burst fractures (e.g., an SLIC score > 4) or injuries with associated potential for progressive neurological injuries should be treated surgically. The chosen approach will vary by specific injury pattern and individual patient characteristics, but options include anterior corpectomy and grafting with plate stabilization or a combined anterior/posterior approach.

Anterior approaches are advantageous in that the supine position and plane of dissection are generally less morbid than the subperiosteal dissection in the prone position for the posterior approach. This approach allows for direct anterior visualization and decompression of the neural elements.[6] If the fracture pattern is associated with retropulsion of fragments into the canal, removal of the fragments and restoration of the anterior column are the primary goals of surgery. Doing so is most efficaciously achieved via an anterior approach with partial or complete corpectomy of the fractured vertebral body.[7,18] Fragments are identified and removed utilizing pituitary or Kerrison rongeurs, and the vertebral foramen are checked for any other fragments or tissues that can cause compression. Discectomy at the level(s) cephalad and caudal to the burst fracture is performed with preparation of the surrounding endplates, followed by grafting with a cortical strut. This technique allows for restoration of the anterior column stability and height, and supplemental anterior plate and screw fixation provides additional support to facilitate arthrodesis.

A posterior approach offers the advantages of rigid fixation with lateral mass and pedicle screws, the ability to rapidly decompress multiple levels, and allows for direct reduction forces to be applied to the cervical spine.[6] If the discoligamentous complex is completely disrupted in addition to a burst fracture, such as in AOSpine type C injuries or if there are associated facet dislocations or fractures, a combined anterior/posterior approach may be required.[7] Direct anterior decompression and anterior column restoration followed by posterior decompression and rigid fixation provides circumferential stabilization for these severely unstable patterns. Biomechanically, combined stabilization has been shown to have the highest stability when compared to anterior-alone or posterior-alone approaches.[4] For the posterior approach, the patient is positioned prone with the head in Mayfield or Doro head pins for stabilization. The approach is carried out in a standard subperiosteal technique, with lateral mass screws placed cephalad and caudal to the injured level(s). When near a junctional level, the posterior cervical construct should be extended to T1 rather than terminating at C7, as multilevel posterior cervical constructs that do not span the junctional region have been shown to have a higher revision rate.[19]

12.5 Conclusion

Despite the relative infrequency with which cervical burst fractures occur, these injuries are typically associated with a high rate of neurological dysfunction and instability. Expeditious emergency evaluation, radiographic diagnosis, classification, and appropriate surgical intervention can yield good results, though neurological outcomes are predicated on the severity of neurological injury at the time of presentation. As with all clinical scenarios, the treating surgeon's judgment, patient characteristics, and injury type should be considered when determining the most appropriate course of intervention.

References

[1] Bensch FV, Koivikko MP, Kiuru MJ, Koskinen SK. The incidence and distribution of burst fractures. Emerg Radiol. 2006; 12(3):124–129

[2] Holdsworth FW. Fractures, dislocations and fracture-dislocations of the spine. Journal of Bone And Joint Surgery. 1963(45):6–20

[3] Denis F. Spinal instability as defined by the three-column spine concept in acute spinal trauma. Clin Orthop Relat Res. 1984(189):65–76

[4] Ianuzzi A, Zambrano I, Tataria J, et al. Biomechanical evaluation of surgical constructs for stabilization of cervical teardrop fractures. Spine J. 2006; 6(5):514–523

[5] Fisher CG, Dvorak MF, Leith J, Wing PC. Comparison of outcomes for unstable lower cervical flexion teardrop fractures managed with halo thoracic vest versus anterior corpectomy and plating. Spine. 2002; 27(2):160–166

[6] Joaquim AF, Patel AA. Subaxial cervical spine trauma: evaluation and surgical decision-making. Global Spine J. 2014; 4(1):63–70

[7] Feuchtbaum E, Buchowski J, Zebala L. Subaxial cervical spine trauma. Curr Rev Musculoskelet Med. 2016; 9(4):496–504

[8] Vaccaro AR, Hulbert RJ, Patel AA, et al. Spine Trauma Study Group. The Subaxial Cervical Spine Injury Classification System: a novel approach to recognize the importance of morphology, neurology, and integrity of the disco-ligamentous complex. Spine. 2007; 32(21):2365–2374

[9] Vaccaro AR, Koerner JD, Radcliff KE, et al. AOSpine subaxial cervical spine injury classification system. Eur Spine J. 2016; 25(7):2173–2184

[10] Lowery DW, Wald MM, Browne BJ, Tigges S, Hoffman JR, Mower WR, NEXUS Group. Epidemiology of cervical spine injury victims. Ann Emerg Med. 2001; 38(1):12–16

[11] Sim V, Bernstein MP, Frangos SG, et al. The (f)utility of flexion-extension C-spine films in the setting of trauma. Am J Surg. 2013; 206(6):929–933, discussion 933–934

[12] Jones C, Jazayeri F. Evolving standards of practice for cervical spine imaging in trauma: a retrospective review. Australas Radiol. 2007; 51(5):420–425

[13] McCulloch PT, France J, Jones DL, et al. Helical computed tomography alone compared with plain radiographs with adjunct computed tomography to evaluate the cervical spine after high-energy trauma. J Bone Joint Surg Am. 2005; 87(11):2388–2394

[14] Schenarts PJ, Diaz J, Kaiser C, Carrillo Y, Eddy V, Morris JA, Jr. Prospective comparison of admission computed tomographic scan and plain films of the upper cervical spine in trauma patients with altered mental status. J Trauma. 2001; 51(4):663–668, discussion 668–669

[15] Schroeder GD, Kepler CK, Koerner JD, et al. A worldwide analysis of the reliability and perceived importance of an injury to the posterior ligamentous complex in AO type A fractures. Global Spine J. 2015; 5(5):378–382

[16] Urrutia J, Zamora T, Yurac R, et al. an independent inter- and intraobserver agreement evaluation of the AOSpine Subaxial Cervical Spine Injury Classification System. Spine. 2017; 42(5):298–303

[17] Silva OT, Sabba MF, Lira HI, et al. Evaluation of the reliability and validity of the newer AOSpine subaxial cervical injury classification (C-3 to C-7). J Neurosurg Spine. 2016; 25(3):303–308

[18] Dvorak MF, Fisher CG, Fehlings MG, et al. The surgical approach to subaxial cervical spine injuries: an evidence-based algorithm based on the SLIC classification system. Spine. 2007; 32(23):2620–2629

[19] Schroeder GD, Kepler CK, Kurd MF, et al. Is it necessary to extend a multilevel posterior cervical decompression and fusion to the upper thoracic spine? Spine. 2016; 41(23):1845–1849

13 Cervical Spine Trauma-Induced Vertebral Artery Injury

Rahul Goel, Hanna Sandhu, I. David Kaye, Hamadi Murphy, Mayan Lendner, and Alexander R. Vaccaro

Abstract

Diagnosis of cervical spine trauma-induced vertebral artery injuries (VAIs) may explain late onset of vertebrobasilar insufficiency (VBI) symptoms and may alter proposed surgical treatment options. Imaging should be strongly considered in case of symptoms of VBI and cervical dislocation or high cervical spine fracture. Although many centers have advocated for computed tomography angiography as a screening tool in the initial screening of trauma patients, further research is needed to fully assess its efficacy in identifying VAI as compared to emerging modalities such as ultrasonography. Treatment may include close observation, administration of anticoagulation and antiplatelet agents, as well as endovascular treatments and surgery depending on the radiological severity and clinical presentation of injury. According to the consensus statement by the American Association of Neurological Surgeons/Congress of Neurological Surgeons Guidelines, anticoagulation is recommended in symptomatic VAI to lessen the risk of early recurrence of stroke. Consultation with vascular neurosurgeons and neurologists may prove beneficial when developing optimal treatment approaches for patients.

Keywords: spine surgery, cervical spine trauma, vertebral artery injury, vertebrobasilar insufficiency, CT angiography, anticoagulation

13.1 Introduction

Vertebral artery injury (VAI) in conjunction with cervical spine trauma can occur secondary to blunt or penetrating injuries of the cervical spine. These injuries, such as thrombi, secondary emboli, or dissections, can often initially present asymptomatically,[1] but their sequelae, such as stroke or even death, can be devastating.[2] The low incidence of these frequently asymptomatic injuries has made diagnosis challenging and the potential for devastating outcomes for both symptomatic and initially asymptomatic injuries, especially in cases requiring surgical management of the spine injury, has made management more nuanced.

13.2 Anatomy

The vertebral arteries arise from the posterosuperior aspect of the first segment of the subclavian arteries, distal to the origin of the common carotid arteries. At times there can be aberrant origination of these arteries, more commonly on the left than the right,[3] and most commonly from the arch of the aorta rather than the subclavian artery. From their origination from the subclavian arteries to their joining at the pontomedullary junction to form the basilar artery, the vertebral arteries can be divided into four segments (V1–V4). The first segment (V1) travels from the origin at the subclavian artery to the transverse process of C6. The second portion (V2) travels cranially through the transverse foramina of C6 to C2. At the level of C2, the artery must course laterally to pass through the foramen transversarium of C1. The third segment (V3) then courses posteromedially along the arch of the atlas prior to turning anteromedially to enter the skull through the foramen magnum. The fourth segment (V4) courses medially once entering the skull to combine with the contralateral vertebral artery to form the basilar artery, which supplies the posterior circulation of the brain through the circle of Willis.

13.3 Epidemiology

Identification of VAIs has steadily increased as imaging modalities for these injuries have improved and are more utilized.[4] Carpenter was the first to describe this injury in association with cervical spine trauma.[5] Subsequently, small cohort studies have reported various rates of VAI with concomitant cervical spine trauma. Weller et al showed a VAI incidence of 33% (4/12) for patients who had a magnetic resonance imaging (MRI) following detection of foramen transversarium fracture on computed tomography (CT) scan.[6] Parbhoo et al found an incidence of 25% (12/47) in a prospective study evaluating cervical trauma patients with MRI and magnetic resonance angiography (MRA).[7]

Larger studies with more extensive screening have found similar results. Miller et al screened all patients with cervical spine fractures, LeFort II or III facial fractures, Horner syndrome, basilar skull fractures involving the foramen lacerum, soft-tissue injuries in the neck, or neurological symptoms otherwise unexplained by intracranial injuries with four vessel cerebral angiography and found a 19% (43/216) incidence of VAI and 11% (24/216) incidence of carotid artery injury (CAI).[8] Ren et al prospectively examined 319 patients with closed cervical trauma with two-dimensional time-of-flight MRA and found an incidence of VAI to be 16% (52/319).[9] Vaccaro et al had previously identified a similar incidence of VAI (19.7%) in cervical spine injuries screened with MRA, although in a smaller cohort (12/61).[10] Ren et al and Vaccaro et al found that 50 to 65% of patients with facet joint dislocation sustained VAI, the most common associated cervical spine injury in their series respectively.

Cothren et al evaluated all blunt trauma admissions in their facility and found that three cervical spine pathologies were associated with a much higher incidence of VAI: subluxations, upper cervical spine fractures (C1–C3), and fractures through the transverse foramen.[11] These findings have been corroborated in various literature.[2,10] Furthermore, large database studies have found that the overall incidence of VAI in all blunt traumas range from 0.075 to 1.14%.[12,13,14,15]

13.4 Mechanism and Types of Arterial Injury

VAI is possible in any of the four segments of vertebral artery; however, the most often injured segment of the vertebral artery is the V2 segment due to its relatively fixed position and the narrow space that it occupies.[16,17,18,19] Chung et al found that the greatest risk factor for injury of the vertebral artery at this segment, V2, was facet fracture with an odds ratio of 20.98 in their multivariate analysis. The authors postulated that the already narrow transforaminal space predisposes the artery to damage with further fracture fragment encroachment.[20]

The most common mechanism associated with VAI has been shown to be a flexion-type force in the cervical spine, most commonly flexion-distraction (▶ Fig. 13.1), but also flexion-compression.[21,22] Sim et al evaluated flexion-type force and its compression of the vertebral artery in cadaveric models, finding that once the physiological flexion range of motion was exceeded, there was impingement upon the vertebral artery.[23] As the flexion force exceeds the physiologic range of motion, the vessel attachments to the surrounding tissues begin to apply shearing forces to the intimal lining. Tears that occur subsequent to this force can lead to thrombus formation and occlusion of the vertebral vessel.

The most common VAI pattern seen is occlusion[24] followed by dissection.[17] The adventitia of the vertebral vessel is relatively resistant to tears as compared to the intima. Due to this, tears within the intima can propagate, creating a dissection plane between these two layers of the vessel. Thrombus formation between these two layers can begin to compress the vessel lumen leading to turbulent flow and occlusion. Occlusion can also occur through direct compression of the vessel from fracture and dislocation fragments.

13.5 Clinical Diagnosis

13.5.1 Presentation

Due to abundant collateral circulation feeding the vertebrobasilar system and posterior circulation of the brain, patients with VAI are often asymptomatic. In the case of atherosclerosis or anatomic variations that cause collateral circulation to be diminished, patients may present with symptoms of vertebrobasilar insufficiency (VBI) such as vertigo, dizziness, dysarthria, blurred vision, tinnitus, dysphagia, and diplopia.[25]

The interval between spinal injury and development of symptoms varies greatly ranging from immediately after the trauma to up to 3 months later.[26] Embolism, thrombus extension, or dissection of the vertebral artery can cause acute or delayed onset of symptoms in initially asymptomatic patients. Heros et al described a patient with VAI who developed a delayed cerebellar infarction in the setting of a normal contralateral artery secondary to a thrombus that had extended distally to the intracranial portion of the vertebral artery.[27] In another case study, Six et al reported a 25-year-old asymptomatic patient who presented with bilateral vertebral artery occlusion and minimal subluxation of C2 on C3.[28] Angiography revealed occlusion of both vertebral arteries but the presence of collateral circulation by the vessels of the thyrocervical trunk and superficial occipital artery. In a retrospective review of 1,283 patients with cervical spine trauma, Blam et al determined that a normal neurological examination was not indicative of vertebral artery patency after cervical spine trauma.[29] Furthermore, VAI was observed in similar frequency among neurologically intact patients as compared with motor incomplete patients.

The late onset of symptoms following VAI suggests that thrombus formation at the injury site followed by clot propagation and subsequent infarction may be the culprit. Therefore, it is important for clinicians to recognize that neurological signs or symptoms of VBI may be delayed, and to consistently monitor a patient's response to treatment both initially and upon subsequent follow-up visits.

13.5.2 Imaging Modalities

Digital subtraction angiography (DSA) is a fluoroscopic technique that allows visualization of blood vessels in contrast with their surrounding bone and soft tissue. DSA has been the "gold

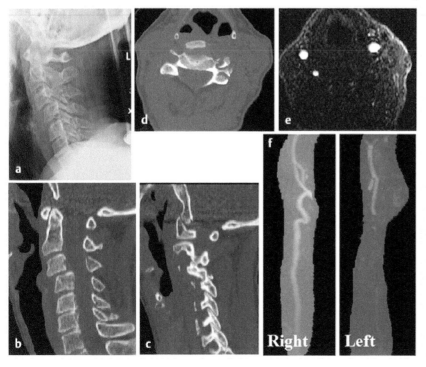

Fig. 13.1 A 42-year-old man presented after a motor vehicle accident with a flexion distraction injury with C3–C4 subluxation. **(a)** Lateral X-ray showing approximately 25% translation of C3 on C4. **(b, c)** Sagittal computed tomography (CT) scan demonstrating C3–C4 translation with facet fracture and impaction. **(d)** Axial CT imaging at C4 demonstrating left facet fracture with a fracture fragment in the left foramen transversarium. **(e)** Axial magnetic resonance angiography (MRA) demonstrating filling defect at the left vertebral artery. **(f)** CT angiography reconstruction demonstrating filling defect at left versus right vertebral artery at the level of the fracture.

standard" for evaluation of residual or recurrent aneurysms after microsurgical clipping.[30] DSA has been proven to be especially useful in detection of vertebral artery abnormalities, including occlusions, ulcerated plaques, aneurysms, and stenoses. DSA systems use X-ray detection to produce 1 to 30 exposures per second of an intra-arterial contrast medium. These arterial images are then converted to digital form and are used to "subtract" the precontrast images from those obtained after injection to visualize arterial structure prior to puncture. DSA examinations can be performed on an outpatient basis and often require 25 to 45 minutes, putting them at a considerable advantage in safety and cost over standard arteriographic examinations, which require overnight observation to detect arterial obstruction or hemorrhage. While there are no randomized clinical studies that document direct or indirect safety effects of DSA, certain complications can arise in DSA exams due to leakage of contrast medium and should be considered in clinical decision-making.

As a less invasive imaging modality, computed tomography angiography (CTA) has begun to replace DSA at many institutions. Unlike DSA, CTA does not require femoral artery puncture or intra-arterial manipulation. In addition, CTA requires fewer personnel, is less time-consuming, requires considerably less contrast, and rarely requires sedation, thereby minimizing anesthesia-related risks. A primary concern with CTA is clip-induced imaging artifacts that may obscure local anatomy and limit analysis of the arterial region of interest.

Imaging modalities used in the radiological examination of high-energy trauma (e.g., fall from a great height, motor vehicle accident, sports-related trauma) often require head and cervical spine CT scans. As a result, many studies have advocated the incorporation of CTA as part of the initial screening of patients presenting with penetrating cervical injury without indication of immediate operation. An 11-month prospective study conducted at the Parkland Memorial Hospital Trauma Center underscored the importance of CTA as a screening tool in addition to CT since it identified 98% of blunt cervical vascular injuries (BCVIs) and provided improved visualization of both normal and abnormal anatomy allowing clinicans to make sound judgments regarding at-risk structures.[31] Eastman et al conducted a study on 162 patients at risk for BCVI which revealed that the results of CTA and DSA were concordant for detection of VAI.[31]

Despite wide acceptance in the radiology literature, many clinicians remain skeptical of CTA.[32] Although CTA is less invasive and provides short examination times, its insufficient sensitivity has made clinicians reluctant to use CTA over DSA as the initial screening modality of choice when identifying VAI. In a 40-month study comprising 7,000 blunt trauma patients, Malhotra et al selected 119 patients for DSA and CTA screening based on criteria including facial and cervical spinal fractures and unexplained neurological deficit.[33] 6 of 62 (10%) CTAs were false positives, which resulted in a sensitivity of 74% and negative predictive value (NPV) of 90%. Factors leading to CTAs being suboptimal include patient factors, such as dental work or foreign metal objects, and technical factors, such as poor contrast in the arteries and motion artifacts. Similarly, Biffl et al found an alarming rate of failures of CTA to detect subtle lesions that were visualized using DSA.[34]

MRA uses MRI and an injection of gadolinium-based contrast material to visualize arterial blood flow. Since the exam does not use ionizing radiation, it is less likely to cause an allergic reaction. Other advantages of MRA include absence of flow-related enhancement of an artery, which may indicate occlusion and presence of pseudoaneurysms (▶ Fig. 13.2). Although a number of studies describe the use of MRA to identify BCVI, there is a paucity of literature regarding the sensitivity and specificity of MRA in patients with VAI.

An emerging imaging modality for VAIs is ultrasonography. Being inexpensive, quick, and noninvasive, this modality may be utlized more in the future as an efficacious screening method. Yang et al provided a case series using this modality where vertebral artery dissection was detected in symptomatic patients even when DSA was negative.[35] Larger series are needed to fully evaluate ultrasonagrapy for diagnosis of VAI.

13.6 Treatment

Traumatic VAI may result in vertebrobasilar infarction. Regardless of the exact mechanism of vertebral artery occlusion, patients with symptoms of posterior circulation ischemia without stroke are treated with intravenous heparin.[36] Schellinger et al recommends prophylaxis of suspected vertebrobasilar ischemia by initial administration of heparin using an effective activated partial thromboplastin time (aPTT) of at least twice the baseline value followed by oral anticoagulation with warfarin for 3 to 6 months in the subacute stage.[37]

Clinical presentation and radiological severity may indicate treatment with antiplatelet agents or endovascular management

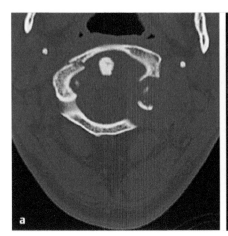
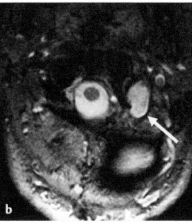

Fig. 13.2 (a) A 54-year-old man with C1 burst fracture (Jefferson fracture) who presented without any neurological deficits. (b) Magnetic resonance imaging (MRI) revealed the presence of a left vertebral artery pseudoaneurysm (*white arrow*).

to lessen the risk of early recurrence of stroke. The American Association of Neurological Surgeons/Congress of Neurological Surgeons Guidelines reported better outcomes in patients with posterior circulation stroke and VAI when treated with intravenously administered heparin or orally administered antiplatelet agents.[38] Spaniolas et al reviewed 574 patients with blunt VAI (BVAI) among the 761,385 blunt trauma admissions in the National Trauma Data Bank (0.075% overall incidence). Asymptomatic patients who were treated with heparin or aspirin had a significantly lower incidence of stroke compared to those who did not receive therapy.[39]

In cases of coexisting traumatic brain injury or polytrauma, anticoagulation may be contraindicated. High-grade, symptomatic injuries in patients with poor collateral supply may require endovascular treatment, the alternative key form of treatment for traumatic VAI. The choice of technique for VAI may vary depending on the grade of VAI, site of injury, and presence of collateral circulation. Endovascular techniques include stenting, vertebral artery occlusion, and pseudoaneurysm coil embolization.[40] The benefits of anticoagulation therapy must be weighed against its pontetial risks. In a review of 24 patients who were fully anticoagulated, Biffl et al reported sources of hemorrhage in the nasopharynx, gastrointestinal tract, liver, and retroperitoneum.[30] The study showed 25 to 54% of the trauma population range experience complications associated with anticoagulation such as hemorrhage, worsening neurological function, and increasing infarction size. Antiplatelet drugs are less hazardous than anticoagulants which can result in intramural hemorrhage in one-third of patients according to MRI.[41] A randomized trial conducted by the Cervical Artery Dissection in Stroke Study (CADISS) investigators revealed that stroke occurred in 1 (2%) of 59 patients treated with antiplatelet drugs and 1 (4%) of 28 patients treated with anticoagulant drugs. There was no significant difference between the two treatments at prevention of recurrent stroke at 3 months. The Cervical Artery Dissection in Ischemic Stroke Patients (CADISP) Study Group has advocated antiplatelet therapy in patients with cervical dissection and anticoagulation in those with free-floating intraluminal thrombus on vascular imaging and occlusion of the dissected artery.[42]

Vertebral artery transection is life threatening and must be selectively managed when accompanied by hemorrhagic shock and respiratory compromise. Patients with suspected cervical spine injury require emergent airway management, resuscitation, and embolization.[43] Early recognition of vertebral vessel disruption is important, particularly in patients with minor ischemic symptoms for which administration of either antiplatelet agents or anticoagulation can reduce risk of posterior circulation infarction.[18]

The treatment for asymptomatic VAI is controversial at this time. There have been no Level 1 or Level 2 studies that have been completed evaluating treatment methods. Miller et al showed in a retrospective chart review that the treatment of asymptomatic VAI helped to reduce the rate of stroke following injury.[44] Anticoagualtion in these patients is not without risk; Biffl et al reported that 2 of the 24 patients treated with heparin developed hemorrhagic stroke requiring cessation of heparin therapy.[34] There are contraindications to anticoagulation and antiplatelet therapy in asymptomatic VAI patients: concurrent bleeding elsewhere, impending surgery, and bleeding disorders such as hemophilia A or B.[45] Sack et al evaluated patients who were treated operatively for cervical spine fractures while not being anticoagulated for an asymptomatic VAI.[46] In this small cohort of seven patients, no patient experienced postoperative stroke symptoms, though three of these patients were started on aspirin following their surgery.

In the case of cervical spine operations, management of VAI typically includes tamponade with a hemostatic agent, direct repair, and postoperative endovascular procedures to prevent delayed complications. When hemostasis by tamponade is used, several studies strongly recommend immediate angiography to confirm adequate collateral circulation to the brain. Further management by embolization and anticoagulation would depend on the etiology detected by the angiographic findings.[47] Although VAI can lead to catastrophic outcomes including death, neurological sequelae attributable to VAI are rare. Miller et al reported an overall stroke rate of 2.6% among 64 patients with varying grades of VAI.[44]

References

[1] Taneichi H, Suda K, Kajino T, Kaneda K. Traumatically induced vertebral artery occlusion associated with cervical spine injuries: prospective study using magnetic resonance angiography. Spine. 2005; 30(17):1955–1962

[2] Fassett DR, Dailey AT, Vaccaro AR. Vertebral artery injuries associated with cervical spine injuries: a review of the literature. J Spinal Disord Tech. 2008; 21(4):252–258

[3] Yuan SM. Aberrant origin of vertebral artery and its clinical implications. Rev Bras Cir Cardiovasc. 2016; 31(1):52–59

[4] Newhall K, Gottlieb DJ, Stone DH, Goodney PP. Trends in the diagnosis and outcomes of traumatic carotid and vertebral artery dissections among Medicare Beneficiaries. Ann Vasc Surg. 2016; 36:145–152

[5] Carpenter S. Injury of neck as cause of vertebral artery thrombosis. J Neurosurg. 1961; 18:849–853

[6] Weller SJ, Rossitch E, Jr, Malek AM. Detection of vertebral artery injury after cervical spine trauma using magnetic resonance angiography. J Trauma. 1999; 46(4):660–666

[7] Parbhoo AH, Govender S, Corr P. Vertebral artery injury in cervical spine trauma. Injury. 2001; 32(7):565–568

[8] Miller PR, Fabian TC, Croce MA, et al. Prospective screening for blunt cerebrovascular injuries: analysis of diagnostic modalities and outcomes. Ann Surg. 2002; 236(3):386–393, discussion 393–395

[9] Ren X, Wang W, Zhang X, Pu Y, Jiang T, Li C. Clinical study and comparison of magnetic resonance angiography (MRA) and angiography diagnosis of blunt vertebral artery injury. J Trauma. 2007; 63(6):1249–1253

[10] Vaccaro AR, Klein GR, Flanders AE, Albert TJ, Balderston RA, Cotler JM. Long-term evaluation of vertebral artery injuries following cervical spine trauma using magnetic resonance angiography. Spine. 1998; 23(7):789–794, discussion 795

[11] Cothren CC, Moore EE, Ray CE, Jr, Johnson JL, Moore JB, Burch JM. Cervical spine fracture patterns mandating screening to rule out blunt cerebrovascular injury. Surgery. 2007; 141(1):76–82

[12] McKevitt EC, Kirkpatrick AW, Vertesi L, Granger R, Simons RK. Blunt vascular neck injuries: diagnosis and outcomes of extracranial vessel injury. J Trauma. 2002; 53(3):472–476

[13] Risgaard O, Sugrue M, D'Amours S, et al. Blunt cerebrovascular injury: an evaluation from a major trauma centre. ANZ J Surg. 2007; 77(8):686–689

[14] Berne JD, Norwood SH, McAuley CE, Villareal DH. Helical computed tomographic angiography: an excellent screening test for blunt cerebrovascular injury. J Trauma. 2004; 57(1):11–17, discussion 17–19

[15] Schneidereit NP, Simons R, Nicolaou S, et al. Utility of screening for blunt vascular neck injuries with computed tomographic angiography. J Trauma. 2006; 60(1):209–215, discussion 215–216

[16] Parent AD, Harkey HL, Touchstone DA, Smith EE, Smith RR. Lateral cervical spine dislocation and vertebral artery injury. Neurosurgery. 1992; 31(3):501–509

[17] Biffl WL, Ray CE, Jr, Moore EE, et al. Treatment-related outcomes from blunt cerebrovascular injuries: importance of routine follow-up arteriography. Ann Surg. 2002; 235(5):699–706, discussion 706–707

[18] Bartels E. Dissection of the extracranial vertebral artery: clinical findings and early noninvasive diagnosis in 24 patients. J Neuroimaging. 2006; 16(1):24–33

[19] Arnold M, Bousser MG, Fahrni G, et al. Vertebral artery dissection: presenting findings and predictors of outcome. Stroke. 2006; 37(10):2499–2503

[20] Chung D, Sung JK, Cho DC, Kang DH. Vertebral artery injury in destabilized midcervical spine trauma; predisposing factors and proposed mechanism. Acta Neurochir (Wien). 2012; 154(11):2091–2098, discussion 2098

[21] Giacobetti FB, Vaccaro AR, Bos-Giacobetti MA, et al. Vertebral artery occlusion associated with cervical spine trauma. A prospective analysis. Spine. 1997; 22(2):188–192

[22] Veras LM, Pedraza-Gutiérrez S, Castellanos J, Capellades J, Casamitjana J, Rovira-Cañellas A. Vertebral artery occlusion after acute cervical spine trauma. Spine. 2000; 25(9):1171–1177

[23] Sim E, Vaccaro AR, Berzlanovich A, Pienaar S. The effects of staged static cervical flexion-distraction deformities on the patency of the vertebral arterial vasculature. Spine. 2000; 25(17):2180–2186

[24] Friedman D, Flanders A, Thomas C, Millar W. Vertebral artery injury after acute cervical spine trauma: rate of occurrence as detected by MR angiography and assessment of clinical consequences. AJR Am J Roentgenol. 1995; 164(2):443–447, discussion 448–449

[25] Deen HG, Jr, McGirr SJ. Vertebral artery injury associated with cervical spine fracture. Report of two cases. Spine. 1992; 17(2):230–234

[26] Quint DJ, Spickler EM. Magnetic resonance demonstration of vertebral artery dissection. Report of two cases. J Neurosurg. 1990; 72(6):964–967

[27] Heros RC. Cerebellar infarction resulting from traumatic occlusion of a vertebral artery. Case report. J Neurosurg. 1979; 51(1):111–113

[28] Six EG, Stringer WL, Cowley AR, Davis CH, Jr. Posttraumatic bilateral vertebral artery occlusion: case report. J Neurosurg. 1981; 54(6):814–817

[29] Torina PJ, Flanders AE, Carrino JA, et al. Incidence of vertebral artery thrombosis in cervical spine trauma: correlation with severity of spinal cord injury. AJNR Am J Neuroradiol. 2005; 26(10):2645–2651

[30] Thaker NG, Turner JD, Cobb WS, et al. Computed tomographic angiography versus digital subtraction angiography for the postoperative detection of residual aneurysms: a single-institution series and meta-analysis. J Neurointerv Surg. 2011

[31] Eastman AL, Chason DP, Perez CL, McAnulty AL, Minei JP. Computed tomographic angiography for the diagnosis of blunt cervical vascular injury: is it ready for primetime? J Trauma. 2006; 60(5):925–929, discussion 929

[32] Lee TS, Ducic Y, Gordin E, Stroman D. Management of carotid artery trauma. Craniomaxillofac Trauma Reconstr. 2014; 7(3):175–189

[33] Malhotra A, Kalra VB, Wu X, Grant R, Bronen RA, Abbed KM. Imaging of lumbar spinal surgery complications. Insights Imaging. 2015; 6(6):579–590

[34] Biffl WL, Moore EE, Elliott JP, et al. The devastating potential of blunt vertebral arterial injuries. Ann Surg. 2000; 231(5):672–681

[35] Yang L, Ran H. The advantage of ultrasonography in the diagnosis of extracranial vertebral artery dissection: two case reports. Medicine (Baltimore). 2017; 96(12):e6379

[36] Thibodeaux LC, Hearn AT, Peschiera JL, et al. Extracranial vertebral artery dissection after trauma: a 5-year review. Br J Surg. 1997; 84(1):94

[37] Schellinger PD, Schwab S, Krieger D, et al. Masking of vertebral artery dissection by severe trauma to the cervical spine. Spine. 2001; 26(3):314–319

[38] Hadley MN, Walters BC, Grabb PA, et al. Management of vertebral artery injuries after nonpenetrating cervical trauma. Neurosurgery. 2002; 50(3) Suppl:S173–S178

[39] Spaniolas K, Velmahos GC, Alam HB, de Moya M, Tabbara M, Sailhamer E. Does improved detection of blunt vertebral artery injuries lead to improved outcomes? Analysis of the National Trauma Data Bank. World J Surg. 2008; 32(10):2190–2194

[40] Desouza RM, Crocker MJ, Haliasos N, Rennie A, Saxena A. Blunt traumatic vertebral artery injury: a clinical review. Eur Spine J. 2011; 20(9):1405–1416

[41] Markus HS, Hayter E, Levi C, Feldman A, Venables G, Norris J, CADISS trial investigators. Antiplatelet treatment compared with anticoagulation treatment for cervical artery dissection (CADISS): a randomised trial. Lancet Neurol. 2015; 14(4):361–367

[42] Engelter ST, Brandt T, Debette S, et al. Cervical Artery Dissection in Ischemic Stroke Patients (CADISP) Study Group. Antiplatelets versus anticoagulation in cervical artery dissection. Stroke. 2007; 38(9):2605–2611

[43] Willis BK, Greiner F, Orrison WW, Benzel EC. The incidence of vertebral artery injury after midcervical spine fracture or subluxation. Neurosurgery. 1994; 34(3):435–441, discussion 441–442

[44] Miller PR, Fabian TC, Bee TK, et al. Blunt cerebrovascular injuries: diagnosis and treatment. J Trauma. 2001; 51(2):279–285, discussion 285–286

[45] Desouza RM, Crocker MJ, Haliasos N, Rennie A, Saxena A. Blunt traumatic vertebral artery injury: a clinical review. Eur Spine J. 2011; 20(9):1405–1416

[46] Sack JA, Etame AB, Shah GV, La Marca F, Park P. Management and outcomes of patients undergoing surgery for traumatic cervical fracture-subluxation associated with an asymptomatic vertebral artery injury. J Spinal Disord Tech. 2009; 22(2):86–90

[47] Park HK, Jho HD. The management of vertebral artery injury in anterior cervical spine operation: a systematic review of published cases. Eur Spine J. 2012; 21(12):2475–2485

14 Sport-Related Cervical Spine Injuries and Return-to-Play Criteria

Amandeep Bhalla and Christopher M. Bono

Abstract

Intimate awareness among players, athletic organizations, and health care providers about sports-related cervical spine injuries is the key for prevention, management, and informed decision-making about return to play. Treatment decisions can have significant health, psychological, and economic implications for scholastic and professional athletes alike. Cervical spine injuries can occur during contact and noncontact sports, ranging from minor muscle strains to catastrophic spinal cord injuries (SCIs). Athletes with underlying cervical canal stenosis are at particular risk for spinal cord neurapraxia, characterized by transient motor and/or sensory deficits in all four extremities. Physicians and first responders at organized sporting events should have established protocols for emergent initial assessment and treatment strategies in the event of an on-field injury. Athletes with suspected cervical spine injuries should undergo neurological evaluation and be handled with spinal precautions to prevent secondary injury. Factors influencing return-to-play decisions should be specific to the athlete, underlying anatomy, injury type, and sport, while considering the degree of ongoing symptoms. Although some injuries can be career ending, many athletes are often able to return to sport after appropriate treatment, provided the potential for substantial reinjury is minimized. Prudently, an athlete should be healed, demonstrate a neurologically intact exam, be free of pain, and have full strength and range of motion prior to returning to sport.

Keywords: spinal cord injury, sport injuries, cervical fractures, sprains and strains, burners, cervical cord neurapraxia, cervical disc herniations

14.1 Epidemiology

Cervical spine injuries are common and range from relatively minor injuries, such as muscle strains, to life-threatening, unstable fractures or dislocations with spinal cord injury (SCI). Although cervical spine injuries are most common in athletes who participate in organized contact and collision sports, such as rugby, American football, and hockey, they frequently occur in those also who participate in noncontact sports, such as baseball, gymnastics, cycling, skiing, snowboarding, and diving. While organized sports injuries are well studied, the injuries that occur during recreational sporting activities are likely underreported but can be just as devastating. Athletes with underlying conditions, such as congenital spinal stenosis, may be more likely to sustain a serious spinal cord injury (SCI).

In the United States, cervical spine injuries are the most common axial skeletal injuries, though less than 1% result in fractures, dislocations, or SCI.[1] Catastrophic cervical SCI, though rare, is an inherent risk of high-velocity collision sports. Sports-related SCI occurs at a mean age of 24 years.[2] While the incidence of sports-related SCI was about 14% in the 1970s,[3] this has decreased over time due to increased public awareness, safer rules governing play, and improved protective equipment. Indicative of the progress made in prevention of sports-related catastrophic cervical spine injuries, recent studies report the rate of all SCI attributable to athletic activities has decreased to 8%.[4,5]

The most common mechanism for cervical SCI in contact supports is applied axial load.[6] Scrum and tackle in rugby account for most of the cervical trauma in that sport. Tackling and blocking are two of the most frequent mechanisms that result in cervical injuries in American football. Unfortunately, an increase in the rate of catastrophic cervical spine injuries coincided with the advent of modern helmets as head protection encouraged playing techniques that enabled use of the top of the helmet as the initial point of contact for blocks and tackles.[7] Similar phenomena have been observed in other sports such as ice hockey.[8]

Increased awareness and public education about the dangers of spear tackling (i.e., tackling with the crown of the head) have led to a marked decrease in the number of serious cervical spine injuries in American football.[6,9] In 1976, the National Collegiate Athletic Association Football Rules Committee and high school football governing bodies banned headfirst contact.[10] Repetitive traumatic axial loads from spear tackling result in loss of normal cervical lordosis, vertebral abnormalities, and eventual cervical spinal stenosis[9] (▶ Fig. 14.1). In the 12 years

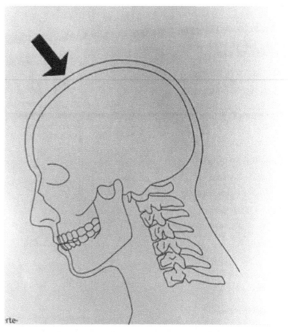

Fig. 14.1 Illustration depicting the mechanism of force of spear tackler spine. The straightened cervical spine (in tackle position) enables axial load to be directly transmitted to the anterior cervical vertebrae which obviates a large degree of posterior soft-tissue energy absorption. (Reproduced from Vaccaro A, Fehlings M, Dvorak M. Spine and Spinal Cord Trauma: Evidence Based Management. Thieme, 2011.)

following the implementation of rules barring headfirst tackling and blocking, the rate of cervical SCIs in scholastic football declined by 70%.[3,6] Changes in rules governing the play of Canadian ice hockey, specifically preventing checking from behind, have also markedly decreased the incidence of cervical injuries.[11]

In a study of spine injuries in the National Football League spanning from 2000 to 2010, 44.7% of injuries were of the cervical spine. The mean time missed for play was 120 days for a cervical fracture and 85 days for cervical disc degeneration/herniation.[1] In an epidemiologic review of catastrophic cervical spine injuries in high school and collegiate athletes between 1989 and 2002, Boden et al[12] noted an average of 15 catastrophic cervical spine injuries per year in scholastic football players, which included transient cord neurapraxia and C1 and C2 fractures. The reported traumatic quadriplegia rate was 5 per 100,000 high school athletes and 1 per 100,000 college athletes. In 2002, the incidence of traumatic quadriplegia for high school athletes and college athletes was down to 0.38 per 100,000 and 1.33 per 100,000, respectively.[7] Although rates of catastrophic injuries have decreased over time, participants in high-energy contact sports continue to be at risk.

14.2 Initial Management

An athlete who reports axial or radiating pain, decreased range of motion of neck, or loss of function should be removed from play and undergo full neurological examination. In the event a structural or neurological injury is suspected, the athlete's neck should be immobilized in a rigid cervical collar. An unconscious player should be treated as though the cervical spine is unstable until proven otherwise. Strict spinal precautions are instituted, including placement on a rigid backboard, while the patient is transferred to a trauma center. Protective helmets and shoulder pads worn by some players can hinder initial evaluation. If the injured athlete is wearing a helmet, the facemask should be removed to facilitate access to the airway, however the helmet itself should remain in place until there are several people available to help with its removal in a controlled environment, usually in a hospital setting. To ensure appropriate alignment, the helmet and shoulder pads should be removed at the same time to avoid undue flexion or extension of the neck. Improper handling of an unstable cervical spine could lead to additional displacement and potentially worsening of neurological injury or even lead to cardiopulmonary compromise.

14.3 Specific Injuries

14.3.1 Strains and Sprains

Injuries to cervical paraspinal muscles and ligaments are commonly encountered in sports. Muscular strains, contusions, and ligamentous sprains are self-limited injuries. Of note, it is imperative to rule out occult destabilizing ligamentous injuries. With a high index of suspicion, stability can be confirmed with further imaging. Dynamic flexion-extension radiographs have played a vital role in the past. Based on classic cadaveric studies, when all cervical spinal ligaments are intact, horizontal movement of one vertebra on the next should not exceed 3.5 mm,

and the angular displacement of one vertebra on the next is typically 11 degrees or less.[13,14] However, many feel these thresholds are too high. Furthermore, distortions in measurements may occur in patients with cervical muscle spasms; while in younger athletes, additional physiologic ligamentous laxity can lead to pseudosubluxation. In cases of pseudosubluxation or significant neck spasm, it is prudent to maintain young athletes within a cervical collar for approximately 3 weeks, after which repeat dynamic cervical radiographs can be performed. At that time, if the athlete is free of pain and has full range of motion without radiographic instability, sports can be resumed.

Though somewhat outside the scope of this chapter, detecting occult cervical ligamentous injuries in obtunded injured athletes deserves some mention. As per general trauma protocols, high-energy injury mechanisms warrant at least computed tomography (CT) imaging to rule out subluxations or fractures not perceptible on plain radiographs. Furthermore, CT scan offers superior visualization of the occipitocervical and cervicothoracic junctions compared to plain radiographs. Though some disagree, magnetic resonance imaging (MRI) might be warranted if further suspicion of ligamentous disruption remains despite a negative CT scan.[15,16]

14.3.2 Cervical Fractures and Dislocations

A broad range of cervical fractures may be sustained during contact sports. Majority of fractures and dislocations occur in the lower cervical spine. Stable cervical spinal fractures involving a spinous process or lamina can be treated symptomatically. In such cases, flexion and extension radiographs should be obtained to rule out ligamentous injury. Sports may be resumed once osseous healing is complete and painless range of motion is restored. Upper cervical spinal fractures are relatively uncommon in this population. Of them, odontoid fractures are the most common in athletes.[17] Many odontoid fractures in the young athletes may be treated with a hard collar or a halo vest, however anterior screw fixation or posterior C1–C2 arthrodesis may be warranted in cases of neurological injury or significant displacement.[15] Most C1 fractures are stable; however, unstable C1 burst fractures associated with C1–C2 instability may require instrumented fusion. The functional limitations and risks of adjacent injury following upper cervical fusion represent one of the absolute contraindications to return-to-play.

Axial load mechanisms are a common cause of sports-related cervical spine morbidity. The response of the spine to applied axial load depends on the position of the neck at the time of injury. Axial forces applied across a relatively flexed neck result in flexion forces on the anterior elements and distractive forces on the posterior elements. Energy from this mechanism may result in a so-called teardrop fracture involving the anteroinferior vertebral body[7] while simultaneously causing distractive injury to the posterior structures. Disruption of the stabilizing posterior soft-tissue elements, including the supraspinous ligament, interspinous ligaments, and facet capsules, is the critical component leading to instability and decisions regarding management.

Disruption of the posterior ligamentous structures without vertebral body fractures can result in bilateral facet subluxation or frank dislocation with or without subsequent SCI. The addition of a rotational movement to an axial load in flexion can lead to unilateral facet dislocations that are inherently more stable than bilateral injuries and are less likely to lead to SCI. Regardless of the exact mechanism, disruption of the posterior ligamentous complex usually necessitates surgical stabilization to restore stability.

Axial load applied across a neutrally aligned neck is more likely to result in a compression fracture of the vertebral body. With greater and more abruptly delivered energy, a burst fracture may result in which there is, by definition, a free fragment of the posterior vertebral body wall. Burst fractures in neurologically intact patients with reasonable alignment are usually treated by a hard collar, unless there is concomitant disruption to the posterior ligamentous complex. Patients with C7 burst fractures, because of their location at the cervicothoracic junction, have a higher risk for developing progressive kyphotic deformity, thereby warranting more diligent radiographic observation and employment of nonoperative treatment regimen[4] (▶ Fig. 14.2). Surgical stabilization may be required to mitigate progressive deformity progression.

Though they can occur from a variety of mechanisms, the smaller articular surface area of cervical facet joints makes them more susceptible to dislocation via a flexion-distraction mechanism. Cervical facet dislocations in the setting of neurological injury warrant urgent reduction at a trauma or SCI center. Given that timely reduction is believed to be a critical factor, particularly for patients with incomplete SCI, it is reasonable to perform a closed reduction with traction in the awake patient who cooperates with serial neurological examinations. MRI is advised prior to any manipulation in obtunded or noncooperative patients. Following reduction in the awake and cooperative patient, MRI may be obtained to rule out intervertebral disc injury and to guide operative decision-making, particularly if posterior surgery is planned.

14.3.3 Burners or Stingers

The terms "burner" and "stinger" are used interchangeably in the literature. While not precisely cervical spine injuries, both describe common athletic injuries from insult to the brachial plexus or an exiting cervical nerve root, resulting in sudden nondermatomal pain and paresthesias in a single extremity. Weakness may or may not be associated with the injury. The defining characteristic that differentiates burners from a central spinal cord process is the involvement of only one extremity. Several mechanisms may cause a burner: stretch injury to the brachial plexus from ipsilateral shoulder depression and contralateral neck flexion, direct blunt trauma to the brachial plexus at Erb's point superior to the clavicle, and compression of the exiting cervical nerve root with neck extension and lateral bending.[4,18]

Symptoms are usually self-limiting and resolve in a short period of time. In athletes with recurrent or chronic burners, the etiology is more likely to be the result of nerve root compression in the intervertebral neuroforamina secondary to cervical disc disease.[19] Younger athletes with a lower prevalence of cervical disc disease are more likely to have sustained trauma outside of the spine and within the brachial plexus itself. It is reasonable in such cases to obtain a cervical spine MRI to rule out the possibility of a significant disc herniation. Electromyography may be considered for athletes with more than several weeks of persistent symptoms to determine the presence of a cervical root injury versus brachial plexopathy. Athletes may return to sport after resolution of symptoms provided they demonstrate full strength and range of motion. The athlete and coaching staff should be counseled that recurrence remains unpredictable and is a risk. Modification of tackling techniques, in conjunction with rehabilitation and paraspinal muscle strengthening, may be effective in preventing or decreasing the rate of recurrence.[20]

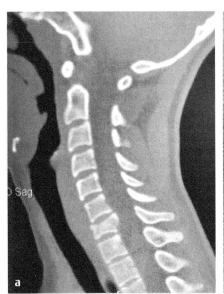
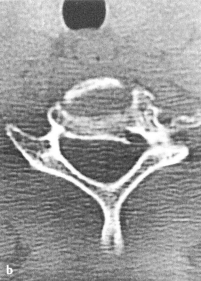
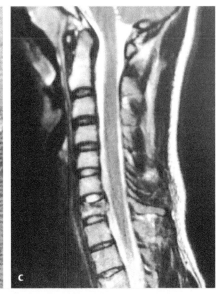

Fig. 14.2 Sagittal **(a)** and axial **(b)** computed tomography (CT) images of the cervical spine and sagittal T2-weighted magnetic resonance imaging (MRI) slice **(c)** demonstrating a traumatic C7 burst fracture following an axial load injury. (Reproduced from: Vaccaro A, Fehlings M, Dvorak M. Spine and Spinal Cord Trauma: Evidence Based Management. Thieme, 2011.)

14.3.4 Cervical Cord Neurapraxia or Transient Quadriplegia

Distinct from burners, a traumatic injury to the neck may result in transient bilateral or sensory or motor deficits which has been termed cervical cord neurapraxia or transient quadriplegia. Neurological symptoms involving more than one extremity should prompt concern for spinal cord involvement. Cervical spinal cord neurapraxia has been estimated to occur in 7 per 10,000 football players.[21] It is thought to be the result of transient spinal cord compression or concussive cord injury causing physiologic conduction block without anatomic disruption of neuronal tracts. Episodes can last from minutes to several days.[22] These injuries may occur from momentary cord compression endured during extreme neck flexion or extension. Hyperextension can cause an inward buckling of the ligamentum flavum resulting in cord compression.

Transient quadriplegia may herald an underlying anatomic abnormality such as congenital, developmental, or degenerative cervical stenosis (▶ Fig. 14.3). Athletes may also have congenital conditions such as Klippel–Feil syndrome which refers to a failure of cervical vertebral segmentation, resulting in a reduced number of segments among which to dissipate load.[23,24] This predisposes the spine to traumatic injury. Developmental dens hypoplasia, or os odontoideum, may contribute to atlantoaxial instability and increase the risk for traumatic upper cervical SCI. Of note, regardless of the presence of transient quadriplegia, both Klippel–Feil syndrome and dens hypoplasia are absolute contraindications to participation in contact sports. Horizontal C3–C4 cervical facet orientation and relative hypermobility of the neck in extension have also been implicated as contributing factors for transient quadriparesis.[25]

In an early, large case series following 110 athletes who sustained cord neurapraxia, a high recurrence rate (56%) was noted. However, no subsequent permanent neurological deficits were reported over the ensuing follow-up period.[26] Given an approximate 50% rate of recurrence, it is advisable for athletes who have experienced a cervical cord neurapraxia event to refrain from contact sports altogether.[4] This, however, remains controversial.

Attempts have been made to identify at-risk players. In a study of National Football League (NFL) predraft athletes, Schroeder et al reported that a diagnosis of cervical spinal pathology had been made in 4.8% of athletes, with the most common diagnoses being spondylosis, stenosis, and disc herniation.[27] However, screening for cervical spinal stenosis in patients who plan to participate in contact sports is not cost effective. Likewise, it is difficult to determine whether an athlete with relative cervical stenosis may be at truly higher risk for neurological injury. Prospectively followed NFL athletes with known absolute cervical spinal stenosis, and a history of previous surgery, have demonstrated no difference in performance-based outcomes and no reports of neurological injury during their careers.[27] Ultimately, it is difficult to know whether an asymptomatic patient with cervical stenosis may be at increased risk for transient neurapraxia and therefore relative stenosis is not considered as a contraindication to play. Athletes with significant cervical spinal stenosis should be counseled on the increased risks for SCI before participation in athletics.

Management of patients who sustain cervical cord neurapraxia differs on the basis of whether there is underlying cervical stenosis or predisposing ligamentous laxity. Athletes who have experienced an episode of transient quadriplegia with known cervical stenosis should not participate in contact sports. These athletes, by virtue of the neuropraxic event, have effectively demonstrated diminished functional neurological capacity for contact sports. Athletes with ligamentous instability and a history of cervical cord neurapraxia without appreciable central stenosis, should also refrain from contact sports. Consideration for return-to-play is given to athletes with full neurological recovery without evidence of spinal stenosis, cord compression/ edema, or ligamentous laxity.[22]

Although there is insufficient evidence correlating spinal canal narrowing and permanent neurological injury,[28] retrospective MRI studies of cervical spinal cord-injured athletes demonstrated statistically significantly smaller space available for the spinal cord. Aebli et al found that patients with a disc-level canal diameter of 8 mm or less measured on MRI are at risk of acute SCI after a minor trauma to the cervical spine.[29] It is worth noting, however, that a diameter of 8 mm or less is already beyond the threshold for absolute stenosis, which is typically defined as a canal diameter < 10 mm.

14.3.5 Cervical Disc Herniations

Acute herniation of the nucleus pulposus of the intervertebral disc through the annulus fibrosus may occur with sports-related neck trauma. There is a higher rate of cervical interver-

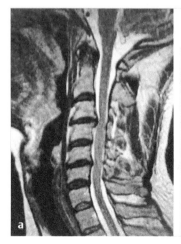
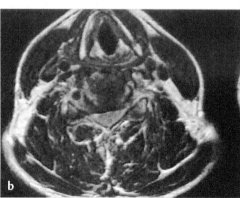

Fig. 14.3 Sagittal (a) and axial (b) T2-weighted magnetic resonance images (MRI) showing congenital cervical stenosis in a patient who sustained a cervical cord neurapraxia. (Reproduced from Vaccaro A, Fehlings M, Dvorak M. Spine and Spinal Cord Trauma: Evidence Based Management. Thieme, 2011.)

tebral disc herniation with contact sports compared to the general population. Noncontact sports may have a protective effect against cervical disc herniations due to increased dynamic muscular support of the cervical spine.[3,30] Symptomatic cervical disc herniations may present with radicular pain, sensory changes, or weakness in the distribution of the affected peripheral nerve. More significant central disc herniations with compression of the cord can lead to acute cervical myelopathy and warrant surgical decompression to mitigate risk for neurological progression. Cervical disc herniations accounted for 5.8% of cervical spine injuries in NFL athletes between 2000 and 2010 and have been found to cause significant morbidity and missed playing time.[1] Hsu et al examined performance-based outcomes of NFL athletes treated for cervical disc herniations, finding that players who undergo surgical treatment have a higher return-to-play-rate and longer careers compared to players treated nonoperatively.[31]

14.4 Return to Play Criteria

Decision-making about return-to-play is focused on optimizing recovery as well as preventing further injury. Unfortunately, current guidelines are based on expert opinion and professional experience. Experts uniformly agree, however, that prior to any player's return to play from a cervical sports injury, the athlete should be neurologically intact and have full strength and range of motion. Given the unique circumstances of each player's injury, symptoms, and underlying anatomy, return-to-play decision-making is complex. It is, therefore, not surprising that there are no well-defined algorithms to which athletic organizations adhere.

In general, the likelihood of return-to-play is high for burners though some practitioners do not allow athletes to return for the remainder of the season if they have sustained three or more burners within 1 year.[32] The likelihood for a safe return-to-play is lower for patients who have sustained episodes of transient cervical neurapraxia. Some experts contend that patients with transient neurapraxia without stenosis or ligamentous laxity may return to play, though this is controversial and continues to be debated. Patients with concomitant stenosis and ligamentous laxity should refrain from play.[22]

In cases necessitating surgical intervention, adequate healing and restoration of spinal structural integrity are important factors in determining safe return-to-play. Contact sports after posterior laminoforaminotomy for cervical root decompression are considered safe as there is minimal surgical alteration of the integrity of the spinal column. Following a single-level anterior cervical discectomy and fusion (ACDF), provided there are no residual neurological deficits, there is good range of motion, and radiographs demonstrate solid fusion, athletes may return to contact sports. There are mixed views on safe return-to-play after two-level ACDF. However, most believe the longer lever arm and biomechanical changes of a three-level ACDF preclude safe return to contact sports.[3]

Succinctly based on a review of the literature and expert opinion, Kepler and Vaccaro proposed nine absolute contraindications to return to intense athletic activity after cervical spine fracture: occipitocervical arthrodesis, atlantoaxial insta-

bility, spear tackler spine, residual subaxial spine instability, substantial sagittal malalignment, narrowing of the spinal canal as a result of retropulsed fragments, residual neurological deficits, loss of normal cervical spine range of motion, and arthrodesis of three or more disc levels.[32] There are limited data on safe return-to-play after cervical disc arthroplasty,[33] a motion-preserving treatment option that is becoming more prevalent.

14.5 Conclusion

Improved posttraumatic care coordination and increased awareness of injury prevention techniques have contributed to the decrease in catastrophic sports-related cervical spine injuries over time. Physicians who cover athletic events must have a thorough knowledge of cervical spine injuries and neurological sequelae and should practice rehearsed protocols for emergent management of these patients. An athlete should be without neurological deficit, pain-free, and with full range of motion and strength prior to returning to sport. Due it its high visibility and significant economic footprint, American football has benefited from significant research to improve participant safety. Additional efforts in research and public education about sports-related cervical spine injuries would be sure to benefit recreational, scholastic, and professional athletic participants across a range of sports.

References

[1] Mall NA, Buchowski J, Zebala L, Brophy RH, Wright RW, Matava MJ. Spine and axial skeleton injuries in the National Football League. Am J Sports Med. 2012; 40(8):1755–1761

[2] DeVivo MJ. Causes and costs of spinal cord injury in the United States. Spinal Cord. 1997; 35(12):809–813

[3] Rosenthal BD, Boody BS, Hsu WK. Return to play for athletes. Neurosurg Clin N Am. 2017; 28(1):163–171

[4] Schroeder GD, Vaccaro AR. Cervical spine injuries in the athlete. J Am Acad Orthop Surg. 2016; 24(9):e122–e133

[5] National Spinal Cord Injury Statistical Center. Spinal cord injury facts and figures at a glance. J Spinal Cord Med. 2013; 36(1):1–2

[6] Torg JS, Vegso JJ, O'Neill MJ, Sennett B. The epidemiologic, pathologic, biomechanical, and cinematographic analysis of football-induced cervical spine trauma. Am J Sports Med. 1990; 18(1):50–57

[7] Banerjee R, Palumbo MA, Fadale PD. Catastrophic cervical spine injuries in the collision sport athlete, part 1: epidemiology, functional anatomy, and diagnosis. Am J Sports Med. 2004; 32(4):1077–1087

[8] Tator CH, Carson JD, Cushman R. Hockey injuries of the spine in Canada, 1966–1996. CMAJ. 2000; 162(6):787–788

[9] Torg JS, Sennett B, Pavlov H, Leventhal MR, Glasgow SG. Spear tackler's spine. An entity precluding participation in tackle football and collision activities that expose the cervical spine to axial energy inputs. Am J Sports Med. 1993; 21(5):640–649

[10] Torg JS, Truex R, Jr, Quedenfeld TC, Burstein A, Spealman A, Nichols C, III. The National Football Head and Neck Injury Registry. Report and conclusions 1978. JAMA. 1979; 241(14):1477–1479

[11] Tator CH, Provvidenza C, Cassidy JD. Spinal injuries in Canadian ice hockey: an update to 2005. Clin J Sport Med. 2009; 19(6):451–456

[12] Boden BP, Tacchetti RL, Cantu RC, Knowles SB, Mueller FO. Catastrophic cervical spine injuries in high school and college football players. Am J Sports Med. 2006; 34(8):1223–1232

[13] Cantu RC, Li YM, Abdulhamid M, Chin LS. Return to play after cervical spine injury in sports. Curr Sports Med Rep. 2013; 12(1):14–17

[14] White AA, III, Panjabi MM. The basic kinematics of the human spine. A review of past and current knowledge. Spine. 1978; 3(1):12–20

[15] Hsu WK, Anderson PA. Odontoid fractures: update on management. J Am Acad Orthop Surg. 2010; 18(7):383–394

[16] Simon JB, Schoenfeld AJ, Katz JN, et al. Are "normal" multidetector computed tomographic scans sufficient to allow collar removal in the trauma patient? J Trauma. 2010; 68(1):103–108

[17] Dodwell ER, Kwon BK, Hughes B, et al. Spinal column and spinal cord injuries in mountainbikers:a13-yearreview.AmJSportsMed.2010;38(8):1647–1652

[18] Meyer SA, Schulte KR, Callaghan JJ, et al. Cervical spinal stenosis and stingers in collegiate football players. Am J Sports Med. 1994; 22(2):158–166

[19] Levitz CL, Reilly PJ, Torg JS. The pathomechanics of chronic, recurrent cervical nerve root neurapraxia. The chronic burner syndrome. Am J Sports Med. 1997; 25(1):73–76

[20] Weinberg J, Rokito S, Silber JS. Etiology, treatment, and prevention of athletic "stingers". Clin Sports Med. 2003; 22(3):493–500, viii

[21] Torg JS, Guille JT, Jaffe S. Injuries to the cervical spine in American football players. J Bone Joint Surg Am. 2002; 84-A(1):112–122

[22] Dailey A, Harrop JS, France JC. High-energy contact sports and cervical spine neuropraxia injuries: what are the criteria for return to participation? Spine. 2010; 35(21) Suppl:S193–S201

[23] Bailes JE. Experience with cervical stenosis and temporary paralysis in athletes. J Neurosurg Spine. 2005; 2(1):11–16

[24] Torg JS, Pavlov H, Genuario SE, et al. Neurapraxia of the cervical spinal cord with transient quadriplegia. J Bone Joint Surg Am. 1986; 68(9):1354–1370

[25] Brigham CD, Capo J. Cervical spinal cord contusion in professional athletes: a case series with implications for return to play. Spine. 2013; 38(4):315–323

[26] Torg JS, Corcoran TA, Thibault LE, et al. Cervical cord neurapraxia: classification, pathomechanics, morbidity, and management guidelines. J Neurosurg. 1997; 87(6):843–850

[27] Schroeder GD, Lynch TS, Gibbs DB, et al. The impact of a cervical spine diagnosis on the careers of National Football League athletes. Spine. 2014; 39(12):947–952

[28] Torg JS, Naranja RJ, Jr, Pavlov H, Galinat BJ, Warren R, Stine RA. The relationship of developmental narrowing of the cervical spinal canal to reversible and irreversible injury of the cervical spinal cord in football players. J Bone Joint Surg Am. 1996; 78(9):1308–1314

[29] Aebli N, Rüegg TB, Wicki AG, Petrou N, Krebs J. Predicting the risk and severity of acute spinal cord injury after a minor trauma to the cervical spine. Spine J. 2013; 13(6):597–604

[30] Zmurko MG, Tannoury TY, Tannoury CA, Anderson DG. Cervical sprains, disc herniations, minor fractures, and other cervical injuries in the athlete. Clin Sports Med. 2003; 22(3):513–521

[31] Hsu WK. Outcomes following nonoperative and operative treatment for cervical disc herniations in National Football League athletes. Spine. 2011; 36(10):800–805

[32] Kepler CK, Vaccaro AR. Injuries and abnormalities of the cervical spine and return to play criteria. Clin Sports Med. 2012; 31(3):499–508

[33] Kang DG, Anderson JC, Lehman RA, Jr. Return to play after cervical disc surgery. Clin Sports Med. 2016; 35(4):529–543

15 Craniovertebral Injuries in Pediatric Patients

A. Karim Ahmed, Randall J. Hlubek, and Nicholas Theodore

Abstract

The craniovertebral junction has a unique and complicated anatomy. The patterns of injury in this location include longitudinal subluxation with failure of stabilization, translational atlantoaxial subluxation, atlantoaxial rotatory fixation, and fractures. However, ligamentous injuries in the absence of fractures are most commonly seen in pediatric patients. The diagnosis and treatment of craniovertebral injuries in pediatric patients are multimodal, requiring an appreciation for the unique anatomy, mechanisms of injury, and developmental considerations of this population.

Keywords: atlantoaxial rotatory fixation, fracture, ligamentous injury, longitudinal, subluxation, translational atlantoaxial

15.1 Craniovertebral Anatomy

The occiput articulates with the cervical spine at C1, the atlas. The bilateral anterior and posterior arches form the ring of the atlas, with the center of each arch indicated by a tubercle (i.e., anterior and posterior tubercles). The lateral edges of the central canal are formed by the lateral masses; the foramen transversarium and the transverse processes are encountered with further lateral progression.

The cervical spine imparts mobility to the head, serves as the point of attachment for key muscles of the back and neck, protects essential vasculature, and houses nerves that innervate critical musculature. Although the cervical spine is not a load-bearing structure at rest, it may function as a shock absorber in cases of blunt force to the skull.

Cephalad to the lateral masses, the atlas contains two large facet joints for the occipital condyles. The occipital condyles are located on the inferior portion of the skull at the occipital bone. Of note, the foramen magnum and medial portion of the posterior fossa are also constituents of the occipital bone. In addition, the basion and opisthion are important landmarks demarcating the midpoint of the anterior and posterior aspects of the foramen magnum, respectively.

The atlanto-occipital joint allows for most of the vertical motion of the head. The posterior surface of the anterior tubercle contains a facet joint to articulate with the dens of C2, the axis. The inferior articulating facets of the atlas and the superior articulating facets of the axis form a synovial joint. The atlantoaxial junction allows for rotational movement of the head and is the only set of two contiguous, unfused vertebrae that does not contain an intervertebral disc. Any load to the atlantoaxial junction is thus transmitted through the lateral masses—unlike in caudal spinal levels, where the load is transmitted through the intervertebral discs and vertebral bodies.[1,2,3,4]

An understanding of the anatomy and function of the ligaments that span from the occiput to the axis is critical for understanding the motion of the head and traumatic injury.

The apical ligament of the dens is a fibrous midline structure connecting the cephalad portion of the dens to the anterior margin of the foramen magnum. The bilateral alar ligaments span superolaterally from the dens to the occipital condyles, restricting excessive rotation of the head. The transverse ligament of the atlas attaches to the medial surfaces of the C1 lateral masses, forming a strong band that prevents dissociation of the dens. The midline of the transverse ligament has both a superior projection, which connects to the foramen magnum, and an inferior projection, which connects to the body of the axis. The entire structure is known as the *cruciform ligament*, or *cruciate ligament,* of the atlas. Furthermore, a ligament known as the *tectorial membrane* descends from the clivus and travels along the anterior aspect of the central canal, eventually becoming the posterior longitudinal ligament.[5]

The axis and each subsequent caudal vertebra down to the sacrum contains an intervertebral disc and bilateral synovial joints articulating two adjacent vertebrae. The foramen transversarium of the first six cervical vertebrae house the vertebral arteries that arise from the first portion of the subclavian artery. The vertebral arteries are divided into four segments: V1 is preforaminal, spanning from its origin at the subclavian artery to the C6 foramen transversarium; V2 is foraminal and extends through the foramina transversaria from C6 to C2; V3 is extradural, spanning from C2 to the dura and V4 is intradural, combining with its contralateral artery to form the basilar artery at the anterior surface of the pons. Caudally, the vertebral arteries have two branches that combine in the midline to form the anterior spinal artery. The dorsal spinal arteries are branches from the posterior inferior cerebellar arteries or, less commonly, direct branches from the vertebral arteries. The single anterior spinal artery and dual posterior spinal arteries supply most of the spinal cord. In the cervical spine, segmental spinal arteries arise from the vertebral and cervical arteries, from posterior intercostal arteries in the thoracic spine, and from lumbar arteries in the abdomen. Branches of the segmental spinal arteries — the anterior and posterior radicular arteries — supply anterior and posterior nerve roots. The segmental spinal arteries further branch into segmental medullary arteries that join the anterior spinal artery. The largest of the segmental medullary arteries is the artery of Adamkiewicz.

Motor innervation from the cervical spine is pivotal for upper extremity mobility and respiration. The phrenic nerve, from C3 to C5, provides motor innervation to the diaphragm. The brachial plexus is from C5 to T1. In addition, C5 and C6 form most of the axillary nerve, C5 to C7 form the musculocutaneous nerve, C6 to T1 form the median nerve, C5 to T1 form the radial nerve, and C8 and T1 form the ulnar nerve. Abduction of the arm is primarily conducted by the C5 nerve, flexion of the elbow by C6, extension of the elbow by C7, flexion of the digits by C8, and adduction and abduction of the digits by T1.[1]

15.2 Embryology and Development

The pattern of ossification that the atlas and axis undergo in early life is an essential consideration in assessing the extent of trauma to the craniovertebral junction. The occipital and first three cervical somites give rise to the craniovertebral junction, with the four occipital somites forming most of the skull base.[2] During embryonic development, the atlas contains a posterior midline synchondrosis between the paired neural arches and paired neurocentral synchondroses between the bilateral neural arches and anterior arch. Ossification of the anterior arch occurs between 3 months and 1 year of age, and ossification of the posterior arch is complete by 3 years of age. The neurocentral synchondroses fuse at about 7 years of age.

The axis undergoes three phases of ossification, with the first at 4 months of fetal life, the second at 6 months of fetal life, and the third at about 3 to 5 years of postnatal life. The first wave of ossification involves the bilateral neural arches and the centrum. The second involves bilateral ossification centers at the basal dental segment. The third ossification center is at the apical dental segment at the tip of the dens.[2]

The axis has paired primary ossification centers that fuse in the midline of the dens, as well as primary ossification centers at the neural arch and the body. In addition, a secondary ossification center is at the apex of the dens.

15.3 Mechanisms of Injury

Four primary injury patterns occur in the craniocervical junction of pediatric patients. These patterns are longitudinal subluxation with failure of stabilization, translational atlantoaxial subluxation, atlantoaxial rotatory fixation, and fractures.[2]

15.3.1 Longitudinal Subluxation

Longitudinal subluxation of the atlanto-occipital joint occurs because of ligamentous injury, often in high-speed motor vehicle collisions, and can lead to severe damage at the cervicomedullary junction. Atlanto-occipital dislocation (AOD) consists of a disarticulation of the occipital condyles from the atlas. AOD is almost always fatal if left untreated, and instrumented arthrodesis is necessary in all patients who survive. AOD accounts for 35% of fatal cervical spine injuries that result from motor vehicle crashes.[6,7] Three main categories of AOD are anterior displacement of the occiput (type I) (▶ Fig. 15.1a), vertical distraction of the occiput with respect to the atlas (type II) (▶ Fig. 15.1b), and posterior displacement of the occiput with respect to the atlas (type III) (▶ Fig. 15.1c).[2,8]

The transverse ligament and the apical ligament of the dens are the strongest ligaments in the atlanto-occipital junction and impart most of its stability.[5,6] Largely due to ligament laxity and the horizontal plane of articular surfaces, AOD is three times more common in pediatric patients than in adults.[2,6,9,10,11,12] Additional predisposing factors may include smaller atlanto-occipital joints and a greater ratio of head weight to body weight, which increases the likelihood of instability at that location.[2,6,7] The diagnosis of AOD is made on the basis of measurement of the basion–dens interval in the sagittal plane or the C1–condyle interval (CCI)—as will be discussed in detail later in this chapter.[2,9]

15.3.2 Translational Atlantoaxial Subluxation

Translational atlantoaxial subluxation is due to ligamentous instability between C1 and C2, resulting in anterior displacement of the atlas, relative to the axis. This subluxation is often attributed to injuries of the transverse ligament and may result in spinal cord compression anteriorly from the dens and posteriorly from the posterior arches of the atlas.[2,13] Translational atlantoaxial subluxation is often accompanied by wide fractures of the C1 ring and can be classified into two broad categories based on location. Differentiating type I from type II injuries is crucial in guiding treatment. Type I translational atlantoaxial subluxation necessitates internal fixation, whereas 74% of patients with type II injuries recover with nonoperative conservative management of the injuries.[2,14] Type I injuries are ligamentous, occurring at the midpoint of the transverse ligament (*type IA*) or at its periosteal insertion site (*type IB*). Type II injuries occur at the insertion sites of the transverse ligament to the C1 lateral masses and consist of a C1 comminuted fracture at the lateral masses (*type IIA*) or an avulsion fracture of the C1 tubercle of the lateral mass (*type IIB*).

15.3.3 Atlantoaxial Rotatory Subluxation

Atlantoaxial rotatory subluxation (AARS) involves varying degrees of atlantal dissociation and rotation and is best described by the Fielding and Hawkins classification, types I to IV (▶ Fig. 15.2).[15] The gold standard for imaging of AARS is three-dimensional computed tomography (CT) that can aid significantly in differentiating each type of AARS. Patients with AARS present with the head tilted toward and rotated away from the affected side. The acute presentation of this deformity must be differentiated from muscular torticollis as well as from possible trauma. In AARS, a reflexive sternocleidomastoid spasm occurs at the side of the chin, whereas in muscular torticollis, a sustained spasm occurs contralaterally.

As described by various authors, the subluxation that occurs in AARS is due to resistance in the natural rotation of the atlantoaxial junction.[2,16,17] The first 23 degrees of rotation in either direction occurs with independent motion of the atlas, relative to the axis. After the initial 23 degrees, tightening of the alar ligaments and nonlinear rotation of the dens accompany the subsequent 42 degrees of rotation. Any rotation after 65 degrees occurs with concurrent motion of the atlas and axis.

Type I Atlantoaxial Rotatory Subluxation

In type I AARS, the atlas has isolated rotation greater than 45 degrees, with the dens functioning as a pivot joint in the absence of any translational displacement. Type I is the most common type of AARS and may be treated by reduction and immobilization alone.

Type II Atlantoaxial Rotatory Subluxation

In type II AARS, the atlas is rotated, with one of the lateral articular processes functioning as the pivot joint and the contralateral articular process being disarticulated. Type II AARS

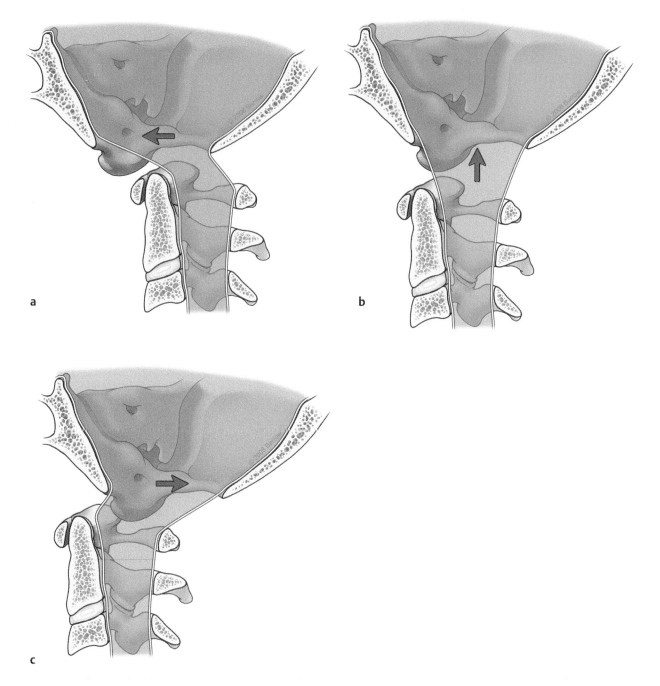

Fig. 15.1 Traynelis classification of atlanto-occipital dislocations. **(a)** Type I illustrates an anterior displacement (*arrow*) of the occiput. **(b)** Type II shows a vertical displacement (*arrow*). **(c)** Type III involves posterior displacement (*arrow*) of the occiput. (Used with permission from Barrow Neurological Institute, Phoenix, AZ.)

involves atlantal rotation exceeding 40 degrees and a defect of the transverse ligament only. Due to the disruption of the anatomic pivot joint in the atlantoaxial junction, type II AARS typically includes 3 to 5 mm of anterior displacement of the atlas relative to the axis. If diagnosed within 14 days, type II AARS may be treated by reduction and halo immobilization. However, diagnosis more than 14 days after an injury necessitates occipitoatlantoaxial or atlantoaxial fusion.

Type III Atlantoaxial Rotatory Subluxation

Type III AARS involves rotation of the atlas, with disarticulation of both lateral masses and anterior displacement of the atlas exceeding 5 mm relative to the axis. In addition, disruptions of both the alar and transverse ligaments are implicated in type III AARS. This category of AARS is treated with reduction and fusion.[2,15]

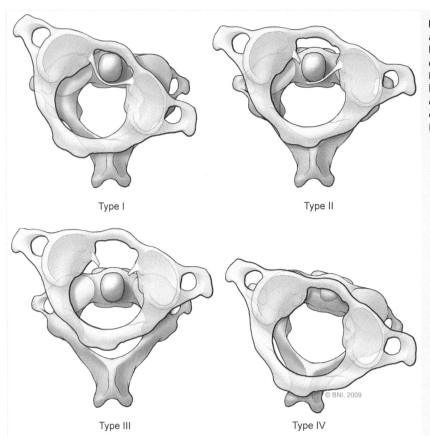

Fig. 15.2 Fielding and Hawkins classification of atlantoaxial rotatory subluxation. Type I is defined by an intact transverse ligament, type II by disruption of the transverse ligament alone, type III by disruption of the transverse and alar ligaments, and type IV by posterior rotatory displacement of the atlas on C2 in patients with odontoid hypoplasia. (Used with permission from Barrow Neurological Institute, Phoenix, AZ.)

Type I

Type II

Type III

Type IV

© BNI, 2009

Type IV Atlantoaxial Rotatory Subluxation

Type IV AARS is similar to type III in that both lateral masses are disarticulated, but type IV involves posterior displacement of the atlas relative to the axis, because of fracture or damage of the dens.[2,15] Similar to type III AARS, type IV is treated with reduction and fusion.[2,15]

15.3.4 Fractures in the Craniovertebral Junction

The craniovertebral junction is susceptible to many fracture patterns because of its complex anatomy and range of motion. Traumatic injury in this location, specific to children, often involves a synchondrosis, which typically fuses by 5 to 7 years of age.[2,18] True fracture of the odontoid synchondrosis results in anterior displacement of the dens with no abnormalities in the atlantodental interval.[2,18,19] Although nondisplaced fractures may be difficult to detect, both displaced and nondisplaced synchondrosis fractures are associated with spinal cord injury 53% of the time.[19,20] Prevertebral soft-tissue abnormality on magnetic resonance imaging (MRI) and evidence of synchondrosis widening on CT may be beneficial to diagnose a synchondrosis fracture. Fractures of the dens, as would be seen in adults, may occur in older children and are the most common fractures of the axis. In accordance with the Anderson and D'Alonzo classification,[21] types I, II, and III odontoid fractures occur at the tip of the dens, at the base, and through the body of C2, respectively.

The bilateral neurocentral synchondroses close between 3 and 6 years of age and should not be mistaken for a hangman fracture (i.e., a pars interarticularis fracture) on plain radiographs. Moreover, fractures of the neurocentral synchondroses are analogous to odontoid epiphysiolysis and can be adequately treated with external immobilization.[2,22]

Fractures of the atlas represent about 15% of fractures in the cervical spine and may accompany ligamentous injuries such as atlanto-occipital dislocation.[23,24] Fractures of the atlas are best appreciated on CT imaging and may include the anterior arch, posterior arch, lateral masses, or combined arch fractures known as the Jefferson fracture. In the absence of instability, isolated C1 fractures may be conservatively treated with halo immobilization.[23]

Pars Interarticularis Fracture

Pars interarticularis fractures, also known as hangman fractures, are injuries that result from hyperextension. Isolated pars fractures do not usually result in neurological injury because the canal typically widens. These fractures are best characterized by anterior or posterior displacement of C2 fragments, based on the Effendi et al[25] classification as modified first in 1985 by Levine and Edwards[26] and then in 2011 by Joaquim and Patel.[23]

Type I pars interarticularis fracture

Type I pars interarticularis fractures are hairline fractures of the pars. They result in minimal (< 3 mm) or no displacement or angulation of the axis.

Type II pars interarticularis fracture

Type II pars interarticularis fractures have more than 3 mm of anterolisthesis of C2 with respect to C3, in addition to severe angulation. Angulation with minimal translation is characterized as type IIA.

Type III pars interarticularis fracture

Type III fractures are relatively rare. They involve anterior displacement, with unilateral or bilateral dislocated facet joints and severe angulation. Present in cases of high-velocity trauma with hyperextension and distraction, this type of fracture is a spondylolisthesis of C2 with bilateral pars fractures. As with most traumatic injuries of the craniovertebral junction, surgical indications for C2 pars fractures are dependent on the amount of instability present. Halo traction reduction or rigid orthosis is indicated for pars fractures in the absence of severe angulation or displacement. Surgery is indicated for wide fractures, severe angulation, and facet joint dislocation.[23,27]

15.4 Special Considerations

Special attention should be paid to pediatric patients with disorders that may involve the craniovertebral junction. Common examples of these disorders are Down syndrome, Morquio syndrome (and other mucopolysaccharidoses), Klippel–Feil syndrome, and others such as Chiari malformation type I, rheumatoid arthritis, and skeletal dysplasias (all of which are beyond the scope of this discussion).

15.4.1 Down Syndrome

Down syndrome, or trisomy 21, is the most frequent chromosomal disorder.[28] Craniovertebral ligament laxity, particularly of the transverse ligament, may lead to progressive atlantoaxial instability in patients with Down syndrome. As a result, 10 to 30% of patients with Down syndrome have widening of the atlantodental interval that exceeds 5 mm.[29,30,31] In addition to atlanto-occipital hypermobility,[32] patients with Down syndrome may be predisposed to os odontoideum or odontoid hypoplasia with canal stenosis.[32,33,34,35]

15.4.2 Morquio Syndrome

Patients with Morquio syndrome (mucopolysaccharidosis type IV) have a mutation in the gene responsible for the production of *N*-acetylgalactosamine-6-sulfatase (type IVA) or in the gene responsible for beta-galactosidase (type IVB), nearly always resulting in involvement of the craniovertebral junction.[36] Patients with Morquio syndrome are predisposed to atlantoaxial instability from dens hypoplasia, similar to a subset of patients with Down syndrome, but they may also have retrodental soft-tissue masses resulting in canal stenosis.[37]

15.4.3 Klippel–Feil Syndrome

This syndrome involves three classic diagnostic criteria: a short neck, a low hairline, and limited neck mobility; all three conditions are present in 50% of patients.[2,38] Klippel–Feil syndrome is a complex disorder that involves vertebral fusion and accelerated spondylosis. Abnormal fusion of the cervical vertebrae increases the moment arm, which may predispose the cervical spine to instability. Patients with Klippel–Feil syndrome, especially those with a traumatic injury, should be carefully evaluated because of the high risk of occipitoatlantoaxial instability and vertebral artery insult.[39,40]

15.4.4 Other Disorders

DiGeorge syndrome is a rare congenital anomaly that affects the craniovertebral junction and many other organ systems. More than one-half (59%) of the patients with DiGeorge syndrome have an open posterior arch of C1, 58% have a dysmorphic dens, and 34% have fusion of C2–C3.[2,41] Notable conditions that may predispose patients to craniovertebral instability include Goldenhar syndrome (oculo-auriculo-vertebral syndrome), spondyloepiphyseal dysplasia congenita, osteogenesis imperfecta, and juvenile idiopathic arthritis.

Os odontoideum is an anatomic abnormality wherein a hypoplastic dens is separated from an ossicle of smooth corticated bone of the C2 body. The two variants of os odontoideum are characterized as orthotopic and dystopic. Differentiating between the two has treatment implications. A dystopic os odontoideum is migrated anteriorly and is functionally fused to the basion, whereas an orthotopic os odontoideum moves alongside the anterior arch of C1.[42] An orthotopic os odontoideum can be reduced for normal alignment with the dens.

15.5 Diagnosis of Craniovertebral Injury

Imaging is the mainstay of pediatric craniovertebral injury assessment. Although plain radiographs precede other imaging techniques, the effective diagnosis of craniovertebral injury involves a combination of imaging techniques and multimodal evaluation. In a notable study by Woodring and Lee[43] of 216 patients with traumatic injury to the cervical spine, 61% of fractures and 36% subluxations/dislocations were undetected on anteroposterior and lateral radiographs and on radiographs of the dens. Alternatively, high-resolution CT imaging offers the most meaningful evaluation of osseous structures and interosseous spaces. However, MRI is superior in assessing soft-tissue structures, ligaments, spinal cord, and nerve roots.[2,44]

When requesting imaging for pediatric patients with suspected craniovertebral trauma, one should consider the mechanisms of trauma and the most common injuries. Most patients under the age of 10 years who have a craniovertebral injury have ligamentous injury in the absence of fractures. In contrast, in older pediatric patients, fractures are seen in 80% of those who have cervical trauma; the rest have ligamentous injury alone, without a fracture.[45,46] Although radiographic evidence of abnormality or fractures may be absent, further evaluation with MRI is warranted for young children because upper cervical spinal cord injury may occur after trauma.[2]

AOD is a potentially life-threatening traumatic condition that warrants careful evaluation. As proposed by Pang, the interval between the CCI should be carefully examined as a site of injury when there is suspicion of traumatic AOD. On a coronal CT, a CCI of 4 mm or greater is an indicator of AOD, with both specificity and sensitivity of 100%.[8,9] Normal CCI joint space is less than 2 mm. The Pang CCI method is preferred over other methods, such as the Sun interspinous ratio, the dens–basion interval, and the Powers ratio, which have sensitivities of 25, 50, and 67%, respectively.[8,9,47]

The atlantodental distance can provide insight into translational atlantoaxial subluxation. In children, a horizontal distance exceeding 4 mm on plain radiographs is cause for concern. Additional imaging modalities such as CT and MRI can be used to further identify traumatic injuries of the C1 lateral mass or transverse ligament, respectively. Hyperintensity of the ligament or loss of continuity would be best appreciated on MRI. As previously described, distinguishing type I from type II translational atlantoaxial subluxation injuries is essential in determining further treatment.[2,14,48]

Stenosis of the cervical spine is not an uncommon condition, especially in older or larger children. Cervical spinal stenosis may contribute to neurapraxia of the cervical spinal cord in young athletes. Cervical spinal stenosis can be assessed by measuring the anteroposterior diameter of the central canal. A normal diameter is considered to be 17 mm, relative stenosis is 10 to 13 mm, and absolute stenosis is any diameter less than 10 mm. However, the diameter of the canal decreases caudally so that the normal value of C1 is 23 mm, C2 is 20 mm, C3 to C6 is 17 mm, and C7 is 15 mm. A more reliable method is the Torg (i.e., Torg–Pavlov) ratio, wherein the diameter of the central canal is compared to the diameter of the respective vertebral body.[49] A ratio less than 0.8 has high sensitivity but low specificity for cervical spinal stenosis.[49,50]

15.6 Treatment

Upper cervical spinal cord injury, or cervicomedullary injury, accompanied by craniovertebral trauma may be life-threatening.

In the acute setting, the mean arterial pressure should be elevated to maintain cord perfusion.[51] Although the data on pediatric patients are limited, the current recommendation is not to administer methylprednisolone to treat spinal cord injury, in accordance with the Third National Acute Spinal Cord Injury Randomized Controlled Trial with adult participants.[52]

Traction with reduction is a particularly powerful tool to use for realigning the craniovertebral junction in chronic injuries. In acute injury to the craniocervical junction, especially with instability, traction is contraindicated as it could lead to stretching of the neural elements and neurological injury. Pharmacologic muscle relaxation in conjunction with traction restored the alignment in 60% of children who had a presumed "irreducible lesion."[53] Because of the stretch on the vasculature and spinal cord, intraoperative traction should always be accompanied by adequate neuromonitoring.

Posterior fixation comprises most cases of surgery for craniovertebral injuries (► Fig. 15.3, ► Fig. 15.4, ► Fig. 15.5, and ► Fig. 15.6).

However, it can be especially challenging in the pediatric population because of skeletal immaturity. The pedicles, facets, and lateral masses of very young children may be too small for screw fixation, which can also cause undue harm to adjacent structures. Steinmann pin and sublaminar wiring fixation may be preferred for use in young children (► Fig. 15.4). The use of a bone graft is also associated with a higher rate of fusion

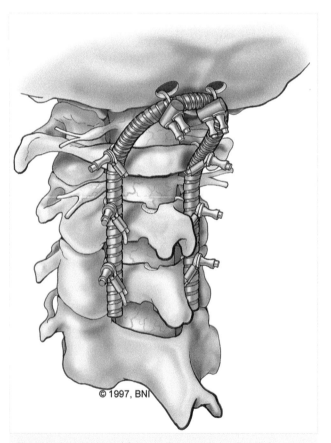

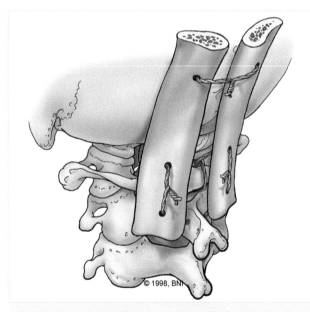

Fig. 15.3 Occipitocervical fusion using bone grafts from the ribs, which are wired to the occiput and the cervical laminae. (Used with permission from Barrow Neurological Institute, Phoenix, AZ.)

Fig. 15.4 Occipitocervical fusion technique using a threaded Steinmann pin wired to the upper cervical spine and occiput. (Used with permission from Barrow Neurological Institute, Phoenix, AZ.)

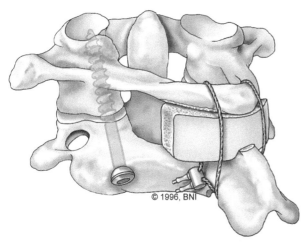

Fig. 15.5 Atlantoaxial fixation with transarticular screws and a strut graft fixed in place with cable or wire looped beneath the C2 spinous process, atlas, axis, and bone graft. (Used with permission from Barrow Neurological Institute, Phoenix, AZ.)

(▶ Fig. 15.3 and ▶ Fig. 15.5).[54] In a study by Ahmed et al,[55] autografted rib grafts were associated with lower morbidity rates than grafts from the iliac crest. The decision to use wired grafts, rods and wires, or screw-based techniques is highly dependent on the anatomy of the patient and the features of the injury (▶ Fig. 15.7). In general, structural bone grafting is absolutely necessary for adequate arthrodesis at the craniocervical junction. The rigid screw-based technique is favorable from a biomechanical standpoint but generally cannot be used in children younger than 3 years of age. Examples include the Brooks and Jenkins[56] fusion and the Dickman–Sonntag[57] interspinous fusion.

Anterior approaches, such as transoral decompression and odontoid screw fixation, may be indicated in certain situations. Irreducible ventral midline extradural compression of the upper cervical cord or cervicomedullary junction requires a transoral approach, but fixation techniques and available space are limited with this technique.[58,59,60] Direct screw fixation of odontoid fractures has several advantages and preserves significant range of motion. However, this technique requires an intact cruciate ligament.[55,58]

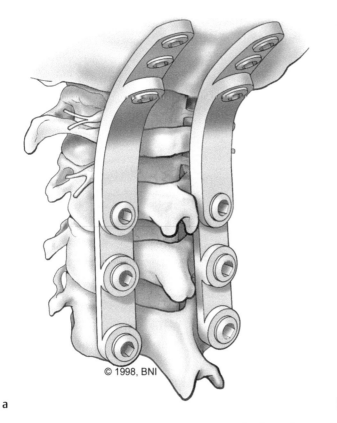

a

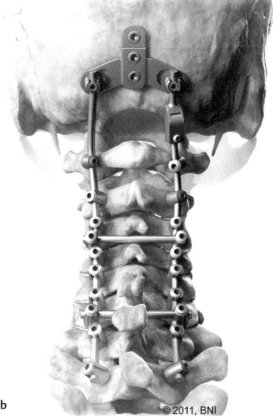

b

Fig. 15.6 **(a)** Occipitocervical screw plates (i.e., Roy-Camille plates). **(b)** A modern construct with polyaxial screws and rods. (Used with permission from Barrow Neurological Institute, Phoenix, AZ.)

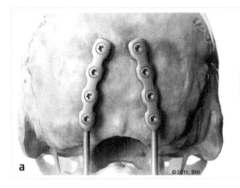
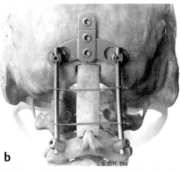

Fig. 15.7 Various options exist for screw fixation to the occiput. **(a)** A disadvantage of lateral fixation is attachment to thin bone, whereas **(b)** a midline occipital plate attaches to thick bone in the keel plate. This illustration of the midline occipital plate depicts the posterior view of an occiput-to-C2 fusion construct after placement of a rib graft, which offers additional stability as positioned between the occiput and the C2 spinous process. (Used with permission from Barrow Neurological Institute, Phoenix, AZ.)

Intraoperative neuronavigation should be considered for arthrodesis of the craniovertebral junction in pediatric patients because of the adjacent critical structures and their anatomic complexity. Malpositioned hardware, neurological injury, and vertebral artery injury have been reported as complications in 31, 5, and 2% of operative cases, respectively.[61,62] Nevertheless, risks can be mitigated with careful preoperative planning and proper surgical technique.

The unique and complex anatomy of the craniovertebral junction makes management of traumatic injuries to this region challenging. Each case is unique, and management must be tailored to the patient and pathology.

References

[1] Drake J, Vogl A, Mitchell A. Gray's Anatomy for Students. 3rd ed. Philadelphia, PA: Elsevier Churchill Livingstone; 2013

[2] Oppenlander M, Clark J, Sonntag VNT. Pediatric craniovertebral junction trauma. In: Schramm J, Di Rocco C, Akalan N, eds. Advances and Technical Standards in Neurosurgery. New York, NY: Springer; 2014:333–353

[3] Vanderah T, Gould D. Nolte's the Human Brain. 7th ed. Philadelphia, PA: Elsevier; 2015

[4] Lang J. Clinical Anatomy of the Cervical Spine. Stuttgart, Germany: Thieme; 1993

[5] Tubbs RS, Hallock JD, Radcliff V, et al. Ligaments of the craniocervical junction. J Neurosurg Spine. 2011; 14(6):697–709

[6] Hall GC, Kinsman MJ, Nazar RG, et al. Atlanto-occipital dislocation. World J Orthop. 2015; 6(2):236–243

[7] Fisher CG, Sun JC, Dvorak M. Recognition and management of atlanto-occipital dislocation: improving survival from an often fatal condition. Can J Surg. 2001; 44(6):412–420

[8] Traynelis VC, Marano GD, Dunker RO, Kaufman HH. Traumatic atlanto-occipital dislocation. Case report. J Neurosurg. 1986; 65(6):863–870

[9] Pang D, Nemzek WR, Zovickian J. Atlanto-occipital dislocation—part 2: the clinical use of (occipital) condyle-C1 interval, comparison with other diagnostic methods, and the manifestation, management, and outcome of atlanto-occipital dislocation in children. Neurosurgery. 2007; 61(5):995–1015, discussion 1015

[10] Garrett M, Consiglieri G, Kakarla UK, Chang SW, Dickman CA. Occipitoatlantal dislocation. Neurosurgery. 2010; 66(3) Suppl:48–55

[11] Bucholz RW, Burkhead WZ. The pathological anatomy of fatal atlanto-occipital dislocations. J Bone Joint Surg Am. 1979; 61(2):248–250

[12] Horn EM, Feiz-Erfan I, Lekovic GP, Dickman CA, Sonntag VK, Theodore N. Survivors of occipitoatlantal dislocation injuries: imaging and clinical correlates. J Neurosurg Spine. 2007; 6(2):113–120

[13] Maiman DJ, Cusick JF. Traumatic atlantoaxial dislocation. Surg Neurol. 1982; 18(5):388–392

[14] Dickman CA, Greene KA, Sonntag VK. Injuries involving the transverse atlantal ligament: classification and treatment guidelines based upon experience with 39 injuries. Neurosurgery. 1996; 38(1):44–50

[15] Fielding JW, Hawkins RJ. Atlanto-axial rotatory fixation. (Fixed rotatory subluxation of the atlanto-axial joint). J Bone Joint Surg Am. 1977; 59(1):37–44

[16] Pang D. Atlantoaxial rotatory fixation. Neurosurgery. 2010; 66(3) Suppl: 161–183

[17] Pang D, Li V. Atlantoaxial rotatory fixation: part 2—new diagnostic paradigm and a new classification based on motion analysis using computed tomographic imaging. Neurosurgery. 2005; 57(5):941–953, discussion 941–953

[18] Bailey DK. The normal cervical spine in infants and children. Radiology. 1952; 59(5):712–719

[19] Connolly B, Emery D, Armstrong D. The odontoid synchondrotic slip: an injury unique to young children. Pediatr Radiol. 1995; 25 Suppl 1: S129–S133

[20] Fassett DR, McCall T, Brockmeyer DL. Odontoid synchondrosis fractures in children. Neurosurg Focus. 2006; 20(2):E7

[21] Anderson LD, D'Alonzo RT. Fractures of the odontoid process of the axis. J Bone Joint Surg Am. 1974; 56(8):1663–1674

[22] Swischuk LE, Hayden CK, Jr, Sarwar M. The dens-arch synchondrosis versus the hangman's fracture. Pediatr Radiol. 1979; 8(2):100–102

[23] Joaquim AF, Patel AA. Craniocervical traumatic injuries: evaluation and surgical decision making. Global Spine J. 2011; 1(1):37–42

[24] Hadley MN, Dickman CA, Browner CM, Sonntag VK. Acute traumatic atlas fractures: management and long term outcome. Neurosurgery. 1988; 23(1):31–35

[25] Effendi B, Roy D, Cornish B, Dussault RG, Laurin CA. Fractures of the ring of the axis. A classification based on the analysis of 131 cases. J Bone Joint Surg Br. 1981; 63-B(3):319–327

[26] Levine AM, Edwards CC. The management of traumatic spondylolisthesis of the axis. J Bone Joint Surg Am. 1985; 67(2):217–226

[27] Hadley MN, Walters BC, Grabb PA, et al. Guidelines for the management of acute cervical spine and spinal cord injuries. Clin Neurosurg. 2002; 49: 407–498

[28] Jones K. Chromosomal abnormality syndromes. In: Jones K, ed. Smith's Recognizable Patterns of Human Malformations. Philadephia, PA: Saunders; 2013:8–10

[29] Caird MS, Wills BP, Dormans JP. Down syndrome in children: the role of the orthopaedic surgeon. J Am Acad Orthop Surg. 2006; 14(11):610–619

[30] Doyle JS, Lauerman WC, Wood KB, Krause DR. Complications and long-term outcome of upper cervical spine arthrodesis in patients with Down syndrome. Spine. 1996; 21(10):1223–1231

[31] Ferguson RL, Putney ME, Allen BL, Jr. Comparison of neurologic deficits with atlanto-dens intervals in patients with Down syndrome. J Spinal Disord. 1997; 10(3):246–252

[32] Wellborn CC, Sturm PF, Hatch RS, Bomze SR, Jablonski K. Intraobserver reproducibility and interobserver reliability of cervical spine measurements. J Pediatr Orthop. 2000; 20(1):66–70

[33] Wiesel SW, Rothman RH. Occipitoatlantal hypermobility. Spine. 1979; 4(3):187–191

[34] Matsunaga S, Imakiire T, Koga H, et al. Occult spinal canal stenosis due to C-1 hypoplasia in children with Down syndrome. J Neurosurg. 2007; 107(6) Suppl:457–459

[35] Segal LS, Drummond DS, Zanotti RM, Ecker ML, Mubarak SJ. Complications of posterior arthrodesis of the cervical spine in patients who have Down syndrome. J Bone Joint Surg Am. 1991; 73(10):1547–1554

[36] Montaño AM, Tomatsu S, Gottesman GS, Smith M, Orii T. International Morquio A Registry: clinical manifestation and natural course of Morquio A disease. J Inherit Metab Dis. 2007; 30(2):165–174

[37] Kulkarni MV, Williams JC, Yeakley JW, et al. Magnetic resonance imaging in the diagnosis of the cranio-cervical manifestations of the mucopolysaccharidoses. Magn Reson Imaging. 1987; 5(5):317–323

[38] Tracy MR, Dormans JP, Kusumi K. Klippel-Feil syndrome: clinical features and current understanding of etiology. Clin Orthop Relat Res. 2004(424):183–190

[39] Hasan I, Wapnick S, Kutscher ML, Couldwell WT. Vertebral arterial dissection associated with Klippel-Feil syndrome in a child. Childs Nerv Syst. 2002; 18(1–2):67–70

[40] Nagib MG, Maxwell RE, Chou SN. Identification and management of high-risk patients with Klippel-Feil syndrome. J Neurosurg. 1984; 61(3):523–530

[41] Ricchetti ET, States L, Hosalkar HS, et al. Radiographic study of the upper cervical spine in the 22q11.2 deletion syndrome. J Bone Joint Surg Am. 2004; 86-A(8):1751–1760

[42] Arvin B, Fournier-Gosselin MP, Fehlings MG. Os odontoideum: etiology and surgical management. Neurosurgery. 2010; 66(3) Suppl:22–31

[43] Woodring JH, Lee C. Limitations of cervical radiography in the evaluation of acute cervical trauma. J Trauma. 1993; 34(1):32–39

[44] Frank JB, Lim CK, Flynn JM, Dormans JP. The efficacy of magnetic resonance imaging in pediatric cervical spine clearance. Spine. 2002; 27(11):1176–1179

[45] Viccellio P, Simon H, Pressman BD, Shah MN, Mower WR, Hoffman JR, NEXUS Group. A prospective multicenter study of cervical spine injury in children. Pediatrics. 2001; 108(2):E20

[46] Evans DL, Bethem D. Cervical spine injuries in children. J Pediatr Orthop. 1989; 9(5):563–568

[47] Dziurzynski K, Anderson PA, Bean DB, et al. A blinded assessment of radiographic criteria for atlanto-occipital dislocation. Spine. 2005; 30(12):1427–1432

[48] Klimo P, Jr, Ware ML, Gupta N, Brockmeyer D. Cervical spine trauma in the pediatric patient. Neurosurg Clin N Am. 2007; 18(4):599–620

[49] Pavlov H, Torg JS, Robie B, Jahre C. Cervical spinal stenosis: determination with vertebral body ratio method. Radiology. 1987; 164(3):771–775

[50] Boockvar JA, Durham SR, Sun PP. Cervical spinal stenosis and sports-related cervical cord neurapraxia in children. Spine. 2001; 26(24):2709–2712, discussion 2713

[51] Vale FL, Burns J, Jackson AB, Hadley MN. Combined medical and surgical treatment after acute spinal cord injury: results of a prospective pilot study to assess the merits of aggressive medical resuscitation and blood pressure management. J Neurosurg. 1997; 87(2):239–246

[52] Bracken MB, Shepard MJ, Holford TR, et al. Administration of methylprednisolone for 24 or 48 hours or tirilazad mesylate for 48 hours in the treatment of acute spinal cord injury. Results of the Third National Acute Spinal Cord Injury Randomized Controlled Trial. National Acute Spinal Cord Injury Study. JAMA. 1997; 277(20):1597–1604

[53] Dahdaleh NS, Dlouhy BJ, Menezes AH. Application of neuromuscular blockade and intraoperative 3D imaging in the reduction of basilar invagination. J Neurosurg Pediatr. 2012; 9(2):119–124

[54] Apostolides PJ, Dickman CA, Golfinos JG, Papadopoulos SM, Sonntag VK. Threaded steinmann pin fusion of the craniovertebral junction. Spine. 1996; 21(14):1630–1637

[55] Ahmed R, Traynelis VC, Menezes AH. Fusions at the craniovertebral junction. Childs Nerv Syst. 2008; 24(10):1209–1224

[56] Brooks AL, Jenkins EB. Atlanto-axial arthrodesis by the wedge compression method. J Bone Joint Surg Am. 1978; 60(3):279–284

[57] Dickman CA, Sonntag VK, Papadopoulos SM, Hadley MN. The interspinous method of posterior atlantoaxial arthrodesis. J Neurosurg. 1991; 74(2): 190–198

[58] Sonntag VK, Dickman CA. Craniocervical stabilization. Clin Neurosurg. 1993; 40:243–272

[59] Oppenlander ME, Kalyvas J, Sonntag VK, Theodore N. Technical advances in pediatric craniovertebral junction surgery. Adv Tech Stand Neurosurg. 2014; 40:201–213

[60] Tuite GF, Veres R, Crockard HA, Sell D. Pediatric transoral surgery: indications, complications, and long-term outcome. J Neurosurg. 1996; 84(4):573–583

[61] Haque A, Price AV, Sklar FH, Swift DM, Weprin BE, Sacco DJ. Screw fixation of the upper cervical spine in the pediatric population. Clinical article. J Neurosurg Pediatr. 2009; 3(6):529–533

[62] Hedequist D, Proctor M. Screw fixation to C2 in children: a case series and technical report. J Pediatr Orthop. 2009; 29(1):21–25

16 Penetrating Injuries to the Cervical Spine

Christine Hammer and James S. Harrop

Abstract

Penetrating injuries to the cervical spine occur most frequently among males in the second to fourth decade of life, generally as a result of interpersonal violence. Mechanisms of injury range from common missile injuries, such as gunshot wounds, to less common missile injuries such as those from nail guns or military-grade explosive devices. Knife stab wounds, or stab wounds, are the most common nonmissile form of penetrating injuries. Less common are accidents or injuries involving objects capable of penetrating the skin (e.g., needles, wood or glass fragments, etc.). Cervical spine instability is relatively uncommon, and thus penetrating injuries to the cervical spine are often able to be treated conservatively without surgery or rigid immobilization. Retained fragments carry some risk of infection, but surgery is reserved for those who have failed conservative antibiotic therapy. Steroid use has been a point of controversy, therefore, routine use of steroids for penetrating injuries to the cervical spine is not recommended.

Keywords: penetrating injuries, cervical spine, stability, instability, immobilization, decompression, fusion, spinal cord injury, gunshot wounds, GSWs, stabbing, knife

16.1 Introduction

The National Spinal Cord Injury Statistics Center (NSCISC) estimates that in the United States, spinal cord injuries (SCI) occur at a rate of 54 cases per one million individuals; there are approximately 17,000 new cases of SCI each year.[1] Injuries involving the cervical spine make up over half of these instances.[2] However, penetrating injuries involving the cervical spine are a relatively uncommon cause of SCI. This is due not only to the rarity of this type of injury, but also to the infrequent association of SCI with penetrating injuries to the cervical spine.[3] For example, at one of the busiest trauma centers in the United States, on average there are only 10 gunshot wounds (GSWs) annually involving the cervical spine, with less than half of victims surviving the initial injury.[4] Furthermore, other studies have shown that less than 10% of all penetrating injuries involving the cervical spine are associated with SCI. Estimates of cervical spine instability range from 0.2 to 4%, a relatively small number of which go on to require immobilization via surgery or orthosis.[4]

Historically, approximately 80% of all new SCI cases occurred in males.[5] In the past few decades, however, there has been a trend toward an increasing incidence of SCIs in females.[5] With regard to data specifically addressing injuries to the cervical spine, including penetrating injuries, males are still most commonly involved.[6] In the United States, non-Hispanic blacks account for a disproportionate fraction of cases of SCI compared to their representation among the general population.[1] While SCI is estimated to occur most commonly during the second to fourth decade, there is a bimodal distribution with a second smaller peak occurring in those over the age of 65 years.[7] The average age of cervical spine injury has been increasing in the recent years, mirroring the steadily increasing average age of the general population. The age distribution of patients with penetrating injuries to the cervical spine is clustered within the second to fourth decade.[8]

Overall, SCIs most commonly result from motor vehicle accidents, falls, acts of violence, and sports/recreation activities in descending order.[9] However, the most commonly reported mechanism of injury among individuals presenting with penetrating injuries to the cervical spine are acts of violence, followed by accidents. Depending on geographic location, this may involve either missile or nonmissile objects, with GSWs being more common in the United States, whereas stab wounds (SWs) predominate in developing countries.[4]

16.2 Mechanisms of Injury

Penetrating injuries to the neck are defined as injuries occurring between the clavicles and the base of the skull. This space is broken down into three zones and injury in any of these three zones may result in injury to the spine (▶ Fig. 16.1).[10]

Zone 2 is the largest and most accessible zone of the neck. Surgical access to zone 3 is limited by the mandible, and access

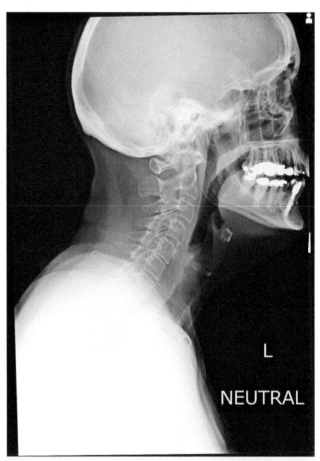

Fig. 16.1 Cervical zones.

to zone 1 may be impeded by the sternum and clavicles. In addition to the spine, mediastinal structures may be at risk of injury when injuries to zone 1 are present. Skull base and craniofacial injuries may accompany penetrating trauma to zone 3. Penetrating injuries involving the cervical spine may be broadly classified into missile (GSWs) or projectile (i.e., non-missile [SWs]) injuries.[11] In layman's terms, missile injuries usually involve bullets or shots, nail guns, or other ballistic sources (e.g., arrows, explosion-related fragments, etc.). Nonmissile injuries include nonballistic SW injuries, including those induced via knives and other objects, which are used intentionally or accidentally.[12]

Classical mechanics relates the kinetic energy of a projectile to its mass and velocity by the formula $KE = 1/2mv^2$; thus, the most important factor predicting the capacity to injure is the projectile's muzzle velocity. Military-grade weapons have a much greater muzzle velocity than civilian weaponry such as the handgun.[13] Beyond the injury caused by the projectile itself, additional kinetic energy is transferred to the tissue in the form of a secondary cavitation wave, causing further destruction in an ellipsoid shape both larger than and remote from the path of the projectile itself. Temporary cavitations are created more commonly by high-velocity projectiles (which travel at 2,000–3,000 feet/second), whereas projectiles from typical civilian handguns and shotguns leave the muzzle at 1,000 to 2,000 feet/second.[13] However, upon striking bone, a projectile typically deforms and expands, leading to increased damage.[14] This is the same principle exploited by the hollow-point bullet. Laboratory studies have shown that energies of 6.8 J are required to penetrate bone; the maximum energy transferred during a stabbing may range from 64 to 115 J.[15]

The material and design of the weapon impacts the extent of injury; from fragments to hollow-point bullets that explode on impact to length and materials involved, the type of bullet, for example, may impact surgical decisions. Most bullets have a lead core, but the jackets can be made of copper, brass, or nickel. Each of these materials are potentially toxic. Lead toxicity from bullets lodged within the spine has been reported. The necrotic effect of copper on brain tissue and rabbit spinal neurons has also been previously described.[16]

16.3 Assessment and Management

16.3.1 Initial Assessment

Patients should be evaluated and stabilized per applicable basic or Advanced Trauma Life Support guidelines. Injury to any of the three zones of the neck may compromise the patient's airway. Furthermore, zone 3 injuries may compromise the integrity of the skull base. Thus, the injury may preclude orotracheal or nasotracheal intubation. Each injury must be evaluated on a case-by-case basis, and the airway must be secured accordingly.

Blood loss may precipitate hypotension which can impact spinal cord perfusion and exacerbate the SCI. Thus, immediate cardiovascular assessment and stabilization is essential. Tetanus prophylaxis should be administered according to current trauma guidelines.[17] A complete neurological assessment should be performed to gain an understanding of the extent of neurological injury, if present. Key elements regarding assessment of penetrating injuries of the cervical spine include motor and sensory

examination of upper and lower extremities as well as an anorectal exam (to assess for sacral involvement). Any obvious retained objects, such as a knife handle and blade, should be left in place until the trajectory, depth, and neurovascular structural involvement are assessed with imaging.[18] In addition, the foreign object may be providing some element of tamponade and, to prevent hemorrhage, should not be removed.[13]

16.3.2 Radiography

X-ray and computed tomography (CT) are the mainstay imaging modalities for the primary evaluation of a penetrating injury to the cervical spine. Furthermore, CT angiography (CTA) may be indicated for evaluation of vascular structures of the neck (e.g., vertebral arteries [VA]/internal and external carotid arteries [ICA/ECA]) and the head. The Denver Screening Criteria (DSC) or the modified Memphis criteria may be used to guide use of CTA.[19] Signs and symptoms on DSC include the following:

- Focal neurological deficits.
- Arterial hemorrhage.
- Cervical bruit or thrill (< 50 years of age).
- Infarct(s) on head CT.
- Expanding neck hematoma.
- Neurological exam inconsistent with head CT findings.

In patients who sustained GSWs, artifacts may limit assessment of bone fractures. Additional evaluation of the discoligamentous complex through magnetic resonance imaging (MRI) may be contraindicated.[4] The safety of MRI is determined by the radiologist who must consider the location of fragments as they relate to veins, arteries, and neural elements.[4] A recent prospective study found that there was no migration of retained fragments in patients with cervical GSWs, thus providing some basis for selecting patients who may benefit from evaluation via MRI.[20] Findings of penetrating SCI on an MRI include those similar to any SCI such as increased T2 signal within the spinal cord or short tau inversion recovery (STIR) signal within the disc or ligaments.[21]

In addition to the spine and spinal cord, penetrating neck injuries pose a risk to the extracranial carotid and vertebral arteries. One should maintain a low threshold for radiographic evaluation of the craniocervical vasculature. Screening may initially be performed via CTA; however, any concerning finding should prompt the use of digital subtraction angiography (DSA). In a case series on 187 US service members that had undergone DSA for blunt or penetrating craniocerebral trauma suffered in the conflict in the Middle East between 2003 and 2008, Bell et al noted a 26.2% incidence of vascular injury.[6] Of the 15 patients that sustained perpetrating injuries to the neck, injuries that were observed included 4 ICA and 1 VA dissections, 5 ICA and 4 VA pseudoaneurysms, 1 ICA and 1 VA arteriovenous (AV) fistula, and 1 pseudoaneurysm of the ECA. Majority of these lesions were amenable to endovascular treatment. In the same series, carotid pseudoaneurysms were the most likely lesions to require open surgical management. In ▸ Fig. 16.2, we show the cervical spine CT images of a 30-year-old male who sustained multiple GSWs to the neck and trunk. Neurologically this patient presented with quadriparesis and was also found to be hemodynamically unstable with concern for possible internal carotid injury in addition to concern for other large vessel injury. In a joint procedure with both vascular and general surgery, the patient had a sternotomy

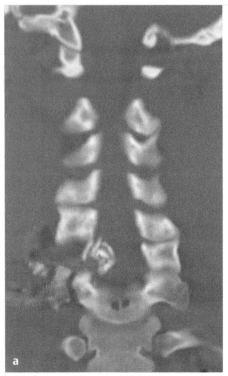
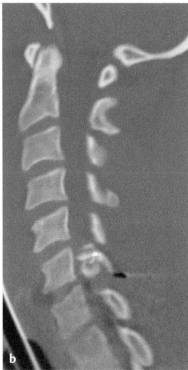

Fig. 16.2 A 30-year-old male presenting with multiple gunshot wounds with injury to the right internal carotid artery. These cervical spine computed tomography (CT) images show multiple views of the gunshot wound injury involving the C6 level including obscuration of the right vertebral artery.

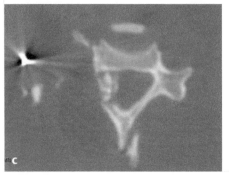

during which bleeding was encountered with concern for innominate versus right common carotid injury. Vascular surgery identified more than 50% injury to the right common carotid; they resected the damaged tissue and reconstructed the vessel with a Dacron graft. Postoperatively, a CTA of the neck was performed which showed the origin of the right vertebral artery was obscured by bullet fragments with reconstitution at V4. This imaging showed that bilateral ECA and ICA were intact without evidence of extravasation.

16.3.3 Medical Management

Controversy exists regarding steroid administration in the setting of acute SCI. Many studies have been done to assess the risks and benefits of steroid use in this patient population. Levy et al found that methylprednisolone neither improved outcomes nor significantly increased complications among patients with SCI and GSWs.[22] Heary et al conducted a retrospective review of patients with GSWs and found that no significant neurological benefits were seen following methylprednisolone or dexamethasone administration.[23]

Infection from external sources of contamination and/or internal sources (e.g., traversing mucosal surfaces) is an inher-

ent risk in cases of penetrating injuries.[16] Prophylactic antibiotics are not indicated and in cases of infection, antibiotics may be used while reserving washout procedures for those cases in which broad-spectrum antibiotics fail.

Immobilization of the cervical spine increases medical costs, limits rehabilitation efforts, and can lead to deconditioning of muscles, while increasing the risk of skin breakdown and pressure ulcer formation. A retrospective study by Eftekhary et al surmised that there is a general overutilization of bracing among patients with GSW-related SCIs, and that cervical orthoses do not improve outcomes in these cases by preventing delayed kyphosis or neurological decline.[3] Other studies similarly found a low incidence of cervical spine instability associated with penetrating injuries and concluded that in the absence of neurological deficits or radiographic evidence of discoligamentous disruption, the use of cervical orthoses for immobilization is not recommended.[24] In another retrospective analysis of patients with penetrating injuries to the neck, the authors noted that instability was present in < 1% of patients with GSWs and was not present in patients presenting with an SW, thus supporting the data that spinal orthoses, in general, are not indicated in the context of penetrating injuries to the cervical spine.[11]

16.3.4 Surgical Management

Cervical spinal instability and SCI is uncommon.[4] The neurologically intact patient presenting without large retained fragments from a penetrating injury to the cervical spine may be managed conservatively, without the need for immobilization.[4]

Decompressive laminectomy may be reserved for cases in which a hematoma, bone fragments, or another foreign body are felt to be the reason for persistent neural compression, in cases of infection, or in instances where a retained penetrating object, such as a knife handle or blade, must be removed in order for the patient to recover.[18] Both the military and civilian literature support the recommendation that while decompressive laminectomy may not improve neurological outcome, surgeons should operate within 24 to 48 hours on patients with incomplete neurological injuries and canal compromise.[25] In patients presenting with GSWs who do not have neurological deficits, or in those patients presenting with a complete SCI, it is not recommended to pursue bony decompression and retrieval of small fragments, or to attempt repair of cerebrospinal fluid (CSF) leaks except in cases where persistent CSF fistulas exist.[4] Attempts to retrieve small fragments invariably involve manipulation of neural elements, risking either worsened edema or extension of the injury without clear benefit of protection or restoration of neurological function. However, in patients presenting with objects that are lodged within the bone, such as a knife, removal is of paramount importance.[26]

Unique circumstances may justify operative intervention. One such circumstance involves barbed projectiles such as nails following nail gun injury or arrows. Attempts at removal have the potential for significant soft-tissue and neurovascular injury secondary to splaying of the barbs.[12] Nathoo et al recommend analyzing a similar nail to educate oneself on the potential position changes of the barbs during removal.[12] Another special circumstance is when one is concerned about the potential for toxicity, as is the case with lead or copper fragments.[23] This may be of particular importance in cases involving military personnel. An improvised explosive device may contain metallic projectiles of unknown or heterogeneous composition, which in some instances may be poisonous or even radioactive.

Repair of a CSF fistula, in cases of any mechanism of penetrating injury to the cervical spine, may be performed through conservative skin closure with a lumbar drain that may be attempted prior to open surgery and primary dural closure or patch with subsequent CSF diversion (e.g., lumbar drain).[27]

As in most cases of penetrating cervical spine injury, ligamentous injury is infrequent, obviating the need for spinal instrumentation. However, if instrumentation is indicated on the basis of instability or secondary to destabilization following decompressive laminectomy, an anterior versus posterior versus combined approach may be decided on after evaluation of the fractures and instability at hand.[3,11,16,24,28,29,30] Although not directly applicable to penetrating spinal trauma, the AOSpine Subaxial Cervical Spine Injury Classification System may provide a conceptual framework to assess for instability after a penetrating injury. Injuries to the articular pillar, capsuloligamentous complex, posterior tension band, or translational injuries following high-impact injuries may require operative intervention.[31] ▶ Fig. 16.3 shows images of a 29-year-old male who was the victim of multiple GSWs during a robbery. On presentation, he was classified as a C5 ASIA A and required an emergent anterior cervical approach at C4–C6 for stabilization.

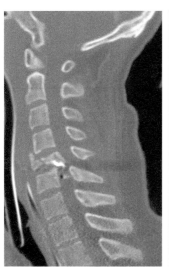
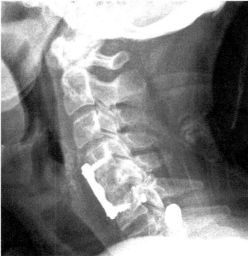
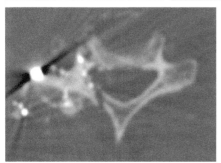

Fig. 16.3 A 29-year-old male, victim of gunshot wounds during a robbery. Extensive fractures of C5 and C6 vertebral bodies related to gunshot injury with retropulsion of C5 vertebral body with near-complete obliteration of the spinal canal as well as disruption of the C5–C6 facet joints bilaterally. Axial images show compression of the left vertebral artery at the level of C4–C5 and the right vertebral artery at the level of C5–C6.

During his workup, a CTA of the neck was performed which showed compression of the left vertebral artery at C4–C5 and the right vertebral artery at C5–C6. Flow was preserved above and below the level of injury, but given the bilateral injury, within 24 hours after surgery he was placed on therapeutic anticoagulation with intravenous heparin. When a therapeutic partial thromboplastin time (PTT) was obtained, he was bridged to long-term anticoagulation with warfarin.

Arterial dissections may often be treated with medical management (anticoagulants) alone. Pseudoaneurysms and AV fistulae are often amenable to endovascular therapy. However, some circumstances involving VA or carotid artery injury may require open surgical repair.[6,18,32] Combat-related VA injuries, similar to civilian injuries, are relatively uncommon. When they do occur, it is often in conjunction with cervical spine fractures.[33] Pseudoaneurysms of the V2 region are more common than occlusion of the VA and other injuries, and may be treated with coil embolization, stent-assisted coil embolization, or with medical management.[6,33,34]

References

[1] National Spinal Cord Injury Statistical Center. Spinal cord injury: facts and figures at a glance from NSCISC Birmingham, AL: University of Alabama at Birmingham, 2016 https://www.nscisc.uab.edu/Public/Facts%202016.pdf

[2] DeVivo MJ, Chen Y. Trends in new injuries, prevalent cases, and aging with spinal cord injury. Arch Phys Med Rehabil. 2011; 92(3):332–338

[3] Eftekhary N, Nwosu K, McCoy E, Fukunaga D, Rolfe K. Overutilization of bracing in the management of penetrating spinal cord injury from gunshot wounds. J Neurosurg Spine. 2016; 25(1):110–113

[4] Beaty N, Slavin J, Diaz C, Zeleznick K, Ibrahimi D, Sansur CA. Cervical spine injury from gunshot wounds. J Neurosurg Spine. 2014; 21(3):442–449

[5] Devivo MJ. Epidemiology of traumatic spinal cord injury: trends and future implications. Spinal Cord. 2012; 50(5):365–372

[6] Bell RS, Vo AH, Roberts R, Wanebo J, Armonda RA. Wartime traumatic aneurysms: acute presentation, diagnosis, and multimodal treatment of 64 craniocervical arterial injuries. Neurosurgery. 2010; 66(1):66–79, discussion 79

[7] Clayton JL, Harris MB, Weintraub SL, et al. Risk factors for cervical spine injury. Injury. 2012; 43(4):431–435

[8] de Barros Filho TE, Cristante AF, Marcon RM, Ono A, Bilhar R. Gunshot injuries in the spine. Spinal Cord. 2014; 52(7):504–510

[9] Fredø HL, Rizvi SA, Lied B, Rønning P, Helseth E. The epidemiology of traumatic cervical spine fractures: a prospective population study from Norway. Scand J Trauma Resusc Emerg Med. 2012; 20:85

[10] Roon AJ, Christensen N. Evaluation and treatment of penetrating cervical injuries. J Trauma. 1979; 19(6):391–397

[11] Lustenberger T, Talving P, Lam L, et al. Unstable cervical spine fracture after penetrating neck injury: a rare entity in an analysis of 1,069 patients. J Trauma. 2011; 70(4):870–872

[12] Nathoo N, Sarkar A, Varma G, Mendel E. Nail-gun injury of the cervical spine: simple technique for removal of a barbed nail. J Neurosurg Spine. 2011; 15(1):60–63

[13] Patil R, Jaiswal G, Gupta TK. Gunshot wound causing complete spinal cord injury without mechanical violation of spinal axis: case report with review of literature. J Craniovertebr Junction Spine. 2015; 6(4):149–157

[14] Healey CD, Spilman SK, King BD, Sherrill JE, II, Pelaez CA. Asymptomatic cervical spine fractures: current guidelines can fail older patients. J Trauma Acute Care Surg. 2017; 83(1):119–125

[15] Horsfall I, Prosser PD, Watson CH, Champion SM. An assessment of human performance in stabbing. Forensic Sci Int. 1999; 102(2–3):79–89

[16] Bono CM, Heary RF. Gunshot wounds to the spine. Spine J. 2004; 4(2):230–240

[17] Rhee P, Nunley MK, Demetriades D, Velmahos G, Doucet JJ. Tetanus and trauma: a review and recommendations. J Trauma. 2005; 58(5):1082–1088

[18] Enicker B, Gonya S, Hardcastle TC. Spinal stab injury with retained knife blades: 51 consecutive patients managed at a regional referral unit. Injury. 2015; 46(9):1726–1733

[19] Harrigan MR, Hadley MN, Dhall SS, et al. Management of vertebral artery injuries following non-penetrating cervical trauma. Neurosurgery. 2013; 72 Suppl 2:234–243

[20] Slavin J, Beaty N, Raghavan P, Sansur C, Aarabi B. Magnetic resonance imaging to evaluate cervical spinal cord injury from gunshot wounds from handguns. World Neurosurg. 2015; 84(6):1916–1922

[21] Gümüş M, Kapan M, Önder A, Böyük A, Girgin S, Taçyıldız I. Factors affecting morbidity in penetrating rectal injuries: a civilian experience. Ulus Travma Acil Cerrahi Derg. 2011; 17(5):401–406

[22] Levy ML, Gans W, Wijesinghe HS, SooHoo WE, Adkins RH, Stillerman CB. Use of methylprednisolone as an adjunct in the management of patients with penetrating spinal cord injury: outcome analysis. Neurosurgery. 1996; 39(6):1141–1148, discussion 1148–1149

[23] Heary RF, Vaccaro AR, Mesa JJ, et al. Steroids and gunshot wounds to the spine. Neurosurgery. 1997; 41(3):576–583, discussion 583–584

[24] Klein Y, Arieli I, Sagiv S, Peleg K, Ben-Galim P. Cervical spine injuries in civilian victims of explosions: should cervical collars be used? J Trauma Acute Care Surg. 2016; 80(6):985–988

[25] Jackson AB, Dijkers M, Devivo MJ, Poczatek RB. A demographic profile of new traumatic spinal cord injuries: change and stability over 30 years. Arch Phys Med Rehabil. 2004; 85(11):1740–1748

[26] Goldberg W, Mueller C, Panacek E, Tigges S, Hoffman JR, Mower WR, NEXUS Group. Distribution and patterns of blunt traumatic cervical spine injury. Ann Emerg Med. 2001; 38(1):17–21

[27] Wang Z, Liu Y, Qu Z, Leng J, Fu C, Liu G. Penetrating injury of the spinal cord treated surgically. Orthopedics. 2012; 35(7):e1136–e1140

[28] Klimo P, Jr, Ragel BT, Rosner M, Gluf W, McCafferty R. Can surgery improve neurological function in penetrating spinal injury? A review of the military and civilian literature and treatment recommendations for military neurosurgeons. Neurosurg Focus. 2010; 28(5):E4

[29] Medzon R, Rothenhaus T, Bono CM, Grindlinger G, Rathlev NK. Stability of cervical spine fractures after gunshot wounds to the head and neck. Spine. 2005; 30(20):2274–2279

[30] Schubl SD, Robitsek RJ, Sommerhalder C, et al. Cervical spine immobilization may be of value following firearm injury to the head and neck. Am J Emerg Med. 2016; 34(4):726–729

[31] Vaccaro AR, Schroeder GD, Kepler CK, et al. The surgical algorithm for the AOSpine thoracolumbar spine injury classification system. Eur Spine J. 2016; 25(4):1087–1094

[32] Xia X, Zhang F, Lu F, Jiang J, Wang L, Ma X. Stab wound with lodged knife tip causing spinal cord and vertebral artery injuries: case report and literature review. Spine. 2012; 37(15):E931–E934

[33] Greer LT, Kuehn RB, Gillespie DL, et al. Contemporary management of combat-related vertebral artery injuries. J Trauma Acute Care Surg. 2013; 74(3):818–824

[34] Tannoury C, Degiacomo A. Fatal vertebral artery injury in penetrating cervical spine trauma. Case Rep Neurol Med. 2015; 2015:571656

17 Cervical Spine Trauma in Patients with Congenital Spinal Stenosis

Colin T. Dunn, Kelley E. Banagan, and Steven C. Ludwig

Abstract

Congenital cervical spinal stenosis is a bony narrowing of the spinal canal that most often presents as cervical myelopathy resulting from degenerative lesions in an already narrowed cervical spinal canal. Several radiographic criteria have traditionally been used to define congenital stenosis, such as midsagittal canal diameter and canal-to-body ratio, but magnetic resonance imaging has emerged as the preferred imaging modality. Patients with congenital stenosis, especially those participating in contact sports, are at elevated risk of neurological injury after cervical spine trauma. Congenital narrowing of the cervical spinal canal is associated with a number of such injuries, including cervical cord neurapraxia, brachial plexus neurapraxia, and central cord syndrome.

Congenital stenosis has implications for return-to-play decisions after cervical spine trauma. Although such decisions should be made on a case-by-case basis, several criteria have been proposed regarding the role congenital stenosis should play in making decisions to permit return to contact activities. Management of cervical spine trauma differs little in patients with congenital spinal stenosis, but there have been questions surrounding the value of prophylactic surgery in patients with congenital stenosis at risk of cervical trauma and how surgical management of stenosis should affect return-to-play decisions.

Keywords: congenital spinal stenosis, cervical spine trauma, Torg ratio, cervical cord neurapraxia, stingers, central cord syndrome

17.1 Introduction

Cervical spinal stenosis can either be degenerative or congenital in origin. Degenerative spinal stenosis generally presents at a later age with myelopathic symptoms resulting from spondylotic encroachment into the cervical spinal canal. In certain patients, symptomatic relief is achieved with decompressive surgery to relieve pressure on the spinal cord.

Congenital spinal stenosis is present from an early age and is generally of unknown etiology. Understanding of the factors that contribute to a congenitally narrow spinal canal is poor, but roles have been proposed for premature closure of ossification centers and neurohormone-mediated negative chemotaxis acting on chondroblasts.[1,2] Most patients with congenital stenosis are asymptotic in the absence of trauma or degenerative changes.

17.2 Congenital Spinal Stenosis

17.2.1 Anatomic Changes in Congenital Spinal Stenosis

Congenital spinal stenosis is characterized by decreased spinal canal areas at multiple levels in the absence of degenerative changes (▶ Fig. 17.1). Patients with congenital spinal stenosis exhibit significantly smaller lateral masses, lamina lengths, and

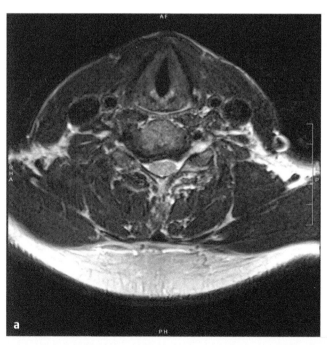
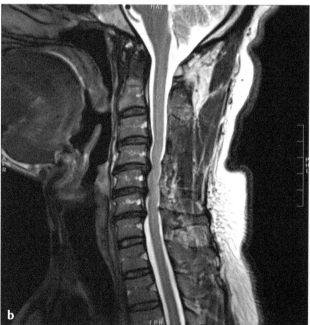

Fig. 17.1 (a) Axial T2-weighted image showing uncovertebral osteophytes causing neural foraminal narrowing, more prominent on the right side and disc bulge causing central canal stenosis. (b) Sagittal T2-weighted image showing cervical canal stenosis at multiple levels. Spinal cord is compressed and deformed but shows no signal changes.

lamina-pedicle angles with larger lamina-disc angles, resulting in a shortened midsagittal canal diameter.[3] Congenital cervical stenosis is strongly associated with decreased sagittal canal diameter and interpedicular distance, but not decreased pedicle length.[4] Congenital stenosis is found in association with a number of syndromic presentations, including achondroplasia, hypochondroplasia, Klippel–Feil syndrome, chondrodysplasia punctata, and brachytelephalangic chondrodysplasia.[1]

17.2.2 Epidemiology

The absence of universally accepted criteria for defining congenital cervical stenosis has complicated the efforts to determine its true prevalence. In one study of skeletal specimens, the prevalence of cervical stenosis in the adult population was estimated at 4.9%.[5] Nakashima et al[6] found narrow cervical canals (< 14 mm anteroposterior diameter on radiograph) in 10.2% of asymptomatic study participants, with greater prevalence in female and older patients. Estimates of the prevalence of congenital cervical spinal stenosis among football players, a population at particular risk of cervical trauma, have varied. Using a Torg ratio < 0.8 at one or more level from C3–C6 to define stenosis, the prevalence of cervical spinal stenosis among professional football players was estimated to be 34%.[7] Another study of college and high school players found congenital cervical stenosis in 7.6% of cases.[8]

17.2.3 Diagnosis

A number of radiological criteria have been proposed for the assessment of congenital cervical stenosis using various imaging techniques. Lateral view radiography of the cervical spine permits assessment of the bony diameter of the spinal canal to identify patients with congenital stenosis. The average values for this measurement range from 17 mm in lower cervical segments to 23 mm at C1. Values below 14 mm at any level are 2 standard deviations below normal, and this cutoff value has often been used to define congenital cervical spinal stenosis.[9,10]

The Torg ratio (▶ Fig. 17.2), calculated as the spinal canal-to-vertebral body ratio on lateral view radiographs, is a frequently used parameter for assessing congenital cervical spinal stenosis. In determining this value, the sagittal diameter of the vertebral body is measured at the mid-point and the sagittal diameter of the spinal canal is measured between the posterior surface of the vertebral body and the posterior margin of the spinal canal. In comparing the use of this ratio with the use of midsagittal canal diameter as diagnostic tools for cervical spinal stenosis, Pavlov et al[11] proposed a cutoff value of 0.82 for identifying congenital cervical stenosis. The use of this measurement rather than midsagittal canal diameter offers the benefit of eliminating magnification errors in radiography caused by differences in target distance, object-to-film distance, and body type.

The use of the Torg ratio for assessing cervical spinal stenosis, particularly in athletes, has received criticism for its poor positive predictive value for finding true stenosis. Blackley et al[12] found a poor correlation between the Torg ratio and canal diameter shown by computed tomography (CT), and Prasad

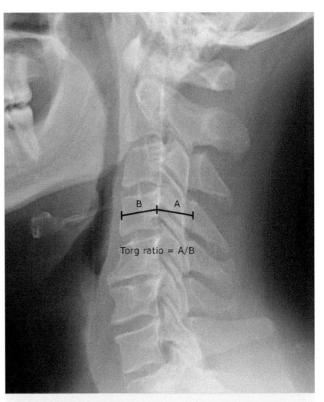

Fig. 17.2 Lateral radiograph of the cervical spine demonstrating calculation of the Torg ratio. *A* is the midsagittal diameter of the spinal canal measured from the posterior surface of the vertebral body to the nearest point of the corresponding lamina. *B* is the midsagittal diameter of the vertebral body as measured at the center of the body.

et al[13] found that Torg ratio correlated poorly with room available for the cord as shown by magnetic resonance imaging (MRI). Herzog et al[14] argue that these criteria have low specificity in determining true stenosis when used among football players because of the players' larger vertebral body diameters; larger vertebral bodies among football players result in smaller Torg ratios, even though their canal diameters may be normal.

Horne et al[15] proposed the lateral mass measurement-to-canal diameter (LM/CD) ratio as a new radiographic indicator of developmental cervical spinal stenosis. In determining this ratio, the LM is measured as the distance between the lateral mass and posterior vertebral body and the CD is measured as the distance between the spinolaminar line and posterior vertebral body. Using an LM/CD ratio ≥ 0.735 at C5 to identify developmental cervical stenosis in the adult population, the authors reported a favorable statistical profile (specificity 80%, sensitivity 76%).[15]

MRI and CT imaging provide better resolution of soft-tissue structures in the spine, allowing for the detection of both developmental and acquired stenosis. These imaging modalities have been used to identify congenital stenosis based on several criteria, including Torg ratio < 0.82[16] and loss of cerebrospinal fluid (CSF) signal surrounding the spinal cord.[17] MRI of the entire cervical spine in both axial and sagittal views using both T1- and T2-weighted images provides comprehensive evaluation of cervical stenosis.[18]

17.3 Risk of Neurological Injury in Cervical Trauma with Congenital Stenosis

17.3.1 Permanent Neurological Injury

Patients with congenital cervical spinal stenosis generally remain asymptomatic until the onset of spondylotic changes leads to further narrowing of the cervical spinal canal. However, patients with congenital stenosis are at greater risk of certain neurological injuries after trauma to the cervical spine.

Numerous studies have reported a link between congenital cervical spinal stenosis and traumatic spinal cord injury (SCI). In 98 patients who had experienced closed cervical spine fractures and/or dislocations, Eismont et al[19] found a correlation between midsagittal canal size as seen on radiographs and the occurrence and degree of neurological impairment after injury. All of the 14 patients in that study with complete quadriplegia had canal diameters less than the average of patients with no neurological deficit. In another study, Kang et al[20] examined the Torg ratio and midsagittal canal diameters on radiographs of 288 patients who had sustained acute fractures or dislocations of the cervical spine. The authors found that a sagittal canal diameter < 13 mm was strongly associated with SCI and that the SCI group had smaller Torg ratios and canal diameters.

Patients with congenital stenosis are also at elevated risk of SCI in cases of structurally insignificant cervical trauma. In patients who had experienced minor cervical trauma, Aebli et al[21] reviewed the radiological characteristics of 45 patients without neurological symptoms and 68 patients suffering from acute cervical SCI and found significantly smaller Torg ratios among the SCI group relative to those without SCI. They did not, however, detect an inverse relationship between Torg ratio and severity of SCI (as assessed by American Spinal Injury Association impairment score), and the Torg ratios did not differ between patients who did or did not fully recover after SCI. The authors propose that patients with a Torg ratio below 0.7 be considered at elevated risk for acute cervical SCI after minor cervical trauma.

In a 2012 study, Takao et al[22] noted that a congenitally narrow spinal canal may be an important risk factor for traumatic cervical SCI. Of the 30 patients with a history of traumatic cervical SCI without major fracture or dislocation at the C3–C4 segment, 27 (90%) had cervical spinal stenosis as determined by sagittal CSF column diameter < 8 mm at this segment, whereas only 61 (6.75%) of 607 healthy volunteers had cervical spinal stenosis at C3–C4. Furthermore, the authors found that the incidence for traumatic cervical SCI without major fracture or dislocation at the C3-C4 segment for patients with cervical spine canal stenosis was 124.5 times higher than those without canal stenosis.

In 53 patients with distractive-extension injuries, Song et al[23] divided patients into one of four categories based on the severity of their SCI: A (complete), B (incomplete), C (radiculopathy), or D (normal). Using this categorization, the authors found an inverse relationship between Torg ratio and severity of symptoms. In another 103 patients with similar injuries, stenosis, as determined by Torg ratio, was found in 20% of patients, and prognosis was worse among patients in this group.[24]

17.3.2 Transient Cervical Neurapraxia

Much of the literature regarding cervical trauma in patients with congenital spinal stenosis focuses on athletes in contact sports and the relative risk for cervical cord neurapraxia (CCN). CCN is an acute transient neurological injury to the cervical cord that involves sensory changes, such as burning pain, numbness, or tingling, with or without motor changes ranging from weakness to complete paralysis. It most often occurs in athletes with congenitally narrow cervical spinal canals as a result of hyperflexion or hyperextension injury.[25] Symptoms generally subside within 15 minutes but can persist for up to 48 hours. Such injuries compress the spinal cord by a "pincer" mechanism in which the spinal cord is pinched between the inferior margin of the one vertebra and lamina of the vertebra below it (▶ Fig. 17.3).[26] The prevalence of these injuries has been estimated at 7 in 10,000 football players.[8]

Among 24 patients with history of CCN, Torg et al[27] found radiographic evidence of congenital cervical stenosis in 17 patients. Relative to a control group, the neurapraxia group had significant stenosis as determined by both sagittal canal diameter and Torg ratio. In a later work, Torg et al[28] conducted an epidemiological study of American football players at various levels of competition and found that 42 of 45 players who had experienced transient neurapraxia of the spinal cord had a Torg–Pavlov ratio < 0.80 at one or more of vertebral levels from C3–C6. The sensitivity of this cutoff value for transient CCN among football players was therefore, determined to be 93%; however, because of the low positive predictive value of this ratio (0.2%), the authors noted that it should not be used as a

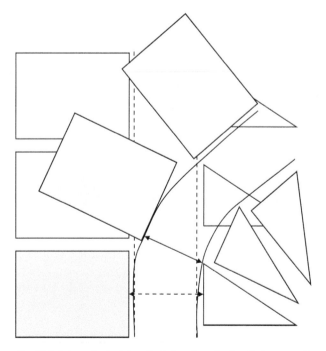

Fig. 17.3 Schematic depicting the "pincer" mechanism that can result in transient cervical neurapraxia. During a hyperextension injury, the spinal canal narrows and the cord becomes pinched between the posteroinferior edge of a vertebral body and the subjacent lamina.

screening mechanism to determine suitability for participation in contact sports.

The effect of CCN on future risk of neurological injury has been questioned. Among 77 players who became permanently quadriplegic from football injuries, none had experienced an episode of CCN before their injury. From the same study, none of 45 players with an episode of CCN became quadriplegic during the follow-up period.[28] In a later study, Torg et al[25] reviewed 110 cases of CCN and confirmed congenital narrowing of the spinal canal as a causative factor. Among the patients who returned to contact activities after an initial episode of CCN, 35 (56%) of 63 experienced a second episode. The patients who experienced a second episode had smaller Torg ratios, smaller disc-level canal diameters, and less space available for the cord. No permanent morbidity occurred in patients who returned to play. These findings led Torg et al[25] to conclude that (1) congenital cervical spinal stenosis does not predispose one to permanent neurological injury, and (2) CCN is unrelated to permanent quadriplegia arising from injury. Reports later emerged, however, of permanent SCI in athletes who returned to play after CCN.[29]

Although CCN is linked to congenital stenosis in adult athletes, this relationship has not been established in the pediatric population. In one case series, each of 13 pediatric patients presenting with sports-related CCN were found to have a normal Torg ratio at C4 and a normal midsagittal canal diameter. Boockvar et al[10] proposed that rather than congenital narrowing of the spinal canal, CCN in pediatric patients might be caused by greater mobility in the pediatric spine, a product of more pliant ligaments, underdeveloped musculature, and immature joints.[30]

17.3.3 "Stinger" Injuries

Stingers are a neurapraxia of the brachial plexus involving transient pain and paresthesias in a single upper extremity. They are most often seen in the setting of football and other collision sports.[31] Associated symptoms include burning and tingling that radiates to the shoulder, arm, and hand. Weakness may also be noted in the deltoid, supraspinatus, and biceps. A number of mechanisms can cause stinger injuries, including (1) lateral flexion of the head away from the affected limb, causing a traction injury of the brachial plexus and/or nerve roots; (2) neck extension and lateral movement toward the side of the symptomatic limb, resulting in compression of nerve roots; and (3) injury from a direct blow to the brachial plexus.[31,32]

Meyer et al[33] retrospectively assessed 266 college football players at the University of Iowa to examine a relationship between cervical spinal stenosis (defined as Torg ratio < 0.8) and stinger injuries. The mean Torg ratio was significantly smaller in players with stingers, and these players were more likely to have cervical spinal stenosis than the asymptomatic patients (47.5 vs. 25.1%). The authors concluded that football players with cervical spinal stenosis have a threefold greater chance of experiencing a stinger. Furthermore, they found cervical spinal stenosis only in players whose stingers were caused by the extension-compression mechanism described above, supporting their claim that a normal Torg ratio may protect athletes from compression-extension mechanism stingers, but not from stingers caused by brachial plexus stretch injury. In another study, Kelly et al[34] used the foramen-to-vertebral body width ratio as seen on radiographs to estimate the degree of foraminal narrowing, finding an association between stinger injuries and both canal and foraminal stenosis.

Other studies helped clarify the relationship between congenital stenosis and stinger injuries, showing that although recurrent stingers are linked to congenital stenosis, players with congenital stenosis may not be at greater risk of a single stinger. Castro et al[35] prospectively assessed 130 college football players using the Torg criteria to determine whether cervical stenosis was predictive of stinger injuries. The authors found that the frequency of a single stinger was no greater among players with cervical stenosis and that players with multiple stingers had smaller Torg ratios than players who had only one. Instead of the Torg ratio of 0.80 proposed by Pavlov et al,[11] Castro et al[35] suggested that a value of 0.70 might be a more clinically appropriate cutoff value. Another study showed that 53% of athletes with chronic recurrent stingers had congenitally narrowed cervical spinal canals by Torg ratio < 0.8.[31]

Page et al[32] reviewed the use of the Torg ratio as a tool to identify players at risk of stinger injuries, finding that a ratio < 0.8 has a sensitivity and specificity of 71% and 68%, respectively, for identifying stingers, with a positive predictive value of 22%. These findings led the authors to conclude that this Torg ratio cutoff was not accurate in predicting stinger experience and, therefore, not clinically useful for asymptomatic players.

17.3.4 Central Cord Syndrome

This syndrome describes an incomplete SCI that presents along a spectrum of neurological deficits ranging from weakness in the hands and forearms to complete quadriparesis with only sacral sparing. It is characterized by greater involvement of the upper extremities. Damage to the cord is localized to the medial portion of the lateral corticospinal tract in the cervical spine.[36] Although it most often occurs among older patients with underlying cervical spondylosis after hyperextension injuries of the head and neck, it is also observed in younger patients with congenitally narrow cervical canals.[37]

Moehl et al[38] presented a report of an 18-year-old patient with central cord syndrome caused by hyperextension injury incurred in a motor vehicle accident. The authors concluded that the patient's congenitally narrow cervical canal predisposed him to this myelopathy in a manner similar to cervical spondylosis. Countee and Vijayanathan[9] provided another report of a patient with congenital cervical stenosis who experienced central cord syndrome after a hyperextension injury. In a case series of 11 patients with acute traumatic central cord syndrome, 10 patients had either spondylosis or stenosis and 2 had congenital stenosis.[39] Finnoff et al[40] reported the case of a college football player who developed central cord syndrome after a hyperextension injury to his cervical spine. The patient was found to have a congenitally narrow cervical spine as determined by the absence of functional reserve around the spinal cord at the level of C3–C4.

17.4 Management

17.4.1 Central Cord Syndrome

Central cord syndrome has traditionally been managed conservatively; substantial neurological recovery is often observed with only careful medical management and early immobilization. Patients with central cord syndrome should be immobilized with a hard collar to prevent further injury, and medical management should entail placement in intensive care, respiratory protection, and maintenance of mean arterial blood pressure at 85 to 90 mm Hg to improve spinal cord perfusion.[41] Once medically stable, if no instability of the axial spine is observed after complete radiographic evaluation, patients should begin mobilization with physical and occupational therapies.

In certain subsets of patients, central cord syndrome can be managed surgically with anterior cervical decompression and fusion, posterior cervical decompression and fusion, or posterior cervical decompression alone.[42] Spinal instability is considered an absolute indication for surgery, whereas underlying spinal stenosis and spondylosis are relative indications for surgery.[37] The value and timing of surgery for patients with spinal stenosis without bony injury is debated.[43] In 24 patients with traumatic central cord syndrome and underlying stenosis or spondylosis, early surgery (< 24 hours of injury) was not found to be associated with greater improvement in motor scores compared with late surgery, although hospital stays were shorter for the early surgery group.[44]

17.4.2 Stingers and Cervical Cord Neurapraxia

Stingers and CCN are transient neurological injuries that usually result in rapid and full recovery. When a stinger is suspected, initial evaluation should include localization of symptoms (unilateral vs. bilateral), assessment of strength, range of motion, reflexes in the neck and upper limb, and performance of the Spurling maneuver to identify injury to the cervical nerve root. If symptoms persist for longer than an hour, imaging including cervical radiography and MRI are recommended to identify instability or foraminal stenosis. If symptoms suggest a transient SCI, acute management should include immediate immobilization until spinal instability can be ruled out. Imaging studies of athletes can be conducted to identify underlying pathological conditions and to inform decisions regarding return to play. Radiography and CT of the cervical spine can identify ligamentous injury, instability, and bony injury, and MRI can reveal damage to the cord and functional stenosis.[45]

17.4.3 Role of Congenital Stenosis in Return-to-Play Guidelines

Numerous guidelines have been proposed for permitting a return to contact activities after neurological injury. Decisions about return to play depend greatly on individual circumstances, but should include consideration of a patient's symptoms, medical history, radiological findings, and sport and position played.[46]

Torg and Ramsey-Emrhein[47] put forth guidelines for participation in collision activities and classified spinal conditions as relative or absolute contraindications to contact sports (▶ Table 17.1). They determined that a Torg ratio < 0.8 in the absence of instability presents no contraindications to participation in contact sports. The following conditions were considered relative contraindications: (1) Torg ratio < 0.8 with one episode of CCN, (2) documented episodes of CCN associated with intervertebral disc disease and/or degenerative disease, and (3) documented episode of CCN associated with MRI evidence of cord defect or cord edema. Documented CCN with ligamentous instability, neurological symptoms lasting > 36 hours, and/or multiple episodes of CCN were considered absolute contraindications.

Cantu et al[48] proposed that decisions regarding return to play involve the consideration of "functional spinal stenosis," defined as the loss of CSF around the spinal cord as shown by MRI, contrast-enhanced CT, or myelography. The authors propose that among patients who have experienced a single episode of transient quadriplegia, there must be a normal spinal canal anteroposterior diameter at all levels and no MRI or CT evidence of functional stenosis or ligamentous injury before return to play.[49]

Surgical management of CCN has implications for return-to-play decisions. Single-level anterior or posterior decompression and fusion, when CSF signal is preserved around the cord, presents no contraindication to return to play. Multilevel decompression and fusion with CSF signal preservation is considered a relative contraindication. However, in patients with congenital narrowing of the spinal canal and absent CSF signal, single-level anterior cervical discectomy and fusion presents an absolute contraindication to return to play.[50]

Table 17.1 Selected guidelines for return-to-play in individuals with cervical stenosis after cervical cord neurapraxia/transient quadriplegia

Torg	Cantu
No contraindication to return-to-play: • Torg ratio ≤ 0.8 in an asymptomatic individual Relative contraindication: • Torg ratio ≤ 0.8 with one episode of cervical cord neurapraxia • Cervical cord neurapraxia associated with intervertebral disc disease and/or degenerative changes • Cervical cord neurapraxia with MRI evidence of cord defect or cord edema Absolute contraindication: • Cervical cord neurapraxia with ligamentous instability, symptoms of neurological findings lasting more than 36 h • Multiple episodes of cervical cord neurapraxia	After one episode of transient quadriplegia, may return to contact sports if each of the following criteria are met: • Full neurological recovery • Full range of cervical spine movement • Normal spinal canal AP diameter at all levels (≥ 13 mm) • No CT or MRI evidence of functional stenosis (loss of CSF signal around cord) or ligamentous injury • No cord compression or edema

Abbreviations: AP, anteroposterior; CSF, cerebrospinal fluid; CT, computed tomography; MRI, magnetic resonance imaging.

17.4.4 Surgical Management

Among 101 study participants with traumatic cervical SCI at the level of C3–C4 without major fracture or dislocation treated nonsurgically at one facility, Takao et al[51] failed to identify a relationship between the rate of spinal canal stenosis at admission and neurological recovery at discharge. Cervical spinal canal stenosis was evaluated by midsagittal diameter of the CSF column shown by MRI, and American Spinal Injury Association motor scores were used to quantify neurological status. On the basis of these results, the authors suggested that decompressive surgery might not be recommended for traumatic cervical SCI without major fracture or dislocation even in the setting of pre-existing stenosis.

Prophylactic Decompression

Prophylactic decompression has been performed on patients with congenital cervical spinal stenosis to prevent neurological injury from minor degenerative lesions that would be insignificant in a nonstenotic canal. The value of prophylactic decompression for the prevention of neurological injury resulting from trauma in patients with congenital stenosis has been questioned.

In their study of the prevalence of cervical spinal stenosis in skeletal specimens, Lee et al[5] noted that although an estimated 4.9% of the adult population has cervical spinal stenosis, spinal trauma is still relatively rare; only approximately 1 in 30,000 Americans become paralyzed due to spinal cord trauma each year. The authors, therefore, recommend that prophylactic decompression should not be performed solely on the basis of radiographic evidence of cervical stenosis. Takao et al[22] also suggested that because of low absolute risk of traumatic cervical SCI, prophylactic surgical management of cervical spinal canal stenosis might not be prudent. Decisions regarding prophylactic decompression should not rely solely on identification of congenital stenosis using the Torg ratio because doing so will fail to identify canal narrowing around the disc caused by spondylosis or soft-tissue protrusion.[52]

17.5 Conclusion

Congenital cervical spinal stenosis is a bony narrowing of the cervical spine that has been linked to a heightened risk for certain types of neurological injuries after trauma to the cervical spine. Participants in contact sports are at particular risk for such injuries such as CCN, stingers, and central cord syndrome. In patients with cervical spine trauma, practitioners should include consideration of congenital stenosis in their decision-making before recommending a return to contact activities.

References

[1] Hulen CA, Herkowitz HN. Congenital spinal stenosis: review, pitfalls, and pearls of management. Semin Spine Surg. 2007; 19(3):177–186

[2] Roth M, Krkoska J, Toman I. Morphogenesis of the spinal canal, normal and stenotic. Neuroradiology. 1976; 10(5):277–286

[3] Jenkins TJ, Mai HT, Burgmeier RJ, Savage JW, Patel AA, Hsu WK. The triangle model of congenital cervical stenosis. Spine. 2016; 41(5):E242–E247

[4] Bajwa NS, Toy JO, Young EY, Ahn NU. Establishment of parameters for congenital stenosis of the cervical spine: an anatomic descriptive analysis of 1,066 cadaveric specimens. Eur Spine J. 2012; 21(12):2467–2474

[5] Lee MJ, Cassinelli EH, Riew KD. Prevalence of cervical spine stenosis. Anatomic study in cadavers. J Bone Joint Surg Am. 2007; 89(2):376–380

[6] Nakashima H, Yukawa Y, Suda K, Yamagata M, Ueta T, Kato F. Narrow cervical canal in 1211 asymptomatic healthy subjects: the relationship with spinal cord compression on MRI. Eur Spine J. 2016; 25(7):2149–2154

[7] Odor JM, Watkins RG, Dillin WH, Dennis S, Saberi M. Incidence of cervical spinal stenosis in professional and rookie football players. Am J Sports Med. 1990; 18(5):507–509

[8] Smith MG, Fulcher M, Shanklin J, Tillett ED. The prevalence of congenital cervical spinal stenosis in 262 college and high school football players. J Ky Med Assoc. 1993; 91(7):273–275

[9] Countee RW, Vijayanathan T. Congenital stenosis of the cervical spine: diagnosis and management. J Natl Med Assoc. 1979; 71(3):257–264

[10] Boockvar JA, Durham SR, Sun PP. Cervical spinal stenosis and sports-related cervical cord neurapraxia in children. Spine. 2001; 26(24):2709–2712, discussion 2713

[11] Pavlov H, Torg JS, Robie B, Jahre C. Cervical spinal stenosis: determination with vertebral body ratio method. Radiology. 1987; 164(3):771–775

[12] Blackley HR, Plank LD, Robertson PA. Determining the sagittal dimensions of the canal of the cervical spine. The reliability of ratios of anatomical measurements. J Bone Joint Surg Br. 1999; 81(1):110–112

[13] Prasad SS, O'Malley M, Caplan M, Shackleford IM, Pydisetty RK. MRI measurements of the cervical spine and their correlation to Pavlov's ratio. Spine. 2003; 28(12):1263–1268

[14] Herzog RJ, Wiens JJ, Dillingham MF, Sontag MJ. Normal cervical spine morphometry and cervical spinal stenosis in asymptomatic professional football players. Plain film radiography, multiplanar computed tomography, and magnetic resonance imaging. Spine. 1991; 16(6) Suppl:S178–S186

[15] Horne PH, Lampe LP, Nguyen JT, Herzog RJ, Albert TJ. A novel radiographic indicator of developmental cervical stenosis. J Bone Joint Surg Am. 2016; 98(14):1206–1214

[16] Yu M, Tang Y, Liu Z, Sun Y, Liu X. The morphological and clinical significance of developmental cervical stenosis. Eur Spine J. 2015; 24(8):1583–1589

[17] Brigham CD, Capo J. Cervical spinal cord contusion in professional athletes: a case series with implications for return to play. Spine. 2013; 38(4):315–323

[18] Lund T, José Santos de Moraes O. Cervical, thoracic, and lumbar stenosis. In: Winn HR, ed. Youmans and Winn Neurological Surgery. Vol 3. 7th ed. Philadelphia, PA: Elsevier; 2017:2373–2383

[19] Eismont FJ, Clifford S, Goldberg M, Green B. Cervical sagittal spinal canal size in spine injury. Spine. 1984; 9(7):663–666

[20] Kang JD, Figgie MP, Bohlman HH. Sagittal measurements of the cervical spine in subaxial fractures and dislocations. An analysis of two hundred and eighty-eight patients with and without neurological deficits. J Bone Joint Surg Am. 1994; 76(11):1617–1628

[21] Aebli N, Wicki AG, Rüegg TB, Petrou N, Eisenlohr H, Krebs J. The Torg-Pavlov ratio for the prediction of acute spinal cord injury after a minor trauma to the cervical spine. Spine J. 2013; 13(6):605–612

[22] Takao T, Morishita Y, Okada S, et al. Clinical relationship between cervical spinal canal stenosis and traumatic cervical spinal cord injury without major fracture or dislocation. Eur Spine J. 2013; 22(10):2228–2231

[23] Song KJ, Choi BW, Kim SJ, Kim GH, Kim YS, Song JH. The relationship between spinal stenosis and neurological outcome in traumatic cervical spine injury: an analysis using Pavlov's ratio, spinal cord area, and spinal canal area. Clin Orthop Surg. 2009; 1(1):11–18

[24] Song KJ, Choi BW, Park CI, Lee KB. Prognostic factors in distractive extension injuries of the subaxial cervical spine. Eur J Orthop Surg Traumatol. 2015; 25 Suppl 1:S101–S106

[25] Torg JS, Corcoran TA, Thibault LE, et al. Cervical cord neurapraxia: classification, pathomechanics, morbidity, and management guidelines. J Neurosurg. 1997; 87(6):843–850

[26] Penning L. Some aspects of plain radiography of the cervical spine in chronic myelopathy. Neurology. 1962; 12:513–519

[27] Torg JS, Pavlov H, Genuario SE, et al. Neurapraxia of the cervical spinal cord with transient quadriplegia. J Bone Joint Surg Am. 1986; 68(9):1354–1370

[28] Torg JS, Naranja RJ, Jr, Pavlov H, Galinat BJ, Warren R, Stine RA. The relationship of developmental narrowing of the cervical spinal canal to reversible and irreversible injury of the cervical spinal cord in football players. J Bone Joint Surg Am. 1996; 78(9):1308–1314

[29] Brigham CD, Adamson TE. Permanent partial cervical spinal cord injury in a professional football player who had only congenital stenosis. A case report. J Bone Joint Surg Am. 2003; 85-A(8):1553–1556

[30] Boden BP, Tacchetti RL, Cantu RC, Knowles SB, Mueller FO. Catastrophic cervical spine injuries in high school and college football players. Am J Sports Med. 2006; 34(8):1223–1232

[31] Levitz CL, Reilly PJ, Torg JS. The pathomechanics of chronic, recurrent cervical nerve root neurapraxia. The chronic burner syndrome. Am J Sports Med. 1997; 25(1):73–76

[32] Page S, Guy JA. Neurapraxia, "stingers," and spinal stenosis in athletes. South Med J. 2004; 97(8):766–769

[33] Meyer SA, Schulte KR, Callaghan JJ, et al. Cervical spinal stenosis and stingers in collegiate football players. Am J Sports Med. 1994; 22(2):158–166

[34] Kelly JD, IV, Aliquo D, Sitler MR, Odgers C, Moyer RA. Association of burners with cervical canal and foraminal stenosis. Am J Sports Med. 2000; 28(2):214–217

[35] Castro FP, Jr, Ricciardi J, Brunet ME, Busch MT, Whitecloud TS, III. Stingers, the Torg ratio, and the cervical spine. Am J Sports Med. 1997; 25(5):603–608

[36] Jimenez O, Marcillo A, Levi AD. A histopathological analysis of the human cervical spinal cord in patients with acute traumatic central cord syndrome. Spinal Cord. 2000; 38(9):532–537

[37] Nowak DD, Lee JK, Gelb DE, Poelstra KA, Ludwig SC. Central cord syndrome. J Am Acad Orthop Surg. 2009; 17(12):756–765

[38] Moiel RH, Raso E, Waltz TA. Central cord syndrome resulting from congenital narrowness of the cervical spinal canal. J Trauma. 1970; 10(6):502–510

[39] Quencer RM, Bunge RP, Egnor M, et al. Acute traumatic central cord syndrome: MRI-pathological correlations. Neuroradiology. 1992; 34(2):85–94

[40] Finnoff JT, Mildenberger D, Cassidy CD. Central cord syndrome in a football player with congenital spinal stenosis: a case report. Am J Sports Med. 2004; 32(2):516–521

[41] Molliqaj G, Payer M, Schaller K, Tessitore E. Acute traumatic central cord syndrome: a comprehensive review. Neurochirurgie. 2014; 60(1–2):5–11

[42] Brodell DW, Jain A, Elfar JC, Mesfin A. National trends in the management of central cord syndrome: an analysis of 16,134 patients. Spine J. 2015; 15(3):435–442

[43] Aarabi B, Hadley MN, Dhall SS, et al. Management of acute traumatic central cord syndrome (ATCCS). Neurosurgery. 2013; 72 Suppl 2:195–204

[44] Guest J, Eleraky MA, Apostolides PJ, Dickman CA, Sonntag VK. Traumatic central cord syndrome: results of surgical management. J Neurosurg. 2002; 97(1) Suppl:25–32

[45] Kurian PA, Light DI, Kerr HA. Burners, stingers, and cervical cord neurapraxia/transient quadriparesis. In: O'Brien M, Meehan WP III, eds. Head and Neck Injuries in Young Athletes. Cham: Springer International Publishing; 2016:129–141

[46] Creighton DW, Shrier I, Shultz R, Meeuwisse WH, Matheson GO. Return-to-play in sport: a decision-based model. Clin J Sport Med. 2010; 20(5):379–385

[47] Torg JS, Ramsey-Emrhein JA. Suggested management guidelines for participation in collision activities with congenital, developmental, or postinjury lesions involving the cervical spine. Med Sci Sports Exerc. 1997; 29(7) Suppl:S256–S272

[48] Cantu RC. Functional cervical spinal stenosis: a contraindication to participation in contact sports. Med Sci Sports Exerc. 1993; 25(3):316–317

[49] Cantu RC, Li YM, Abdulhamid M, Chin LS. Return to play after cervical spine injury in sports. Curr Sports Med Rep. 2013; 12(1):14–17

[50] Maroon JC, El-Kadi H, Abla AA, et al. Cervical neurapraxia in elite athletes: evaluation and surgical treatment. Report of five cases. J Neurosurg Spine. 2007; 6(4):356–363

[51] Takao T, Okada S, Morishita Y, et al. Clinical influence of cervical spinal canal stenosis on neurological outcome after traumatic cervical spinal cord injury without major fracture or dislocation. Asian Spine J. 2016; 10(3):536–542

[52] Aebli N, Rüegg TB, Wicki AG, Petrou N, Krebs J. Predicting the risk and severity of acute spinal cord injury after a minor trauma to the cervical spine. Spine J. 2013; 13(6):597–604

18 Trauma in Patients with Rheumatoid Arthritis of the Cervical Spine

Joseph D. Smucker and Rick C. Sasso

Abstract

Patients with rheumatoid arthritis (RA) have a predisposition to nontraumatic cervical spine disorders and neurological concerns that may result from these changes. With improvements in medical treatment of RA, the incidence of significant cervical spine involvement appears to be declining and/or may be less significant when present. Medical management of RA may predispose this patient population to unique challenges that may necessitate unique perioperative morbidity related to wound healing, instrumentation placement and bone quality, healing of arthrodesis, and bracing requirements. Nonsurgical and surgical management of traumatic injuries in the cervical spine must account not only for the nature of the traumatic concern, but also baseline changes in the cervical spine related to RA and ongoing medical management of RA. With careful consideration of the patient and these principles, successful management of traumatic injuries in the cervical spine can be effectively accomplished.

Keywords: cervical spine, trauma, rheumatoid arthritis, nonoperative management, operative management, spinal instrumentation, case examples

18.1 Introduction

Over past two decades, treatment of rheumatoid arthritis (RA) has advanced to a degree that has allowed less frequent involvement of cervical spine pathology in RA patients.[1,2] While patients with RA always benefit from careful consideration with respect to cervical spine concerns, neck pain, and neurological issues, many of the former concerns with this disease process were nontraumatic in nature and were more frequently related to the progressive changes associated with the inflammatory rheumatologic concern.[2]

RA does predispose patients to cervical spine concerns including C1–C2 instability, subaxial spondylolisthesis, pannus formation, destructive joint disease, diminished bone quality, and nontraumatic cervical radiculopathy, and/or cervical myelopathy.[1,2,3,4,5,6,7] In addition, treatments for RA have a potential to create negative effects on the patient's bone health, soft-tissue healing characteristics, bone healing characteristics, and perioperative morbidity.[1,8,9] For this reason, any surgical intervention on a patient with RA does have the potential for increased morbidity either secondary to the disease process or to the treatment of the disease process over time. These same characteristics, therefore, affect a surgeon's consideration of treatment of a patient with a traumatic lesion to the cervical spine who has baseline RA.

Despite the potential for decreasing rheumatoid cervical spine lesions with medical management over time, a physician evaluating a patient with a history of RA must recognize the difference between baseline rheumatologic cervical spine disease and acute traumatic lesions.[2,3,5,8,9,10,11,12,13,14] In addition, subsequent treatment must take into consideration the potential for increased morbidity in this unique patient population.

18.2 Incidence of Injury

To the authors' knowledge, there has been no definitive account of the incidence of traumatic cervical spine injuries in patients who also have RA. It is appropriate to consider these two populations' patients as intersecting only with a potential traumatic event. It is, therefore, incumbent upon evaluating health care providers to obtain an appropriate patient history including past medical history and medication history, in addition to the standard trauma history that accompanies a recent history of injury.[1,2,3,5,11,12,13,14,15] This has the potential to affect not only the treating physicians, but also those who are involved in interpreting radiographic studies and assessing the potential for perioperative risk, including the risk of infection and anesthesia risks and complications.

18.3 Patient Assessment

The assessment of the cervical spine in the setting of trauma has been well described.[16,17,18,19,20,21,22,23] Assessments of patients with a history of RA require a similar, prescribed, workup.[3,4,5,14] This includes a thorough history, a comprehensive physical examination, and appropriate radiographic evaluation. Computed tomography (CT) imaging of the spine has increased the sensitivity and specificity of diagnosis of traumatic cervical spine injury in the acute setting. This same imaging technology is appropriate for an initial assessment of patients with RA as well. However, a negative CT scan may not be appropriate for final assessment or exclusion of injury in patients with trauma and a history of RA. Consideration of dynamic CT examinations may be of importance in this unique population of patients.[24] Rheumatoid concerns in the cervical spine are well known to produce compressive pathology including the possibility of retrodental pannus.[6] In addition, spondylolisthesis maybe underappreciated on supine imaging, or CT only imaging. A low threshold for magnetic resonance imaging (MRI) and awake, active, upright dynamic radiographs should be present in a patient with trauma and known RA. Patients with new or increased neck pain should always be carefully screened both clinically and radiographically as part of a complete spine workup. In the context of RA, the threshold for consultation of a spine specialist may be diminished in this same, unique, patient population.[1,3,11,25] For example, the difference between rheumatologic instability at C1–C2 and traumatic instability may be difficult to distinguish in even the most skilled hands.[24,26] Serial follow-up and appropriate initial immobilization may be the key to safe patient care following the index injury.

Outside of imaging assessments, repeat clinical and neurological assessments have a potential to play a key role in patients with traumatic injuries. Distracting injuries should be successfully treated and appropriately managed prior to full clearance of the cervical spine in this unique patient population. In addition, if rheumatoid pathology is discovered in the cervical spine, this may play a role in anesthesia care and careful intubation, even if no traumatic injury is ultimately identified in the cervical spine.[27,28,29,30,31,32,33]

18.4 Nonoperative Management

Nonoperative management of patients with cervical spine trauma and RA is directed in accordance with the potential for bone healing.[4,34] If no traumatic injury is identified yet patients continue to have cervical spine pain, clearance in the Emergency Department or hospital setting may not be indicated in this patient population. In this circumstance, delayed dynamic radiographs at the discretion of a spine-care specialist are often considered, even to complement a normal appearing CT or MR scan.

Discontinuation of cervical immobilization may proceed at the discretion of the treating physician when acute, dynamic instability has been effectively ruled out. This may be a difficult threshold to reach. If the patient has baseline pain, new or increased pain must be carefully evaluated. Acute, muscular injury/strain or "whiplash" is a diagnosis of exclusion rather than an assumption in all patients. This is especially true in patients with RA. A concerted effort should be made in this circumstance to identify any former imaging that may have been performed in a patient with trauma, prior to the traumatic event. This has the potential to differentiate an acute injury from baseline concerns. Awake patient assessments over time are also critical to immobilization discontinuation and progression to additional nonsurgical care.

In the absence of an acute fracture and at the exclusion of an acute ligamentous instability, gentle and active (nonpassive, nonmanipulative) physical therapy and close clinical assessments may proceed with a focus on appropriate pain management and nonsteroidal anti-inflammatory drug (NSAID) utilization. Certain medications may be excluded from consideration based upon the patient's innate risk for medication-induced complications and baseline use of NSAIDS. Serial assessments of progress are made over time in the clinical setting, and time can allow for improvement in patient-reported pain and function.

Clinical and/or radiographic follow-up of patients may be discontinued when pain has returned either to baseline or has resolved, and when function has returned to baseline and neurological assessments have remained stable. Coordination and communication with the patient's rheumatologist is critical over the course of posttrauma treatment and at the time of discontinuation of posttrauma follow-up. Patient education and communication remains critical in continued index suspicion for a new concern over time.

18.5 Operative Management

With very few exceptions, operative treatment of traumatic injuries in the cervical spine in patients with RA is similar in principle and design to treatment of patients with cervical spine trauma in the absence of RA. Modern cervical instrumentation has revolutionized the treatment of patients with cervical spine disorders including patients with cervical trauma, rheumatologic diseases of the cervical spine, and degenerative diseases of the cervical spine (▸ Fig. 18.1). Moving beyond single plane wiring techniques, multipoint posterior screw/rod fixation systems using the novel screw placement is now the standard of care. Anterior only versus anterior/posterior treatment is of consideration in all patients, but may be especially important to consider in patients with diminished bone quality or bone healing potential. Posterior instrumentation currently includes consideration of powerful fixation techniques such as pedicle screw placement, translaminar screw placement, and C1 lateral mass screw fixation. The cranial and caudal aspects of instrumentation must be especially secure in this patient population. Attachment of these novel bone/screw techniques to a vertical, rod-based stabilization system is currently facilitated by modern instrumentation systems by way of polyaxial screw heads, novel offset connection systems, articulated vertical rod and screw systems, prebent vertical rod systems, multidiameter rod systems, and improved surgical techniques. Computer-assisted spinal navigation has revolutionized the surgeon's understanding of cervical spine anatomy, traumatic injury anatomy, and instrumentation placement.

At the time of writing, the Food and Drug Administration (FDA) approval does exist for multipoint/segmental instrumentation systems, as well as computer-assisted instrumentation techniques in posterior treatment of the cervical spine. The workhorse of multilevel cervical spine instrumentation in the setting of traumatic injury is the posterior cervical approach. Both segmental instrumentation and multilevel decompression may be accomplished via a single surgical incision with posterior techniques. Indeed, many of the approaches that are currently utilized for treatment of rheumatoid pathology of the cervical spine are also posteriorly based and can easily be adapted for the same patient population in the context of trauma.

A low threshold should exist for multi-segment instrumentation in patients with RA. Bone quality and instrumentation fixation must also be considered. This is at the potential expense of an increased risk of infection and a decreased incidence of bone healing with the same posterior cervical techniques (in patients with RA). Supplemental anterior and/or external immobilization is of significant consideration in segmental instrumentation of the cervical spine.

18.5.1 Surgical Techniques: Anterior-only

Anterior-only surgical stabilization and/or decompression is a powerful technique in many patients with cervical spine trauma.[35,36,37,38] Though it is beyond the specific scope of this chapter, anterior techniques offer the advantage of direct decompression of the burden of discogenic and vertebral body fracture-related pathology that may be present in patients with traumatic injury. Partial and/or complete corpectomy and anterior fusion with instrumentation may be performed in a stand-alone mode, if the number of levels is carefully taken into consideration.[39,40] Combination of this method of decompression with discectomy and fusion offers the opportunity to avoid combined posterior procedures. Bone quality is of consideration with respect to graft settling and instrumentation purchase.

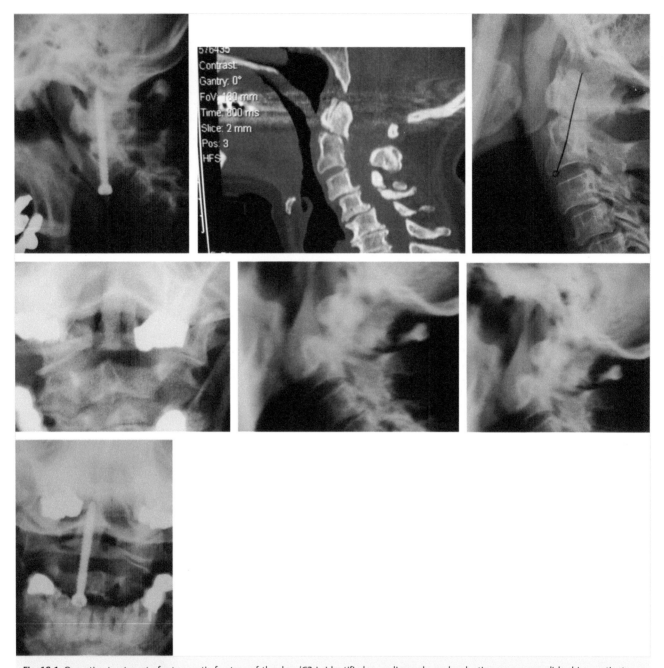

Fig. 18.1 Operative treatment of a traumatic fracture of the dens/C2 is identified on radiographs and reduction was accomplished in a patient with baseline rheumatoid arthritis. Treatment was performed with a single odontoid screw technique resulting in initially diminished pain but, progressing later to pseudoarthrosis.

Anterior procedures certainly have an advantage with respect to surface area and vascular perfusion as these factors relate to bone healing. Anterior cervical discectomy and fusion (ACDF) may offer the opportunity to correct deformity at the expense of the challenges associated with multilevel healing of ACDF. These techniques also offer the opportunity to obtain multipoint fixation with a plate/screw system. Although beyond the scope of this text, compression plating techniques and variable-angle screw use may provide for consistent instrumentation purchase and graft compressive properties in contrast to traditional anterior plating techniques.

18.5.2 Surgical Techniques: Posterior-only

Posterior spinal decompression is often considered to be an indirect method of addressing compressive, traumatic spinal pathology (▶ Fig. 18.2). In the authors' opinion, these techniques are of little utility in the treatment of trauma in the absence of instrumentation and fusion. Patients with RA may have existing pathology that is poorly addressed with decompression alone. Fusion in isolation may be of consideration in traumatic C1–C2 pathology and in numerous neurologically

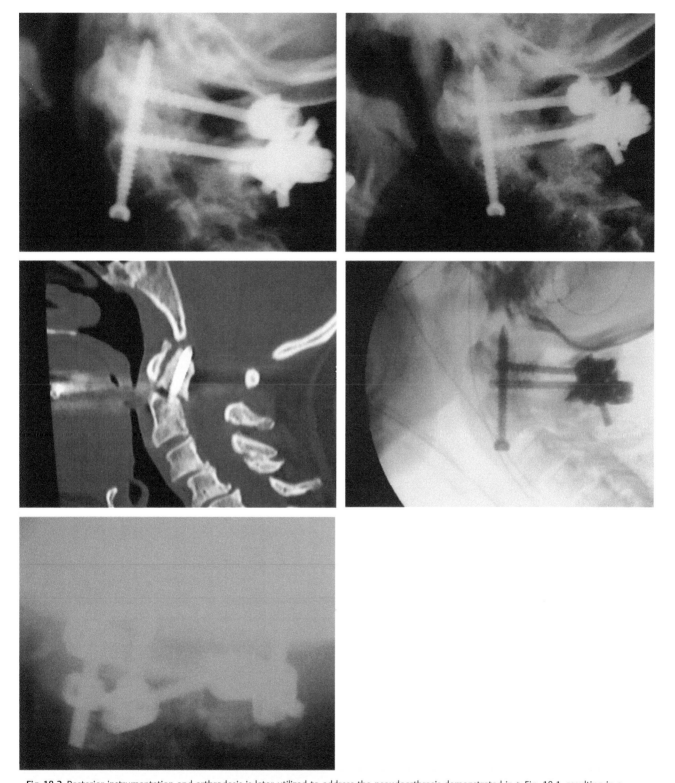

Fig. 18.2 Posterior instrumentation and arthrodesis is later utilized to address the pseudoarthrosis demonstrated in ▶ Fig. 18.1, resulting in a stable arthrodesis and diminished pain.

intact injuries. Posterior fusion without decompression increases the bone-healing surface area and potential instrumentation options, especially with respect to translaminar techniques of instrumentation.

Posterior instrumentation and fusion remains a workhorse technique for the treatment of patients with traumatic injury to the cervical spine. These techniques allow for a multiplicity of fixation techniques via powerful fixation methods such as pedicle screw fixation, translaminar screws, and transarticular C1–C2 fixation. In contrast to lateral mass fixation, these techniques have the potential to provide for immediately stable fixation in patients with diminished bone quality or healing potential. These techniques are performed at an increased risk of infection in contrast to anterior-only surgery. In addition, they are performed at the potential expense of the ability to directly decompress levels of the spine affected by discogenic or vertebral body pathology.

With respect to patients with RA, bone quality, fusion healing potential, and infection risk must be carefully considered with posterior-only and with anterior techniques that are combined with posterior fixation. All posterior techniques are based upon the ability of the surgeon to achieve stable fixation above and below the region of injury. This may be especially important in patients with RA, where pedicle screw and translaminar techniques offer excellent options at cranial and/or caudal fixation levels.[41] Every effort should be made to utilize these techniques at the cranial and caudal fixation levels, including the addition of levels of fixation that would otherwise not be included for decompressive-only purposes from a posterior-only approach. Extension cranially to C2 with translaminar screws or pedicle screws and caudally to C7 with pedicle or translaminar techniques versus to T1 or T2 with pedicle screws, are excellent options.

Computer-assisted spinal navigation may play a role in a surgeon's ability to successfully visualize points of fixation and place instrumentation in patients undergoing multipoint posterior cervical instrumentation. In the absence of a surgeon's ability to utilize navigation, intraoperative CT-like imaging also provides the ability to guide the surgeon's assessment of instrumentation placement prior to completion of the surgical procedure. This is an evolving component of spine surgical practice, and while not the standard of care at the time of this writing, it has powerful potential for use in posterior approaches in instances of trauma to the axial skeleton.

18.5.3 Anterior-Posterior Considerations

The threshold to perform anterior and posterior treatment of traumatic injuries to the cervical spine in patients with RA should be decreased. This is not only a preoperative judgment, but also an intraoperative and postoperative assessment. The drivers of this consideration are bone quality and bone healing potential. Secondary considerations include surgical complexity and the ability of the surgeon to achieve multipoint fixation above and below the level(s) of injury. Theoretically, the ability to achieve multiple points of fixation at a given level while at the same time provide for multiple bone healing surfaces is the primary consideration behind a surgeon's planning for anterior and posterior combined techniques.

References

[1] Thonse R, Belthur M. Rheumatoid arthritis and neck pain. Postgrad Med J. 2003; 79(938):711

[2] Wasserman BR, Moskovich R, Razi AE. Rheumatoid arthritis of the cervical spine—clinical considerations. Bull NYU Hosp Jt Dis. 2011; 69(2):136–148

[3] Ambrose NL, Cunnane G. Importance of full evaluation in patients who complain of neck pain. Ir J Med Sci. 2009; 178(2):209–210

[4] Bréban S, Briot K, Kolta S, et al. Identification of rheumatoid arthritis patients with vertebral fractures using bone mineral density and trabecular bone score. J Clin Densitom. 2012; 15(3):260–266

[5] de Souza MC, de Ávila Fernandes E, Jones A, Lombardi I, Jr, Natour J. Assessment of cervical pain and function in patients with rheumatoid arthritis. Clin Rheumatol. 2011; 30(6):831–836

[6] Grob D, Würsch R, Grauer W, Sturzenegger J, Dvorak J. Atlantoaxial fusion and retrodental pannus in rheumatoid arthritis. Spine. 1997; 22(14):1580–1583, discussion 1584

[7] Mahajan R, Huisa BN. Vertebral artery dissection in rheumatoid arthritis with cervical spine disease. J Stroke Cerebrovasc Dis. 2013; 22(7):e245–e246

[8] Bouchaud-Chabot A, Lioté F. Cervical spine involvement in rheumatoid arthritis. A review. Joint Bone Spine. 2002; 69(2):141–154

[9] Joaquim AF, Appenzeller S. Cervical spine involvement in rheumatoid arthritis—a systematic review. Autoimmun Rev. 2014; 13(12):1195–1202

[10] Dreyer SJ, Boden SD. Natural history of rheumatoid arthritis of the cervical spine. Clin Orthop Relat Res. 1999(366):98–106

[11] Kauppi MJ, Barcelos A, da Silva JA. Cervical complications of rheumatoid arthritis. Ann Rheum Dis. 2005; 64(3):355–358

[12] Kopacz KJ, Connolly PJ. The prevalence of cervical spondylolisthesis. Orthopedics. 1999; 22(7):677–679

[13] Narváez J, Narváez JA, Serrallonga M, et al. Subaxial cervical spine involvement in symptomatic rheumatoid arthritis patients: comparison with cervical spondylosis. Semin Arthritis Rheum. 2015; 45(1):9–17

[14] Zhang T, Pope J. Cervical spine involvement in rheumatoid arthritis over time: results from a meta-analysis. Arthritis Res Ther. 2015; 17:148

[15] Shen FH, Samartzis D, Jenis LG, An HS. Rheumatoid arthritis: evaluation and surgical management of the cervical spine. Spine J. 2004; 4(6):689–700

[16] Chew BG, Swartz C, Quigley MR, Altman DT, Daffner RH, Wilberger JE. Cervical spine clearance in the traumatically injured patient: is multidetector CT scanning sufficient alone? Clinical article. J Neurosurg Spine. 2013; 19(5):576–581

[17] Darras K, Andrews GT, McLaughlin PD, et al. Pearls for interpreting computed tomography of the cervical spine in trauma. Radiol Clin North Am. 2015; 53(4):657–674, vii

[18] Griffith B, Vallee P, Krupp S, et al. Screening cervical spine CT in the emergency department, phase 3: increasing effectiveness of imaging. J Am Coll Radiol. 2014; 11(2):139–144

[19] Haris AM, Vasu C, Kanthila M, Ravichandra G, Acharya KD, Hussain MM. Assessment of MRI as a modality for evaluation of soft tissue injuries of the spine as compared to intraoperative assessment. J Clin Diagn Res. 2016; 10(3):TC01–TC05

[20] Joaquim AF, Patel AA. Subaxial cervical spine trauma: evaluation and surgical decision-making. Global Spine J. 2014; 4(1):63–70

[21] Tran B, Saxe JM, Ekeh AP. Are flexion extension films necessary for cervical spine clearance in patients with neck pain after negative cervical CT scan? J Surg Res. 2013; 184(1):411–413

[22] Ulbrich EJ, Carrino JA, Sturzenegger M, Farshad M. Imaging of acute cervical spine trauma: when to obtain which modality. Semin Musculoskelet Radiol. 2013; 17(4):380–388

[23] Utz M, Khan S, O'Connor D, Meyers S. MDCT and MRI evaluation of cervical spine trauma. Insights Imaging. 2014; 5(1):67–75

[24] Söderman T, Olerud C, Shalabi A, Alavi K, Sundin A. Static and dynamic CT imaging of the cervical spine in patients with rheumatoid arthritis. Skeletal Radiol. 2015; 44(2):241–248

[25] Roche CJ, Eyes BE, Whitehouse GH. The rheumatoid cervical spine: signs of instability on plain cervical radiographs. Clin Radiol. 2002; 57(4):241–249

[26] Ecker RD, Dekutoski MB, Ebersold MJ. Symptomatic C1–2 fusion failure due to a fracture of the lateral C-1 posterior arch in a patient with rheumatoid arthritis. Case report and review of the literature. J Neurosurg. 2001; 94(1) Suppl:137–139

[27] Asano N, Ishiguro S, Sudo A. Head positioning for reduction and stabilization of the cervical spine during anesthetic induction in a patient with subaxial subluxation. J Neurosurg Anesthesiol. 2012; 24(2):164–165

[28] Cagla Ozbakis Akkurt B, Guler H, Inanoglu K, Dicle Turhanoglu A, Turhanoglu S, Asfuroglu Z. Disease activity in rheumatoid arthritis as a predictor of difficult intubation? Eur J Anaesthesiol. 2008; 25(10):800–804

[29] Cooper RM. Rheumatoid arthritis is a common disease with clinically important implications for the airway. J Bone Joint Surg Am. 1995; 77(9):1463–1465

[30] Hakala P, Randell T. Intubation difficulties in patients with rheumatoid arthritis. A retrospective analysis. Acta Anaesthesiol Scand. 1998; 42(2):195–198

[31] Lopez-Olivo MA, Andrabi TR, Palla SL, Suarez-Almazor ME. Cervical spine radiographs in patients with rheumatoid arthritis undergoing anesthesia. J Clin Rheumatol. 2012; 18(2):61–66

[32] Takenaka I, Aoyama K, Iwagaki T, Ishimura H, Takenaka Y, Kadoya T. Fluoroscopic observation of the occipitoatlantoaxial complex during intubation attempt in a rheumatoid patient with severe atlantoaxial subluxation. Anesthesiology. 2009; 111(4):917–919

[33] Tokunaga D, Hase H, Mikami Y, et al. Atlantoaxial subluxation in different intraoperative head positions in patients with rheumatoid arthritis. Anesthesiology. 2006; 104(4):675–679

[34] Ørstavik RE, Haugeberg G, Uhlig T, et al. Self reported non-vertebral fractures in rheumatoid arthritis and population based controls: incidence and relationship with bone mineral density and clinical variables. Ann Rheum Dis. 2004; 63(2):177–182

[35] Alves PL, Martins DE, Ueta RH, Del Curto D, Wajchenberg M, Puertas EB. Options for surgical treatment of cervical fractures in patients with spondylotic spine: a case series and review of the literature. J Med Case Reports. 2015; 9:234

[36] Feuchtbaum E, Buchowski J, Zebala L. Subaxial cervical spine trauma. Curr Rev Musculoskelet Med. 2016; 9(4):496–504

[37] Jack A, Hardy-St-Pierre G, Wilson M, Choy G, Fox R, Nataraj A. Anterior surgical fixation for cervical spine flexion-distraction injuries. World Neurosurg. 2017; 101:365–371

[38] Lins CC, Prado DT, Joaquim AF. Surgical treatment of traumatic cervical facet dislocation: anterior, posterior or combined approaches? Arq Neuropsiquiatr. 2016; 74(9):745–749

[39] Sasso RC, Ruggiero RA, Jr, Reilly TM, Hall PV. Early reconstruction failures after multilevel cervical corpectomy. Spine. 2003; 28(2):140–142

[40] Singh K, Vaccaro AR, Kim J, Lorenz EP, Lim TH, An HS. Biomechanical comparison of cervical spine reconstructive techniques after a multilevel corpectomy of the cervical spine. Spine. 2003; 28(20):2352–2358, discussion 2358

[41] Ilgenfritz RM, Gandhi AA, Fredericks DC, Grosland NM, Smucker JD. Considerations for the use of C7 crossing laminar screws in subaxial and cervicothoracic instrumentation. Spine. 2013; 38(4):E199–E204

19 Traumatic Cervical Myelopathy

Robert F. Heary and Raghav Gupta

Abstract

Traumatic cervical spinal cord injury (SCI) occurs in patients presenting with blunt trauma due to motor vehicle accidents (MVAs), sports-related injuries, falls, and injuries related to interpersonal violence. Cervical SCI can present with symptoms of myelopathy secondary to compression of the cervical spinal cord. A decrease in the sagittal diameter of the spinal canal has been found to correlate with an increased incidence of cervical myelopathy following trauma. Multiple conditions, such as spondylosis, ossification of the posterior longitudinal ligament (OPLL), and congenital spinal stenosis, can increase the risk for presentation with myelopathic symptoms after cervical trauma. These conditions are characterized in this chapter with respect to the mechanisms of injury, clinical presentations, and resulting patient outcomes that have been reported in the context of cervical trauma.

Keywords: cervical trauma, myelopathy, spondylosis, OPLL, SCI, spinal stenosis

19.1 Traumatic Cervical Spinal Cord Injury

The epidemiology of traumatic spinal cord injury (SCI) has been well characterized in the neurosurgical literature. It has an estimated annual incidence of 25 to 59 new cases per million individuals in the United States and occurs 3 to 4 times more commonly in men than in women.[1] The underlying etiology for traumatic SCI varies and can include motor vehicle accidents (MVAs), acts of violence, sports-related injuries, falls, and other miscellaneous causes. MVAs are the leading cause of SCIs in the United States. Falls, meanwhile, account for most cases of SCI in elderly individuals (defined as adults over the age of 60 years).[2] Traumatic cervical SCI is fairly common with 2.4% of patients who present with blunt trauma suffering from cervical spine injuries.[3]

Acute traumatic cervical SCI can result in a clinical syndrome termed myelopathy resulting from compression of the spinal cord. While symptoms of cervical myelopathy can vary depending on the location and severity of cord compression, patients commonly present with disturbances in balance and/or gait, decreased hand dexterity, numbness in the hands and/or feet, bowel and bladder incontinence, and signs of upper and/or lower motor neuron dysfunction. Signs of myelopathy are detected on physical examination and include the presence of pathological reflexes including a positive Babinski sign, Hoffman sign, as well as ankle clonus and lower extremity hyperreflexia.[4] Increased lower extremity muscle tone, or spasticity, is another sign of myelopathy. While the most common etiology for cervical myelopathy is spondylosis, other etiologies can include, but are not limited to spinal neoplasms, ossification of the posterior longitudinal ligaments (OPLL), and congenitally narrowed spinal canals (▶ Fig. 19.1). A decrease in the sagittal diameter of the spinal canal has been found to correlate with an

increased incidence of cervical myelopathy.[5] Given that each of the aforementioned etiologies of cervical myelopathy can result in a decrease in the sagittal diameter of the spinal canal, when superimposed upon trauma, these conditions can predispose one to presentation with myelopathy resulting from spinal cord compression.

19.2 Sagittal Diameter of the Spinal Canal and Torg–Pavlov Ratios

In the past, the anteroposterior diameter (or sagittal diameter) of the spinal canal on lateral radiographs has been used to diagnose critical cervical canal stenosis. A diameter < 13 mm had been proposed as the threshold under which pathological changes in the intervertebral discs have been observed.[6] However, given discrepancies in the canal diameter between patients of different ethnic backgrounds[7] and radiographic magnification variability,[4] the Torg–Pavlov ratio was developed for making the diagnosis of critical spinal canal stenosis. Here, the sagittal diameter of the spinal canal is divided by the sagittal diameter of the vertebral body at the same level.[8] In the original study where this ratio was proposed, a value of < 0.82 diagnosed cervical canal stenosis in 92% of cases.[8] When Torg–Pavlov ratios in patients with and without cervical spondylotic myelopathy were compared, the mean Torg–Pavlov ratio was found to be significantly smaller in patients with spondylotic myelopathy (0.72 vs. 0.95; $p < 0.001$).[9] In patients presenting with minor trauma to the cervical spine, a Torg–Pavlov ratio < 0.70 has been found to have the greatest positive likelihood ratio for predicting SCI.[10]

19.3 Trauma in Patients with Cervical Spondylosis

Cervical spondylosis (or osteoarthritis) refers to a pair of entities including degenerative disc disease (DDD) and facet joint degeneration, which are both commonly observed in elderly patients. DDD results from compromised diffusion of oxygen and nutrients through the intervertebral discs over time leading to a radial redistribution of compressive forces within the vertebral column. This can present radiographically as a herniated disc, decreased intervertebral disc height, hypertrophy of the ligamentum flavum (▶ Fig. 19.2), and/or osteophyte formation. Osteophyte formation along the ventral aspect of the spinal canal is a physiological response to the increased stress on the vertebral endplates and stabilizes the neighboring vertebrae by increasing the surface area of the vertebral endplates. Myelopathy and radiculopathy can result from compression of the cervical spinal cord and cervical nerve roots, respectively, by these bony spurs. Clinical symptoms of cervical spondylosis can include neck pain, arm pain, upper extremity weakness, and/or neurological symptoms resulting from spinal cord or nerve root compression. The prevalence of radiographically

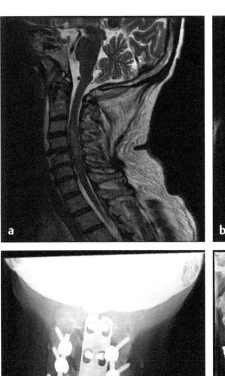

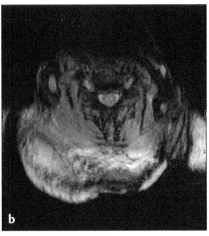

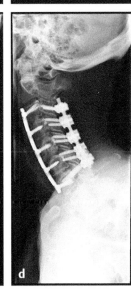

Fig. 19.1 A 61-year-old woman with no known history of cervical spine disease was involved in a fall. She presented to the emergency department with symptoms consistent with a central cord syndrome including profound hand weakness and diminished sensation in the hands, trunk, and lower extremities. **(a)** Magnetic resonance imaging (MRI; T2-weighted sagittal) study obtained at the time of admission. Congenitally narrowed spinal canal with abnormal signal extending from C3 to C6 within the cord parenchyma. Also, abnormal signal is evident in the C4–C5 intervertebral disc with questionable fracture of the superior aspect of the C5 vertebra. **(b)** MRI (T2-weighted axial) images at the C4–C5 level demonstrate markedly narrowed spinal canal with increased signal within the cord parenchyma. **(c, d)** Plain film images (antero-posterior and lateral) obtained 6 months following the injury demonstrate solid fusions from C3 to C7 with anterior/posterior stabilization having been performed. The rationale for this single-setting, anteroposterior surgery was to increase the space available for the swollen spinal cord and improve the odds of neurological recovery. At 6 months out from surgery, she had improved hand function although weakness of the opponens and intrinsic muscles persisted to a moderate degree. Lower extremity power was within normal limits and some gait spasticity persisted. Sensory examination had gradually improved but was not yet normal in the hands or lower extremities.

determined cervical DDD in men and women above the age of 40 years has been estimated to be 21.7%.[11,12] Meanwhile, the incidence of myelopathy resulting from cervical spondylosis has been estimated to be 4 per 100,000 person-years. Elderly male patients, however, are disproportionately affected more frequently in relation to other patient demographics.

Trauma in a patient with underlying cervical spondylosis can present paradoxically with a neurological deficit but little or no radiographic abnormalities.[13] In this subpopulation of patients, the traumatic event preceding the presentation with myelopathy is often minor. This underscores the disparity between the clinical presentation and the associated imaging findings. The mechanism by which SCI occurs is believed to be through bulging of the ligamentum flavum anteriorly into the spinal canal upon cervical spine extension. Posteriorly directed bone spurs and herniated discs, therefore, can compress the cord anteriorly while the ligamentum flavum enfolding does so posteriorly. In addition, hypertrophy of the laterally located uncovertebral facet joints can also contribute to narrowing of the overall spinal canal space. However, ligamentous and disc injury can occur if there is a rotational component to the extension. This can lead to intervertebral disc rupture and compression of the cord from the posteroinferior segment of the vertebral body above the ruptured disc (which has been displaced posteriorly), as well as the lamina of the vertebra at the level of the ruptured

disc.[13,14] Patients may be essentially asymptomatic, with previously unidentified spondylosis, and they may present with cervical myelopathy following a relatively minor traumatic episode. This leads to issues regarding insurance payments for spinal care as the patients clearly have abnormalities prior to the traumatic event but they are not symptomatic, and usually not even aware of any cervical pathology being present. In this scenario, the coverage by insurers for spine care is usually the responsibility of the motor vehicle insurance coverage.

In a series reported by Koyanagi et al on 42 patients who presented with acute traumatic cervical SCI over a 9-year period, and who had no evidence of fracture or dislocation, 38 patients (90.5%) were found to have degenerative changes of the cervical spine.[15] The most commonly affected vertebral levels were C3–C4, C4–C5, and C5–C6, in that order. Protruded discs and/or osteophytes were observed in 32 of these patients on magnetic resonance imaging (MRI). Of note, the mean sagittal diameter, on computed tomography (CT) imaging, of the cervical spinal canal in patients presenting with SCI was substantially lower than in comparison to a control group: the mean diameter at C5, for example, was 13.2 mm in the asymptomatic group and 11.0 mm in patients with cervical SCI ($p < 0.001$).[15] Similarly, in a series by Regenbogen et al on 42 patients who presented with traumatic cervical SCI and had minimal or no evidence of bony injury, 38 (90.5%) had moderate to severe cervical spondylosis

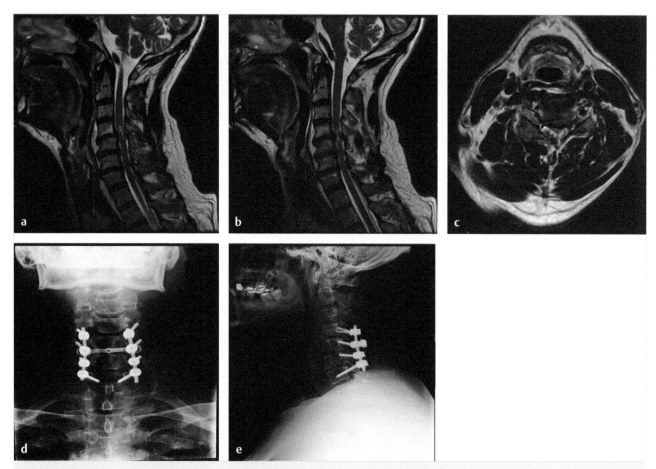

Fig. 19.2 A 63-year-old male with no known history of pathology in the cervical spine was involved in a motor vehicle accident as the driver and he developed signs and symptoms of myelopathy. Upon presentation to the emergency department, his neurological examination was consistent with an ASIA D spinal cord injury. **(a, b)** Magnetic resonance imaging (MRI; T2-weighted sagittal) study (two images) demonstrates a minimal degree of subluxation at the C4–C5 level with a herniated disc compressing the spinal cord. Evidence of ligamentum flavum hypertrophy causing canal narrowing was present at the C4–C6 levels. **(c)** MRI (T2-weighted axial) demonstrates marked canal narrowing at the C4–C5 level with bright signal in the cord proper. **(d, e)** Plain film imaging (anteroposterior and lateral) obtained 6 months following posterior decompression and fusion surgery with lateral mass fixation at C4–C6 and bilateral pedicle screw fixation at the C7 level confirms successful fusion and satisfactory alignment. The rationale for this surgery was to decompress the neural elements and provide stabilization to prevent further cord impairment. At 6 months out from surgery, the patient made a complete recovery with no deficits evident on a detailed neurological examination.

(defined as the presence of anterior or posterior osteophytes and/or narrowing of the intervertebral disc space).[13] Ironically, these numbers are identical to the previously cited study by Koyanagi et al.

The pattern of neurological injury noted in 40% of patients in the series reported by Regenbogen et al was consistent with acute traumatic central cord syndrome (CCS).[13,16] CCS was first described in 1954 by Schneider et al and it is the most frequently encountered incomplete SCI.[13,16] Traumatic CCS typically presents with disproportionately greater motor impairment in the upper extremities compared to the lower extremities, bladder dysfunction, and variable sensory loss below the level of the lesion. Nearly half of CCS cases result from hyperextension in patients with underlying congenital or degenerative spinal stenosis.[16,17] The role and timing of surgical intervention in patients with CCS, in whom there is no evidence of fracture/dislocation or disc herniation, remains unclear. Guest et al have reported no overall improvements in motor outcomes in patients who underwent early (< 24 hours after initial injury) or late surgery (> 24 hours after initial injury).[18]

Whether surgical intervention is beneficial in this subset of patients is not clearly understood. Aito et al, for example, have previously reported no differences in functional outcomes in 44 patients with hyperextension injuries and underlying cervical canal stenosis (due to either spondylosis or congenital causes) who were conservatively managed and 38 patients with skeletal and discoligamentous injuries who underwent surgical intervention.[19] On the other hand, traditional neurosurgical training has called for removal of ongoing neural compressive lesions when the patient is medically stabilized (▶ Fig. 19.1). The exact timing of any surgery, if it is to be performed, remains controversial.

19.4 Trauma in Patients with Ossification of the Posterior Longitudinal Ligament

OPLL is an age-related degenerative condition which has an increased prevalence in Asian patients (in whom the incidence is 2.4%). In addition, the prevalence is higher in men and elderly individuals. Symptomatic patients usually present in either the fifth or sixth decades of life.[20] OPLL most commonly affects the cervical spine[21] and is presumed to be a sequela of herniation of the nucleus pulposus into the PLL, although the exact pathogenesis of this condition is unclear.[22] Genetic, dietary, and metabolic factors have been implicated.[23] Ossification is believed to follow hypertrophy of the PLL, which is histologically characterized by proliferating chondrocytes and spindle cells as well as calcification.[24] Cervical myelopathy, as a consequence of OPLL, was first described in 1960 although the number of reports published since then has steadily increased.[23]

OPLL is believed to increase the risk for cervical SCI following minor trauma.[25] In their series of 231 patients with cervical SCIs, Endo et al reported that 6.5% of these patients had cervical OPLL.[26] In patients with acute cervical SCI without associated fractures and/or dislocations in an Asian population, the incidence of OPLL was estimated to be as high as 38%.[15] An increased risk of developing OPLL-related traumatic myelopathy has been observed in patients with a narrowed spinal canal (< 10 mm),[23] as well as in patients with mixed-type OPLL rather than segmental- or continuous-type OPLL as per the CT-based classification system first described by the Japanese Ministry of Public Health and Welfare.[27,28] In a study by Matsunaga et al, in which the authors prospectively followed 368 patients with cervical OPLL, all 45 patients who had 60% or greater spinal canal stenosis on lateral radiographs, developed myelopathy during the follow-up period, regardless of whether the patients had a history of cervical trauma or not.[27] Below this threshold, however, no difference in the maximum percent stenosis was observed in patients with and without traumatic myelopathy.[27]

Graham et al and Lee et al have previously reported that the most commonly observed form of minor trauma in patients with cervical OPLL, in their series, was a fall.[25,29] The clinical presentation was most often in the form of CCS (defined previously by disproportionately greater motor impairment of the upper extremities).[30,31] Given that neurological injury can result from low-energy trauma to the cervical spine in patients with OPLL, and that SCI often occurs in the absence of bony fractures, a high index of suspicion must be maintained to prevent diagnostic delay and/or delay in surgical intervention. Both MR and CT imaging, if possible, should be performed in the initial imaging workup of these OPLL patients. Removal of the ossified mass via an anterior approach may be preferred in patients with segmental OPLL; however, issues related to excessive bleeding and the increased possibility of dural violations with cerebrospinal fluid (CSF) leaks, has led numerous spine surgeons in the Asia-Pacific region, who frequently care for OPLL patients, to favor posterior surgical approaches. In general, a posterior approach is usually preferred in patients with multilevel OPLL. Regardless of the surgical approach chosen (anterior vs. posterior vs. combined anterior-posterior), the postoperative transverse area of the narrowest part of the spinal cord on T1-weighted MRI correlates strongly with neurological recovery in patients with cervical stenotic myelopathy.[23,32,33]

Data supporting the use of preventative surgery in asymptomatic patients with OPLL is limited. In a prospective study by Matsunaga et al on 368 asymptomatic patients with OPLL, the authors noted a significant decrease in the incidence of minor cervical trauma once patients had been informed about their OPLL condition and had been warned about the possibility of developing traumatic cervical myelopathy. The authors noted that all traumatic episodes, thereafter, were due to MVAs.[27] They recommended only performing preventative surgery in patients who have ≥ 60% canal stenosis, who have lifestyles which predispose them to an increased risk of cervical trauma secondary to MVAs, or who have mixed-type OPLL (which was the most frequently observed ossification type in patients who developed traumatic myelopathy in their series). Katoh and colleagues similarly cautioned against employing surgical intervention in patients without neurological symptoms. Thus, the risks associated with surgery must be weighed against the potential for the development of severe neurological deficits following minor cervical trauma in patients with OPLL.[34]

19.5 Trauma in Patients with Congenital Cervical Spinal Stenosis

Congenital cervical spinal stenosis has an estimated prevalence of 4.9% in adults in United States and is characterized by a multilevel decrease in spinal canal area in the absence of associated spondylotic changes.[35] The condition is associated with several syndromes, including Klippel–Feil syndrome,[36] achondroplasia,[37] and hypochondroplasia.[37] While its etiology is unknown, congenital stenosis can present with multiple anatomical changes to the cervical spine[38] including decreases in the interpedicular distance, the lamina length, and the lateral mass size. These changes result in a decreased sagittal canal diameter. Consequently, patients with congenital cervical spinal stenosis are at an increased risk of developing myelopathy following major or minor trauma to the cervical spine.[39] Multiple radiological criteria can be used for the diagnosis of congenital cervical spinal stenosis including the Torg–Pavlov ratio on CT imaging (< 0.82), or the sagittal canal diameter (< 14 mm), and C5 lateral mass-to-canal diameter ratio (LM/CD; ≥ 0.735) on lateral radiographs.[40]

Athletes in contact sports (i.e., football, rugby, etc.) who have congenital spinal stenosis are at an increased risk of incurring SCI from cervical trauma. The characterization of neurological injuries in patients with congenital spinal stenosis has, therefore, been described extensively within this patient demographic in the neurosurgical literature. These injuries can include transient cervical neurapraxia, stingers (transient neurapraxia of the brachial plexus), and traumatic CCS secondary to cervical spine extension injuries. A description of these injuries as well as a characterization of neurological injuries in patients with congenital cervical spinal stenosis, however, is outside of the scope of this chapter and has been well described elsewhere within this text (see Chapter 17, Cervical Spine Trauma in Patients with Congenital Spinal Stenosis).

19.6 Conclusion

Cervical spondylosis, OPLL, and congenital spinal stenosis can each increase the risk for SCI and presentation with myelopathy following cervical trauma by decreasing the sagittal diameter of the cervical spinal canal and increasing the risk for cervical spinal cord compression. In patients who have had myelopathic symptoms prior to a traumatic episode or who have been previously diagnosed with cervical spondylosis, OPLL, or congenital spinal stenosis, our philosophy is that the resulting health insurance claims should be handled by the individual's health insurance policy. Conversely, patients who *have not* had documented neurological symptoms prior to the traumatic incident and who *have* been diagnosed with one of the conditions listed above at the time of a traumatic cervical event, can apply for workman's compensation (if injured while on the job) or for compensation from their car insurance company (if injured during a car accident). In such cases, the underlying spondylosis, OPLL, or congenital stenosis do not qualify as "pre-existing conditions" from an insurance coverage standpoint, particularly if the patients had not been informed of their conditions (or their increased risk for developing SCI following trauma) prior to the traumatic incident itself.

19.7 Note

There are marked differences in the reported occurrences of spinal cord compression and congenital and acquired spinal canal narrowing based on the region of the world where the reports originate. In particular, incidence and prevalence rates in the Asia-Pacific region often differ appreciably from the United States, and as such, any descriptions must be evaluated carefully for the area from which the published article originated.

References

[1] Devivo MJ. Epidemiology of traumatic spinal cord injury: trends and future implications. Spinal Cord. 2012; 50(5):365–372

[2] Price C, Makintubee S, Herndon W, Istre GR. Epidemiology of traumatic spinal cord injury and acute hospitalization and rehabilitation charges for spinal cord injuries in Oklahoma, 1988–1990. Am J Epidemiol. 1994; 139(1):37–47

[3] Goldberg W, Mueller C, Panacek E, Tigges S, Hoffman JR, Mower WR, NEXUS Group. Distribution and patterns of blunt traumatic cervical spine injury. Ann Emerg Med. 2001; 38(1):17–21

[4] Edwards CC, II, Riew KD, Anderson PA, Hilibrand AS, Vaccaro AF. Cervical myelopathy. current diagnostic and treatment strategies. Spine J. 2003; 3(1):68–81

[5] Eismont FJ, Clifford S, Goldberg M, Green B. Cervical sagittal spinal canal size in spine injury. Spine. 1984; 9(7):663–666

[6] Morishita Y, Naito M, Hymanson H, Miyazaki M, Wu G, Wang JC. The relationship between the cervical spinal canal diameter and the pathological changes in the cervical spine. Eur Spine J. 2009; 18(6):877–883

[7] Murone I. The importance of the sagittal diameters of the cervical spinal canal in relation to spondylosis and myelopathy. J Bone Joint Surg Br. 1974; 56(1):30–36

[8] Pavlov H, Torg JS, Robie B, Jahre C. Cervical spinal stenosis: determination with vertebral body ratio method. Radiology. 1987; 164(3):771–775

[9] Yue WM, Tan SB, Tan MH, Koh DC, Tan CT. The Torg–Pavlov ratio in cervical spondylotic myelopathy: a comparative study between patients with cervical spondylotic myelopathy and a nonspondylotic, nonmyelopathic population. Spine. 2001; 26(16):1760–1764

[10] Aebli N, Wicki AG, Rüegg TB, Petrou N, Eisenlohr H, Krebs J. The Torg-Pavlov ratio for the prediction of acute spinal cord injury after a minor trauma to the cervical spine. Spine J. 2013; 13(6):605–612

[11] Wilder FV, Hall BJ, Barrett JP. Smoking and osteoarthritis: is there an association? The Clearwater Osteoarthritis Study. Osteoarthritis Cartilage. 2003; 11(1):29–35

[12] Lee MJ, Dettori JR, Standaert CJ, Brodt ED, Chapman JR. The natural history of degeneration of the lumbar and cervical spines: a systematic review. Spine. 2012; 37(22) Suppl:S18–S30

[13] Regenbogen VS, Rogers LF, Atlas SW, Kim KS. Cervical spinal cord injuries in patients with cervical spondylosis. AJR Am J Roentgenol. 1986; 146(2):277–284

[14] Forsyth HF. Extension Injuries of the Cervical Spine. J Bone Joint Surg Am. 1964; 46:1792–1797

[15] Koyanagi I, Iwasaki Y, Hida K, Akino M, Imamura H, Abe H. Acute cervical cord injury without fracture or dislocation of the spinal column. J Neurosurg. 2000; 93(1) Suppl:15–20

[16] Schneider RC, Cherry G, Pantek H. The syndrome of acute central cervical spinal cord injury; with special reference to the mechanisms involved in hyperextension injuries of cervical spine. J Neurosurg. 1954; 11(6):546–577

[17] Aarabi B, Koltz M, Ibrahimi D. Hyperextension cervical spine injuries and traumatic central cord syndrome. Neurosurg Focus. 2008; 25(5):E9

[18] Guest J, Eleraky MA, Apostolides PJ, Dickman CA, Sonntag VK. Traumatic central cord syndrome: results of surgical management. J Neurosurg. 2002; 97(1) Suppl:25–32

[19] Aito S, D'Andrea M, Werhagen L, et al. Neurological and functional outcome in traumatic central cord syndrome. Spinal Cord. 2007; 45(4):292–297

[20] Choi BW, Song KJ, Chang H. Ossification of the posterior longitudinal ligament: a review of literature. Asian Spine J. 2011; 5(4):267–276

[21] Saetia K, Cho D, Lee S, Kim DH, Kim SD. Ossification of the posterior longitudinal ligament: a review. Neurosurg Focus. 2011; 30(3):E1

[22] Hirakawa H, Kusumi T, Nitobe T, et al. An immunohistochemical evaluation of extracellular matrix components in the spinal posterior longitudinal ligament and intervertebral disc of the tiptoe walking mouse. J Orthop Sci. 2004; 9(6):591–597

[23] Katoh S, Ikata T, Hirai N, Okada Y, Nakauchi K. Influence of minor trauma to the neck on the neurological outcome in patients with ossification of the posterior longitudinal ligament (OPLL) of the cervical spine. Paraplegia. 1995; 33(6):330–333

[24] Song J, Mizuno J, Hashizume Y, Nakagawa H. Immunohistochemistry of symptomatic hypertrophy of the posterior longitudinal ligament with special reference to ligamentous ossification. Spinal Cord. 2006; 44(9):576–581

[25] Lee CK, Yoon DH, Kim KN, et al. Characteristics of cervical spine trauma in patients with ankylosing spondylitis and ossification of the posterior longitudinal ligament. World Neurosurg. 2016; 96:202–208

[26] Endo S, Shimamura T, Nakae H, et al. Cervical spinal cord injury associated with ossification of the posterior longitudinal ligament. Arch Orthop Trauma Surg. 1994; 113(4):218–221

[27] Matsunaga S, Sakou T, Hayashi K, Ishidou Y, Hirotsu M, Komiya S. Trauma-induced myelopathy in patients with ossification of the posterior longitudinal ligament. J Neurosurg. 2002; 97(2) Suppl:172–175

[28] Abiola R, Rubery P, Mesfin A. Ossification of the posterior longitudinal ligament: etiology, diagnosis, and outcomes of nonoperative and operative management. Global Spine J. 2016; 6(2):195–204

[29] Graham B, Van Peteghem PK. Fractures of the spine in ankylosing spondylitis. Diagnosis, treatment, and complications. Spine. 1989; 14(8):803–807

[30] Murray GC, Persellin RH. Cervical fracture complicating ankylosing spondylitis: a report of eight cases and review of the literature. Am J Med. 1981; 70(5):1033–1041

[31] Kewalramani LS, Taylor RG, Albrand OW. Cervical spine injury in patients with ankylosing spondylitis. J Trauma. 1975; 15(10):931–934

[32] Okada Y, Ikata T, Yamada H, Sakamoto R, Katoh S. Magnetic resonance imaging study on the results of surgery for cervical compression myelopathy. Spine. 1993; 18(14):2024–2029

[33] Fujiwara K, Yonenobu K, Hiroshima K, Ebara S, Yamashita K, Ono K. Morphometry of the cervical spinal cord and its relation to pathology in cases with compression myelopathy. Spine. 1988; 13(11):1212–1216

[34] Mizuno J, Nakagawa H. Ossified posterior longitudinal ligament: management strategies and outcomes. Spine J. 2006; 6(6) Suppl:282S–288S

[35] Lee MJ, Cassinelli EH, Riew KD. Prevalence of cervical spine stenosis. Anatomic study in cadavers. J Bone Joint Surg Am. 2007; 89(2):376–380

[36] Hensinger RN, Lang JE, MacEwen GD. Klippel-Feil syndrome: a constellation of associated anomalies. J Bone Joint Surg Am. 1974; 56(6):1246–1253

[37] Bhattacharjee S, Mudumba V, Aniruddh PK. Spinal canal stenosis at the level of Atlas. J Craniovertebr Junction Spine. 2011; 2(1):38–40

[38] Jenkins TJ, Mai HT, Burgmeier RJ, Savage JW, Patel AA, Hsu WK. The Triangle Model of congenital cervical stenosis. Spine. 2016; 41(5):E242–E247

[39] Stratford J. Congenital cervical spinal stenosis: a factor in myelopathy. Acta Neurochir (Wien). 1978; 41(1–3):101–106

[40] Horne PH, Lampe LP, Nguyen JT, Herzog RJ, Albert TJ. A novel radiographic indicator of developmental cervical stenosis. J Bone Joint Surg Am. 2016; 98(14):1206–1214

20 Minimally Invasive Spine Surgery

Tyler Atkins and Domagoj Coric

Abstract

Over the past 10 years several authors have published several anatomic feasibility studies, case reports, and small case series regarding minimally invasive spine (MIS) treatment of some specific cervical traumatic injuries. This chapter represents a review of current specific cervical traumatic pathologies that have begun to be treated via MIS techniques and discusses the approaches being utilized. Many of the common upper cervical spine fractures, including odontoid fracture, C2 pars fracture, C2 body fracture, and combined C1–C2 injuries, have been treated with variable anterior and posterior (or combination) MIS techniques as modifications of open approaches, often utilizing intraoperative navigation. In addition to summarizing the published techniques, we have included two simple case examples with imaging. Subaxial cervical fractures can also be treated in select cases with MIS instrumentation such as percutaneous lateral mass or pedicle screws. We summarize these techniques and results currently described in the spine literature. In an era of medicine with much focus on limiting morbidity due to interventions, advancements in instrumentation as well as image guidance is leading to ongoing development of MIS operations. Further utilization and future study of MIS techniques in the cervical spine is likely.

Keywords: minimally invasive, MIS, cervical trauma, fracture, percutaneous, odontoid, C1, C2, subaxial

20.1 Role for Minimally Invasive Surgery in Cervical Trauma

Minimally invasive spine (MIS) techniques have been gaining increasing popularity over the past few decades, with most attention paid to the lumbar spine. This has included treatment of a range of pathologies including traumatic injuries, perhaps most popularly with the use of percutaneous pedicle screw-rod systems for thoracolumbar fractures that do not require open reduction or decompression. MIS cervical techniques have similarly been gaining traction, but certainly less so in regard to instrumentation, with most attention being paid to minimally invasive decompression surgeries for degenerative spine pathology. Within the past 10 years, there have been several published anatomic feasibility studies, case reports, and small case series regarding minimally invasive treatment of some specific cervical traumatic injuries. We will review the common MIS principles among these techniques and discuss specific cervical traumatic pathologies where they may be utilized.

Adopting minimally invasive fixation techniques to the cervical spine comes with slightly more trepidation to the surgeon owing to a higher potential for significant complication and injury. This is due to the complex anatomy of the cervical spine. These anatomic considerations include the relative prominence of the cervical spinal cord, presence of the vertebral arteries, as well as the unique bony anatomy of the high cervical and subaxial spine in regard to these structures.

Despite these risks, some attractive considerations of MIS fixation for cervical injuries include the relatively high prevalence of these types of injuries in the elderly population from ground level falls as well as high-impact trauma. Traditional nonoperative interventions of rigid cervical collars or halo immobilization (which offers a higher rate of immobilization of the higher cervical spine) have a relatively high morbidity in the elderly population and are generally less efficacious and more morbid in this patient population. Similarly, traditional open procedures, such as posterior C1–C2 fusions or high cervical anterior cervical discectomy and fusions (ACDFs), in these patients carry significant morbidity.[1,2,3] The ability to perform a minimally invasive surgery obviating the need for prolonged bracing in this patient population is particularly desirable.

Much of the cervical percutaneous MIS screw technology is derived from the techniques developed for the lumbar spine. The increased popularity and sophistication of intraoperative image-guided navigation systems have facilitated the safety and efficacy of percutaneous placement of cervical instrumentation and the overall adoption of MIS techniques in the cervical spine.

20.2 Injuries Treated by MIS Fixation

20.2.1 Odontoid Fracture

Placement of an odontoid screw via a minimally invasive technique has been investigated with good preliminary results. Although the traditional open technique involves relatively little exposure and soft-tissue dissection, there have been several reports of modifying the procedure to make it even less invasive with decreased morbidity. Wang and associates reported on 19 patients who underwent percutaneous odontoid screw placement for treatment of type II and rostral type III odontoid fractures.[4] The overall procedure is quite similar to open odontoid screw placement with only a few differences. The authors report placing the patients in Gardner–Wells tongs with 2 kg of traction. Then, utilizing two c-arms for precise anteroposterior and lateral fluoroscopy to make a 1-cm unilateral horizontal incision at the medial border of the sternocleidomastoid at the C5–C6 level. Dissection is taken to the medial border of the sternocleidomastoid at which point a blunt guide-tube dissector is advanced through the deep tissues to the anterior–superior border of the C2–C3 disc space. A sharp guide wire is placed through the tube once in ideal position, thereafter allowing passing of instruments over the wire in the same sequence as done for open screw placement (drilling, tapping, and screw placement while controlling the guide wire under fluoroscopy). The authors report no surgical complications, specifically no injury to the nonvisualized at-risk visceral and vascular structures of the anterior neck. In this prospective study comparing the percutaneous screw to 23 patients receiving an open operation, they report similar success in fusion with less operating room time and fewer cases of postoperative dysphagia. Images from a similar approach to odontoid screw placement can be seen in ▶ Fig. 20.1, ▶ Fig. 20.2, ▶ Fig. 20.3, and ▶ Fig. 20.4.

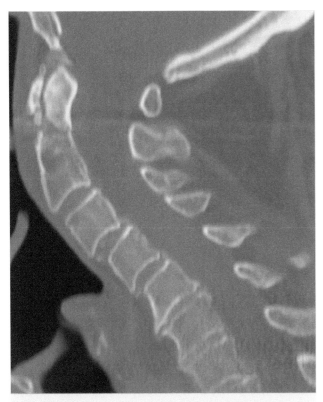

Fig. 20.1 Sagittal reconstruction of cervical spine computed tomography (CT) showing type II odontoid fracture with minimal extension-distraction, ideal for anterior odontoid screw placement.

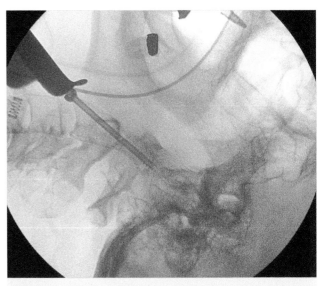

Fig. 20.2 Intraoperative lateral fluoroscopy showing retractor in position in low anterior neck soft tissues, and screw entering C2 body at its inferior border.

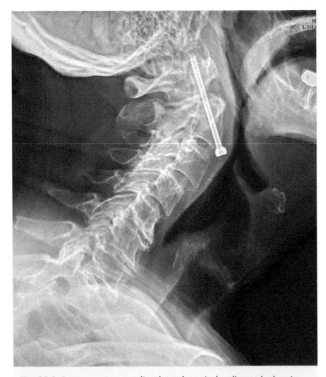

Fig. 20.3 Postoperative standing lateral cervical radiograph showing odontoid screw.

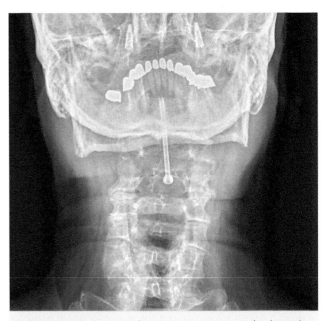

Fig. 20.4 Postoperative standing anteroposterior cervical radiograph showing odontoid screw in ideal midline position.

Holly et al describe an alternative minimally invasive approach to fixation of type II odontoid fractures by utilizing dilating tubular retractors and fluoroscopy for a posterior C1–C2 fusion.[5] Their report includes five patients with type II odontoid fractures. The patients were all positioned prone in Mayfield pins with a 2 cm incision made bilaterally centered over C2. The authors were able to place C1 lateral mass and C2 pedicle screws with this exposure, as well as decorticate the articular surface, place allograft and demineralized bone, and place an appropriate sized rod on either side. No complications are reported and fusion rates of 100% were noted at an average of 32-months follow-up. Images utilizing intraoperative computed tomography (CT) guidance for a posterior hybrid fusion of ante-rolisthesed odontoid fracture can be seen in ▸ Fig. 20.5, ▸ Fig. 20.6, and ▸ Fig. 20.7 (one side with C1 and C3 lateral mass screw and other side C1–2 transarticular screw and C4 lateral mass screw).

20.2.2 Traumatic Spondylolisthesis of the Axis

The hangman fracture, particularly the Levine–Edwards type II (> 3 mm of displacement with < 10 degree of angulation) is an intuitively appropriate candidate for MIS fixation. This common

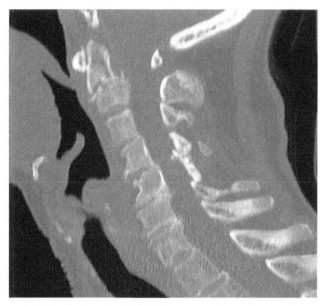

Fig. 20.5 Sagittal reconstruction of cervical spine computed tomography (CT) shows nonhealing type II odontoid fracture with minimal anterior displacement. Patient also has anterior and posterior C1 ring fractures without displacement. Poor candidate for continued conservative management, also not a candidate for isolated anterior odontoid screw placement.

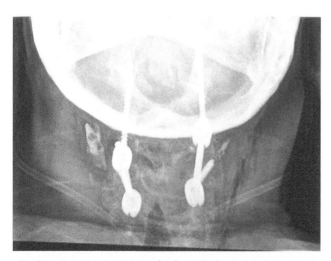

Fig. 20.6 Anteroposterior cervical radiograph showing postoperative result after using intraoperative computed tomography (CT) image guidance for mini-open placement of right C1–C2 transarticular screw and C4 lateral mass screw and left-sided C1 and C3 lateral mass screws.

fracture type could feasibly be treated with two screws placed directly across the fracture line through the C2 pars interarticularis. Two separate groups have published recent reports of this MIS technique. Wu and colleagues reported on 10 patients with hangman fracture treated in this fashion.[6] They utilized nasotracheal intubation, Mayfield skull clamp for positioning with intraoperative fluoroscopy utilizing coronal, lateral, and open-mouth views to guide bilateral percutaneously placed C2 pedicle screws to reduce and secure the fracture. Buchholz et al reported the results of five patients treated with a similar technique, but also utilized intraoperative CT image navigation with the registration star attached to the Mayfield skull clamp.[7] Neither author reported any complications. All patients received postoperative CT scans to assess screw positions. Bucholz et al reported no malpositioning and Wu et al noted 3 of 20 screws with less than 2 mm breach of the pedicle wall (2 medial and 1 lateral).

20.2.3 C2 Body Fracture

At least one case of a complicated C2 vertebral body fracture treated with percutaneous technique has been reported by Kantelhardt et al as part of a larger series of patients with cervical fractures treated with MIS techniques.[8] These authors utilized intraoperative CT image guidance technology with the registration star attached to the Mayfield skull clamp followed by percutaneous placement of bilateral C2 pedicle screws and bilateral C3 lateral mass screws, with a short rod placed down a tubular retractor through which the C2–C3 joint was also decorticated and filled with synthetic bone graft substitutes. The authors reported no complications.

20.2.4 Combined C1–C2 Injuries

There are many variations of combined fractures and ligamentous injuries of the atlas and axis that are typically addressed

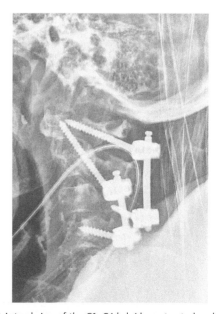

Fig. 20.7 Lateral view of the C1–C4 hybrid construct placed via mini-open technique using intraoperative computed tomography (CT) guidance.

surgically with C1–C2 arthrodesis. Wu and associates describe seven patients with various combinations of C1 ring and odontoid fractures who were all treated with three anteriorly placed percutaneous screws.[9] The authors utilized Gardner–Wells tongs, fluoroscopy, and a similar technique as described previously for percutaneous odontoid screws for anterior access to the high cervical spine. They report placing a single, midline odontoid screw, followed with bilateral transarticular screws into the C1 lateral masses through a single 10-mm incision. No surgical complications are reported.

The same primary author of the above triple-anterior screw technique has also reported using a combination front/back approach with anterior bilateral transarticular screws (same technique as described above) and a posterior mini-open C1–C2 wiring.[10] This was performed for more complex C1–C2 injuries: three cases of Jefferson fracture plus ruptured transverse ligament, one Jefferson fracture plus type II odontoid fracture, and one case of atlantoaxial dislocation. Again, the authors report no surgical complications. Images utilizing intraoperative CT guidance for a posterior hybrid fusion of anteriorly displaced type II odontoid fracture with combined C1 ring fracture can be seen in ▶ Fig. 20.5, ▶ Fig. 20.6, and ▶ Fig. 20.7 (one side with C1 and C3 lateral mass screw and other side C1–C2 transarticular screw and C4 lateral mass screw).

20.2.5 Subaxial Cervical Fracture

Posterior approaches for surgical treatment of traumatic injuries of the subaxial cervical spine most often entail lateral mass screws and less frequently pedicle screws (based on surgeon's preference and experience). A few surgeons have published reports on MIS approaches to placing posterior cervical screws both as a sole treatment for traumatic injuries as well as for posterior stabilization following an anterior cervical operation.

Lateral Mass Screws

Two small case series published by Wang et al of 3 patients in 2003 and a separate larger case series by Wang et al in 2006 with a total of 18 patients (10 being trauma patients) describe the use of the same MIS technique for lateral mass screw placement using tubular retractors in the subaxial cervical spine.[11,12] They fused a maximum of two segments over C3–C7 using their published technique. Cumulatively between these two studies there are 5 patients who received posterior-only surgery (including two neurologically intact patients with bilateral jumped facets, two neurologically intact patients with unilateral jumped facet, and one patient with a fracture dislocation and incomplete quadriplegia.) The remaining eight patients were treated with anterior decompression and fusion (ACDF or corpectomy) followed by the posterior MIS instrumentation. The injuries treated with the 360-degree surgery included burst fractures as well as fracture-dislocations. The authors describe the following surgical technique: patient prone in pins, midline 2 cm incision, fluoroscopically guided tubular retractor placement docking on the lateral mass, denuding of the posterior surface of the lateral mass as well as the facet articular surface, placement of polyaxial screw using fluoroscopy and a modified Magerl technique, and placement of the top loading rod through the tubular retractor. Of their total of 21 cases, the authors converted to open instrumentation on 2 patients for placement of lower screws due to inadequate fluoroscopic visualization of the lower cervical spine. They report no neurological complications and successful fusion in all cases.

A slight variation on the above technique has been separately reported by Fang et al who utilized low-profile plates instead of polyaxial screws and rods with caps.[13] These authors describe two case reports of posterior MIS stabilization following anterior fusion: one bilateral facet dislocation and one burst fracture with posterior distraction. The position, localization, and use of tubular retractor are nearly identical with the difference being use of a plate with screws placed secondarily though the plate once in position. The authors describe easier adjustment of the tubular retractor position with this construct than when trying to move the tube over prominent polyaxial screw heads while placing a rod using the technique described above.

Pedicle Screws

In a comparison study including 56 patients who received either open or MIS surgery for cervical fracture, Komatsubara et al report the use of intraoperative CT navigation and self-retaining tubular retractors for placement of cervical pedicle screws in 37 patients.[14] Their operative time and bleeding were less in the MIS group, as was their reported incidence of clinically significant screw deviation. Their technique includes a laterally placed small skin incision as directed by CT navigation, docking of the self-retaining tubular retractor on the lateral mass, placement of a k-wire for screw guidance, and ultimate placement of a rod for each set of screws down the same retractor. Schaefer et al provide another case series on MIS cervical pedicle screws in the subaxial spine, using fluoroscopy alone without CT navigation.[15] Of the 15 included patients, only 3 were treated for trauma. The majority of patients (i.e., 11 of 15) received both anterior and posterior operations. However, specifically regarding the posterior MIS instrumentation, they had no major complications or need to convert to open surgery. Based on postoperative CT imaging, the authors did have a relatively high (23.6%) rate of suboptimal position of the screws with perforation of the pedicle wall. The majority of these breaches were lateral toward the vertebral artery (18.1%). This rate of undesirable screw position is indicative of the technically challenging nature of MIS approach for these types of screws, and perhaps suggests the technique should be of limited use when not using intraoperative navigation.

Collectively, the authors reporting on subaxial cervical MIS instrumentation discuss a common set of technical challenges. The anatomy of select patients makes fluoroscopic visualization of the lower cervical spine very challenging if not impossible. Placement of the rod or plate down a tubular retractor appears to be a common struggle and somewhat of a limitation on the number of treated segments using these techniques. Moreover, the lateral mass screw placement specifically has a potential limitation in achieving an appropriate lateral trajectory due to abutting of the tubular retractor against the midline spinous process which can be bifid and very wide. Without an open midline incision, this challenge cannot be addressed by simply removing the restrictive spinous process.

20.3 Conclusions and Further Investigations

The literature to date on MIS treatment of cervical trauma is certainly limited and mostly consists of small case series for any given pathology. As such, the role of this information serves largely as proof of concept. Currently lacking is the adequate comparison to standard open operations for each pathology and formal assessment of any potential advantages of MIS (lower operative morbidity, less postop pain, etc.). However, even without the benefit of larger studies a few points of similarity and limitations regarding these MIS techniques can be made. There is certainly a steep learning curve in the percutaneous instrumentation, intraoperative image guidance, and unique fluoroscopy angles for those not accustomed to them. Many of the authors are noted to use intraoperative guidance for screw placement. Some of these authors performed two or sometimes three separate intraoperative CTs, which created a rather high dose of radiation to the patient and added notable length to the overall surgical procedure, both of which obviate some of the proposed advantages of MIS approaches.

Relative contraindications to MIS techniques include significant kyphosis or aberrant bony or vascular anatomy as well as previous surgery in the planned operative approach.

Given the increasing popularity of MIS techniques for thoracolumbar pathologies including trauma, it is reasonable to assume that there will be continued adoption of minimally invasive surgery for cervical trauma indications. The growing prevalence of these conditions in the aging population as well as progressive sophistication of intraoperative navigation will continue to make MIS techniques, including muscle splitting approaches with tubular retractors and percutaneous screw fixation, both desirable and feasible in the future.

References

[1] Daentzer D, Flörkemeier T. Conservative treatment of upper cervical spine injuries with the halo vest: an appropriate option for all patients independent of their age? J Neurosurg Spine. 2009; 10(6):543–550

[2] Delcourt T, Bégué T, Saintyves G, Mebtouche N, Cottin P. Management of upper cervical spine fractures in elderly patients: current trends and outcomes. Injury. 2015; 46 Suppl 1:S24–S27

[3] Jackson AP, Haak MH, Khan N, Meyer PR. Cervical spine injuries in the elderly: acute postoperative mortality. Spine. 2005; 30(13):1524–1527

[4] Wang J, Zhou Y, Zhang ZF, Li CQ, Zheng WJ, Liu J. Comparison of percutaneous and open anterior screw fixation in the treatment of type II and rostral type III odontoid fractures. Spine. 2011; 36(18):1459–1463

[5] Holly LT, Isaacs RE, Frempong-Boadu AK. Minimally invasive atlantoaxial fusion. Neurosurgery. 2010; 66(3) Suppl:193–197

[6] Wu YS, Lin Y, Zhang XL, et al. Management of hangman's fracture with percutaneous transpedicular screw fixation. Eur Spine J. 2013; 22(1):79–86

[7] Buchholz AL, Morgan SL, Robinson LC, Frankel BM. Minimally invasive percutaneous screw fixation of traumatic spondylolisthesis of the axis. J Neurosurg Spine. 2015; 22(5):459–465

[8] Kantelhardt SR, Keric N, Conrad J, Archavlis E, Giese A. Minimally invasive instrumentation of uncomplicated cervical fractures. Eur Spine J. 2016; 25(1):127–133

[9] Wu AM, Wang XY, Chi YL, et al. Management of acute combination atlas-axis fractures with percutaneous triple anterior screw fixation in elderly patients. Orthop Traumatol Surg Res. 2012; 98(8):894–899

[10] Wu AM, Wang XY, Zhou F, Zhang XL, Xu HZ, Chi YL. Percutaneous atlantoaxial anterior transarticular screw fixation combined with mini-open posterior C1/2 wire fusion for patients with a high-riding vertebral artery. J Spinal Cord Med. 2016; 39(2):234–239

[11] Wang MY, Prusmack CJ, Green BA, Gruen JP, Levi AD. Minimally invasive lateral mass screws in the treatment of cervical facet dislocations: technical note. Neurosurgery. 2003; 52(2):444–447, discussion 447–448

[12] Wang MY, Levi AD. Minimally invasive lateral mass screw fixation in the cervical spine: initial clinical experience with long-term follow-up. Neurosurgery. 2006; 58(5):907–912, discussion 907–912

[13] Fong S, Duplessis S. Minimally invasive lateral mass plating in the treatment of posterior cervical trauma: surgical technique. J Spinal Disord Tech. 2005; 18(3):224–228

[14] Schaefer C, Begemann P, Fuhrhop I, et al. Percutaneous instrumentation of the cervical and cervico-thoracic spine using pedicle screws: preliminary clinical results and analysis of accuracy. Eur Spine J. 2011; 20(6):977–985

[15] Komatsubara T, Tokioka T, Sugimoto Y, Ozaki T. Minimally Invasive Cervical Pedicle Screw Fixation by a Posterolateral Approach for Acute Cervical Injury. Clin Spine Surg. 2016 Epub ahead of print

21 Role of Neurointerventional Techniques in Cervical Trauma

Neil Majmundar, Fawaz Al-Mufti, Michael Nosko, Anil Nanda, Sudipta Roychowdhury, and Gaurav Gupta

Abstract

Endovascular techniques, when indicated in the treatment of arterial injuries following cervical trauma, have become more common due to advances in imaging, improvements in the safety profiles of the devices used, and low complication rates. Treatments for penetrating and nonpenetrating injuries include medical management, embolization, and stent placement. In this chapter, we discuss the types of arterial injuries that occur following cervical trauma, the natural history of untreated dissections, their medical management, the imaging modalities used for initial diagnosis, and the role of neurointerventional/endovascular techniques.

Keywords: carotid artery injury, vertebral artery injury, blunt cerebrovascular injury, endovascular, neurointerventional

21.1 Introduction

Traumatic injuries involving the carotid and vertebral arteries following cervical trauma can have devastating neurological outcomes.[1] The incidence of carotid and vertebral artery injuries following cervical trauma has increased as comprehensive screening protocols with more specific and less invasive imaging methods have developed. The primary management of uncomplicated extracranial carotid/vertebral arterial injuries associated with trauma is mainly anticoagulation/antiplatelet therapy, the goal of which is to avoid potential ischemic complications. Neurointerventional techniques are generally reserved for more complicated and refractory injuries in cases where medical management fails or when systemic anticoagulation is contraindicated. These endovascular techniques, when indicated in the treatment of arterial injuries following cervical trauma, have become more common due to advances in imaging, improvements in the safety profiles of the devices used, and low complication rates.

21.2 Types of Vascular Injury After Cervical Trauma

21.2.1 Penetrating Injury

Penetrating trauma to the neck and cervical region, defined as violation of the platysma, is generally divided into three zones, with each zone mandating different management strategies. *Zone 1* is defined as the region from the clavicle/sternum to the cricoid cartilage, *zone 2* is the region from the cricoid cartilage to the angle of mandible, and *zone 3* is the region from the angle of the mandible to the skull base.[2] Carotid injury occurs in approximately 4.9 to 6% of penetrating neck trauma cases.[3,4] Penetrating injury to either the carotid or vertebral arteries carries a mortality of 10%, while combined injuries carry a mortality of 50%.[5] These injuries can be highly lethal if left untreated, approaching a mortality rate of 100%.[6]

Penetrating arterial injuries are most common secondary to gunshot or stab wounds and can result in extracranial carotid or vertebral artery pseudoaneurysms.[7] Although spontaneous resolution of these pseudoaneurysms has been described,[8] this pathology may result in stroke and if untreated, can enlarge and result in compression of local structures, regional pain, and arteriovenous (AV) fistulas.[9,10,11,12]

21.2.2 Nonpenetrating Injury

Blunt Cerebrovascular Trauma

Blunt trauma to the cervical spine can result in blunt cerebrovascular injury (BCVI) from high-energy nonpenetrating blunt force injury.[13] BCVI is seen in approximately 1 to 2% of blunt trauma patients,[14,15,16] and in 2.4% of trauma patients who remain in the hospital over 24 hours.[15] The incidence of BCVI has significantly risen likely due to the development of improved screening protocols as well as advances in and availability of sophisticated noninvasive imaging.[17,18] Comprehensive screening protocols resulting in earlier initiation of anticoagulation in patients diagnosed with BCVI have been shown to result in a significant reduction in stroke risk.[1] The incidence of BCVI in the cervical internal carotid artery (ICA; 0.019–0.8%) is slightly higher than in the vertebral arteries (0.09–0.71%).[14,19,20,21,22]

BCVI carries significant neurosurgical morbidity and mortality rates of 56 and 30%, respectively.[14] The risk of ischemic stroke in patients with BCVI is 9 to 12%, and it typically occurs in patients who have not been started on anticoagulation or antiplatelet therapy.[15,16]

BCVI generally occurs secondary to a high energy transfer mechanism. Injuries which carry considerable risk of BCVI include Le Fort type 2 or 3 fractures, basilar skull fractures involving the carotid canal, traumatic brain injuries with diffuse axonal injury (with Glasgow Coma Scale < 6), cervical vertebral body or transverse foramen fractures/subluxations, cervical ligamentous injuries, near hanging injuries with anoxic brain injury, and clothesline/seat belt abrasions where the patient has local swelling, pain, and mental status change.[20,23,24,25] Crissey and Bernstein identified four fundamental traumatic mechanisms which result in BCVI (▶ Table 21.1). Type 2 injuries, resulting from hyperextension and contralateral rotation of the head and neck, are the most common.[26]

Table 21.1 Crissey and Bernstein traumatic mechanisms[26]

Injury type	Mechanism of injury
Type 1	Direct blow to the neck
Type 2	Hyperextension and contralateral rotation of head and neck
Type 3	Intraoral trauma
Type 4	Skull base fractures involving the sphenoid or petrous bones

The signs and symptoms of BCVI may not always be obvious in trauma patients who generally present with a complex picture. These patients often arrive intubated (precluding an accurate neurological assessment) and generally have multisystem injuries. Signs and symptoms of BCVI include hemorrhage from the nose, mouth, or neck, a cervical bruit in patients aged less than 50 years, a rapidly expanding cervical hematoma, a region of stroke on computed tomography (CT) or magnetic resonance imaging (MRI), Horner syndrome, hemiparesis, vertebrobasilar insufficiency, and a neurological deficit which is inconsistent with imaging findings.[25] As mentioned earlier in the chapter, early and comprehensive screening protocols have led to an increase in the frequency with which BCVI is diagnosed and, in turn, earlier treatment and better prognoses for patients with this injury. Screening protocols developed at the University of Colorado and the University of Tennessee in Memphis have assisted in identifying risk factors, presenting signs and symptoms, and treatment paradigms.[20,23,24]

Stretch injuries to the cervical vessels may result in intimal injuries leading to vessel wall dissection. These injuries can occur secondary to cervical chiropractic manipulation and generally follow hyperextension and rotation of the neck.[6,27]

Occlusive injuries to the carotid or vertebral arties can occur secondary to fractures resulting in subluxation or dislocation. The vertebral artery may be occluded secondary to external force from fractures of the transverse foramen or in cases where the facets are jumped or perched. These injuries are not typically dealt directly via neurointerventional procedures, but they may require proximal occlusion if the patient has active extravasation of blood, or if open reduction will result in further injury to the vessel.

21.3 Pathophysiology of Vascular Injury

21.3.1 Mechanism

Blunt vascular injuries result from high energy transfer after trauma.[28] The injury can result in the development of an intimal flap, which in turn can lead to a dissection of the vessel. The denuded subintimal layer provides a nidus for platelets to aggregate, initiating a series of events resulting in the formation of a thrombus. The thrombus can cause occlusion of the vessel, stenosis of the vessel, or embolization distally resulting in an infarction.[28]

Dissections of the extracranial carotid and vertebral arteries are more common than intracranial dissections as the cervical segments are longer and dissections occur more frequently where a relatively mobile segment of the artery is stretched against an immobile/relatively fixed segment at the base of the skull.[29] Arterial dissection involves the creation of a false lumen due to the extravasation of blood secondary to an intimal tear. As the media and adventitia of the intracranial segments of the vessels weaken, dissection can lead to intradural subarachnoid hemorrhage (SAH) and/or extradural hematomas. Subintimal dissections are more common with intracranial dissections, whereas extracranial vessels usually dissect at the media or between the media and adventitia.

21.3.2 Pseudoaneurysms

Also referred to as "traumatic aneurysms," these result from a disruption of the internal elastic lamina and eventually all layers of the arterial wall.[28] This results in the formation of another channel within the arterial wall which causes the adventitia to expand. Pseudoaneurysms, lacking the normal layers of the vessel wall, are formed when the intramural thrombus weakens the vessel wall and allows for the hematoma to extravasate into the surrounding tissue. A hematoma forms within the false lumen, thus compressing the true lumen of the vessel resulting in stenosis.

These traumatic aneurysms account for approximately 10% of all patients presenting with BCVI.[30] Pseudoaneurysms can form in the acute setting or later as the initial injury to the vessel wall progresses. Approximately 8% of carotid injuries, which initially only consist of a luminal irregularity, may later progress to form a pseudoaneurysm.[31] Extracranial carotid artery pseudoaneurysms reportedly form in 10.3 to 23% of BCVI patients, primarily affecting the upper and middle parts of the vessel.[15,30,32] Pseudoaneurysms of the vertebral artery are not as common and are found in 3.7 to 6.5% of BCVI patients.[15,30]

Pseudoaneurysms may have two different basic structures: saccular and fusiform. Saccular pseudoaneurysms are less common, but have a greater potential to enlarge (33.3%). These form secondary to any mechanism causing a tear or other disruption in the normal vascular wall anatomy.[28] They also have a higher risk of leading to ischemic complications.[28] Fusiform aneurysms form secondary to an arterial stretch injury. They are relatively more benign and approximately half of all can be treated and resolve with antiplatelet therapy.[28,30]

21.3.3 Stroke

In cases of arterial injury, mechanisms completely disrupting blood flow, such as total occlusion of the vessel or transection, have the highest risk of resulting in ischemic stroke.[15,32,33] Although complete occlusions and transections of the cervical vessels are relatively rare, the most common cause of ischemic strokes in patients with cervical trauma is thromboembolism resulting from injury to the arterial wall.[16,34] In these cases patients can develop ischemic stroke from thrombosis/stenosis causing a significant reduction in blood flow, embolization from a thrombus formed after intimal injury, or SAH which is more common in posterior circulation injuries. Pseudoaneurysms carry a significant risk of ischemic stroke (15.4%) due to the potential for distal emboli.[30] The individual risks of stroke with carotid and vertebral artery injuries will be discussed in the upcoming sections (▶ Table 21.2).

Table 21.2 BCVI grading scale[32]

Grade	Description
1	Vessel wall irregularity; < 25% stenosis
2	Intraluminal thrombus or raised intimal flap; ≥ 25% stenosis
3	Pseudoaneurysm
4	Occlusion of the artery
5	Transection of the artery with free extravasation

21.4 Injury to the Carotid Artery

A basilar skull fracture is the strongest predictor of blunt injury to the carotid artery.[20,24] Motor vehicle collisions are by far the most common etiology of blunt carotid injuries, accounting for more than half of the cases.[23,35,36] Other less common etiologies include strangulation and spinal chiropractic manipulation therapy, although vertebral artery dissection is more common following manipulation.[37] Patients with fibromuscular dysplasia are also predisposed to multiple extracranial dissections.

The cervical ICA is most prone to injury over the second and third cervical vertebrae, especially in cases of hyperextension, lateral flexion, and rotation.[28] In cases of significant hyperextension, the ICA can be compressed by the angle of the mandible, and in cases of rotation, by the styloid process.[36,38] The distal cervical ICA can also be injured in cervical trauma resulting in stretching over the lateral masses of the cervical vertebrae.[39]

The risk of stroke with ICA dissection varies with the grade of injury. The grading scale is summarized in ▶ Table 21.3. Grade 1 injuries carry a 3% risk of stroke, and most injuries (70%) will resolve with or without anticoagulation. Approximately 4 to 12% will persist, and progress to a higher grade of injury.[27,28] The use of anticoagulation lowers the risk of progression.[27,40] Approximately 70% of grade 2 injuries, which carry an 11% risk of stroke, progress to a higher grade of injury despite anticoagulation with heparin. Most grade 3 and 4 injuries will persist despite medical treatment. Over time, patients may develop neurological deficits as the initial injury develops. Neurological sequelae develop within 1 to 24 hours of injury in 57 to 75% of cases, explaining the higher rate of BCVI seen in trauma patients hospitalized for greater than 24 hours.[27] Management of these injuries is discussed later in this chapter.

21.5 Injury to the Vertebral Artery

BCVIs involving the vertebral arteries affect 0.5 to 2% of patients who present with blunt trauma to treatment centers with aggressive screening protocols.[25,41,42,43,44] Most blunt vertebral artery injuries are caused by motor vehicle collisions. Chiropractic spinal manipulation therapy, sudden neck turning, and direct trauma to the back of the neck can also result in BCVI of the vertebral artery.[27,45,46]

Vertebral artery injuries generally occur in the V2 and V3 segments of the vertebral artery, as these are the fixed segments.[47] These segments correspond to the artery's location within the transverse foramina, and as it exits the transverse foramina of C1 and travels around the occipitocervical junction.

The risk of stroke following blunt injury to the vertebral artery is listed in ▶ Table 21.4. Unlike the increasing risk of stroke seen with grade of injury, the risk of stroke in vertebral artery injuries is highest (40%) with grade 2 injuries.[40] Grade 1 injuries carry a relatively high risk of 19%, when compared with grade 1 carotid injuries that carry a 3% risk of stroke. Vertebral artery injuries usually do not have a warning sign, such as a transient ischemic attack, prior to a stroke.[27] The average time from injury to stroke is 4 days, ranging from 8 hours to 12 days.[27]

C-spine injuries, most frequently transverse foramina fractures, facet fracture-dislocations, and vertebral subluxations, are the strongest risk factors for vertebral artery injury.[20,23,24,48] The incidence of vertebral artery injury jumps to 6% in cases of cervical spine fractures or ligamentous injuries, although this number varies and has been reported to be as high as 70%.[40,41,48] The overall mortality associated with single vertebral artery BCVI is 16%; bilateral vertebral artery injury is always almost fatal.[41] In certain extreme cases, a vertebrovenous fistula has been reported to form between the vertebral artery and its surrounding venous plexus.[49,50,51]

21.6 Imaging

CT of the head and cervical spine are generally the initial imaging modalities ordered in trauma patients presenting after mechanisms concerning for head and neck injuries. CT angiography (CTA) of the head and neck follows noncontrast imaging as the primary screening modality for vascular injury. SAH secondary to intracranial extension of an extracranial dissection must be ruled out in the presence of traumatic SAH on CT scan following trauma. In all cases of suspected vascular injuries, CTA of the head and neck must be performed.

21.6.1 Computed Tomography

CT scans of the head and neck are useful in identifying strokes, fractures, and grossly obvious hematomas. Rarely, arterial injuries can be seen on noncontrast scans as crescent shaped thickenings in the arterial wall secondary to hematoma formation.[52] Vertebral artery dissections (20%) may also present with posterior fossa SAH.[53]

21.6.2 Computed Tomographic Angiography

CTA of the head and neck is the preferred screening tool for vascular injuries in trauma patients, as it is relatively quick, sensitive, specific, and provides a prompt diagnosis.[44,54] In addition to the vasculature, CTA provides relevant bone and soft-tissue anatomy. In many cases, digital subtraction angiography (DSA) may not need to be performed in addition to CTA imaging.

Table 21.3 Risk of stroke with internal carotid artery blunt cerebrovascular injury[27]

Grade	Stroke risk
1	3%
2	11%
3	33%
4	44%

Table 21.4 Risk of stroke with vertebral artery blunt cerebrovascular injury[27]

Grade	Stroke risk
1	19%
2	40%
3	13%
4	33%

21.6.3 Magnetic Resonance Imaging

MRI of the head and neck is not as accurate as CTA or DSA. The optimal MRI study is axial T1-weighted imaging (T1WI) with fat suppression. This sequence is helpful in differentiating an intimal flap from a fusiform aneurysm. On T2-weighted imaging (T2WI), a hematoma in the wall can be seen as a bright signal in the vessel wall, referred to as the "crescent sign." The most effective use of MRI is to investigate for regions of infarction, not readily visualized on CTA as MRI is more effective in visualizing potential regions affected by embolic phenomenon. The ideal MRI for a dissection includes a magnetic resonance angiography (MRA) of the neck and/or brain with and without contrast with axial black blood sequences.[55]

In the setting of trauma, MRI is not utilized frequently due to the amount of time required for the study. In patients who do not have any obvious signs or symptoms of vascular injury and are undergoing an MRI of the cervical spine to investigate for ligamentous injury, MRA (comparable to CTA) can be performed in combination with the MRI of the cervical spine.

21.6.4 Digital Subtraction Angiography

DSA is the gold standard for diagnosing carotid and vertebral artery injury following trauma. DSA provides both a superior anatomical visualization of the artery itself in an individual frame and an exceptional visualization of real-time flow of blood within the artery allowing the physician to visualize both obvious injury to the vessel wall and more subtle flow-altering injuries. It offers the ability to treat the lesion during the same exam and afford visualization of the contralateral and anterior/posterior circulation collaterals, which is extremely important in deciding upon a particular treatment modality.

In cases of dissection, the intimal flap is usually seen at the most proximal portion of the dissection. The false lumen exists within the intimal flap and will have slower flow of contrast, which will remain within the false lumen well into the venous phase of the study. Dissections may also change configuration on repeat angiograms.[53] In cases of occlusion, the injured artery will taper to the point of occlusion, resulting in stagnation of

blood flow at that point. Kinking of the vessels can be seen with mass effect from a coexisting fracture or subluxation. Suspicious traumatic vascular lesions (pseudoaneurysms) must be followed with a repeat CTA or DSA in 7 to 10 days and at the 6-week interval.

21.7 Management of Vascular Injuries in Cervical Trauma

Several treatment modalities are available for patients presenting with vascular injuries following cervical trauma. Treatment options include conservative management/observation, anticoagulation, antiplatelet therapy, neuroendovascular intervention, and surgery. In cases of penetrating injury to the carotid/vertebral artery, there is a limited role for medical management. ▶ Fig. 21.1 and ▶ Fig. 21.2 provide a basic algorithm for treatment of uncomplicated injuries involving the carotid and vertebral arteries.

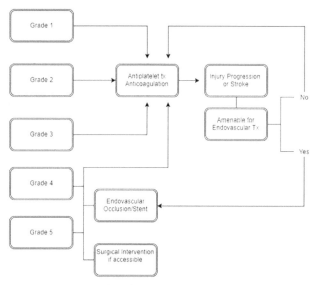

Fig. 21.2 Treatment algorithm for vertebral artery injury.

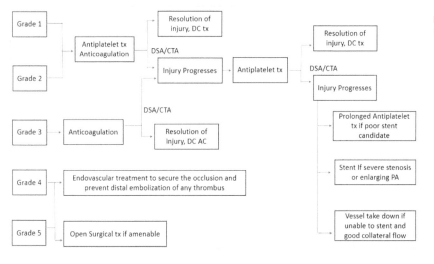

Fig. 21.1 Treatment algorithm for carotid artery injury.

21.7.1 Management of Penetrating Trauma

The management of penetrating neck trauma is guided by initial patient presentation and the anatomic zone of injury. In patients who present with signs of major vascular or aerodigestive tract injuries, emergent airway management and surgical intervention is indicated.[2] Patients who present with zone 1 or 3 injuries should be treated with endovascular intervention, especially if a neurointerventionalist is available in the acute setting.[56,57] The management of zone 2 injuries is debatable; these generally require surgical exploration during which any vascular injury can be addressed.[2,57] As a generalization, the endovascular role in these cases includes assisting in identifying the site of injury with temporary balloon occlusion, vessel take down in cases where the artery is not surgically accessible, and stent reconstruction in cases where the artery can be preserved (▶ Fig. 21.3 and ▶ Fig. 21.4).[6,50] The use of endovascular techniques for other vascular injuries, including AV fistulas, will be discussed later in this chapter.

21.7.2 Management of Nonpenetrating Trauma

Management of patients with BCVI is dictated by the grade and progression of injury, as well as the risk of stroke. The goal of treatment with antithrombotic medications (anticoagulation and antiplatelet therapy) is to prevent thromboembolic events, thereby reducing the risk of stroke.[16,34] The management of these patients is complicated by the risk of hemorrhagic complications that can be quite high in patients with multisystem injuries. The outcomes in patients with arterial injuries secondary to cervical trauma greatly depend on the existing neurological deficits when treatment is initiated.[58,59,60] Several studies have demonstrated that patients with low-grade injuries who are neurologically intact have a minimal risk of stroke and have favorable outcomes.[61,62,63]

As discussed in the previous sections, the umbrella term of nonpenetrating injuries includes BCVI, stretch injury causing arterial dissection, and kinking of the artery secondary to compression. Kinking of the artery is generally addressed during surgical decompression in cases of subluxation, and a DSA should be performed once the fracture is stabilized. If open neurosurgical intervention is anticipated in patients with concurrent vascular injury, endovascular intervention with possible vessel take down must be discussed preoperatively as the release of the "tamponading" effect of muscle and bone can cause massive intraoperative bleeding from a ruptured or dissected carotid or vertebral artery.

If CTA is negative or equivocal and there is a very high suspicion of injury, DSA should be performed. Depending upon the location and grade of injury on CTA, patients who do not have any contraindications to anticoagulation should be started on either antiplatelet or anticoagulation therapy, both of which are equally effective in preventing stroke.[64,65] Patients on antiplatelet therapy have 1.8 to 3.7% risk of stroke, and those receiving anticoagulation therapy have a 1.2% risk of stroke.[66,67]

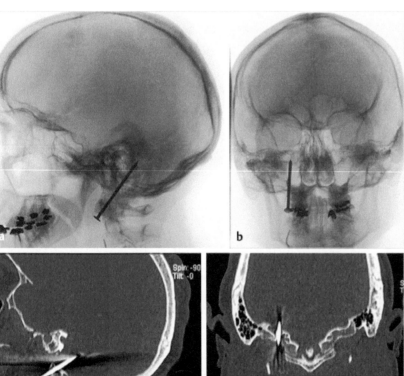

Fig. 21.3 A 52-year-old male who fell off the roof holding a nail gun accidentally shot himself through the neck with a nail. The nail extends through the neck, through the right occipital condyle with the tip embedded within the cerebellum. (a) Lateral view in the angiography suite showing the nail. (b) Anteroposterior view. (c) Computed tomography (CT) C-spine sagittal view showing nail through the occipital condyle next to the jugular foramen. (d) CT C-spine coronal view showing nail through the jugular foramen.

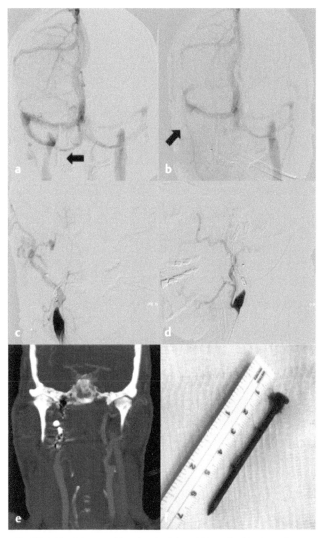

Fig. 21.4 The 52-year-old male who injured himself with the nail gun was brought to the angiography suite due to concern for vascular injury following the computed tomography angiography (CTA). The nail was barbed, so injury to the right sigmoid sinus and internal jugular vein were suspected. Therefore, prior to attempted removal of the barbed nail, the right sigmoid sinus and right internal jugular vein were occluded. During removal of the nail under fluoroscopic guidance, one of the barbs injured the right internal carotid artery (ICA). The right ICA was then occluded with balloon-assisted coiling. (**a**) Digital subtraction angiography (DSA) anteroposterior (AP) view showing the proximity of the nail (*arrow*) to the venous structures. (**b**) DSA AP view after embolization of the right sigmoid sinus (*arrow*) and jugular vein. (**c**) DSA AP view after coil embolization of the right ICA. (**d**) DSA lateral view after coil embolization of the right ICA. (**e**) CTA coronal view showing the coils used to embolize the right ICA. The lack of contrast filling the right internal jugular vein can also be appreciated in this image. Note the adequate filling of contrast in the right ICA, ACA, and MCA despite coil embolization of the right ICA. (**f**) Nail after it was removed.

The partial thromboplastin time (PTT) goal for patients started on heparin therapy should be 40 to 50 seconds.[27] Heparinization should be avoided in patients who are at high risk of bleeding. These include patients affected by intracranial hemor-

rhage, intra-abdominal injuries (spleen/liver), pelvic fractures, and impending operative interventions.

Management of Carotid Artery Injuries

Patients with grade 1 or 2 injuries, carrying a 3 to 11% risk of stroke, respectively, should be started on heparin or aspirin. Grade 1 injuries generally resolve on their own, while the majority of grade 2 injuries (70%) will progress to a more severe grade despite treatment with heparin. Aspirin is preferred as it is easier to administer in the outpatient setting.

Patients with grade 3 injuries/pseudoaneurysms should be started on heparin, and reevaluated with CTA or DSA 7 to 10 days after injury to assess for resolution or evolution.[31] If the pseudoaneurysm has resolved, anticoagulation can be discontinued. For patients with pseudoaneurysms that have not resolved, heparin should be transitioned to antiplatelet therapy with aspirin. Stent placement can be considered in patients who have severe stenosis or an enlarging pseudoaneurysm. If there is sufficient collateral flow, endovascular take down/ occlusion of the vessel can be performed. Patients who are maintained on aspirin should be reevaluated after 3 months from injury with CTA or DSA. If the pseudoaneurysm has resolved, aspirin may be discontinued. Patients who are not candidates for stent placement should be kept on prolonged aspirin or clopidogrel therapy.[25]

Patients with grade 4 injuries should undergo endovascular treatment to secure the occlusion and prevent distal embolization of any thrombus.

Grade 5 injuries carry a high rate of mortality. Patients with surgically accessible injuries should undergo open surgical repair. Patients with both complete or incomplete transections may be treated with via endovascular intervention. In patients with complete transection, the artery should be occluded; in patients with incomplete transection, stenting can be performed.

Management of Vertebral Artery Injuries

As with the management of carotid artery injuries, evaluation of the contralateral vertebral artery is an essential first step after identification of the injury on CTA or DSA. Vertebral artery dominance, collateral circulation, and grade of injury all affect overall management of the injury.

While there are no specific guidelines for treatment options in vertebral artery injuries, patients with extracranial vertebral artery injury seen on CTA or DSA, who are not at high risk for hemorrhagic complications, should be started on intravenous heparin or aspirin therapy immediately. Asymptomatic patients with extracranial dissections are generally treated with antiplatelet agents with low dose aspirin being the drug of choice. Patients with intracranial dissection require intervention with either arterial occlusion if the anatomy allows for it or stent placement in the presence of a dissection or pseudoaneurysm. Patients with a large infarction should be maintained on anticoagulants for 6 months following injury. CTA, MRA, or DSA should be performed at 3 months after initial injury to reevaluate the lesion. If the lesion has not healed, or the patient is symptomatic, endovascular intervention must be considered. At times, patients may present with dissections resulting in acute thrombi formation which can be seen on DSA. While there are no specific recommendations for managing these rare cases, neurointerventional techniques may play a role in preventing catastrophic basilar artery occlusion (▶ Fig. 21.5).

21.7.3 The Role of Endovascular Therapy

Indications

The goal of endovascular therapy is to prevent a thromboembolic stroke and/or progression of the arterial injury, in conjunction with standard medical therapy. Neurointerventional options include temporary balloon occlusions to verify adequacy of collateral circulations, vessel take downs, vessel embolizations, and stent/flow diverter placement procedures. Patients with higher-grade lesions or for whom medical management is contraindicated due to the potential for hemorrhagic complications may be candidates for endovascular embolization, but not stents in the acute period. One must keep in mind that certain endovascular interventions rely on concomitant initiation of antiplatelet therapy and may significantly increase the risk of hemorrhagic complications.

Indications for endovascular intervention in cases of carotid artery injury include the following:
1. Higher-grade lesions which require occlusion (grades 4 and 5).
2. Enlarging/expanding pseudoaneurysms.

3. Dissections which progress on DSA or remain symptomatic despite medical treatment.
4. Recurrent stroke from thromboembolism.

Indications for endovascular intervention in cases of vertebral artery injury include the following:
1. Intradural dissections with SAH.
2. Extradural dissections which progress on DSA or continue to be symptomatic despite medical treatment.
3. Enlarging/expanding pseudoaneurysms.
4. Strokes secondary to thromboembolism.

Patients who present with an acute occlusion or stenosis in the dominant vertebral artery are at considerable risk of stroke and should undergo emergent endovascular intervention in order to restore flow.

Embolization

The goal of embolization in the acute setting is to control and prevent active hemorrhage from an injured vessel. In cases where the parent artery must be embolized, balloon test occlusions can be performed prior to sacrificing a vessel.

As described earlier in the chapter, a traumatic fistula may form following penetrating injury.[50,51] Embolization has been described in the literature for use in the treatment of traumatic AV fistulas involving the nondominant vertebral artery; good outcomes and resolution of the pathology

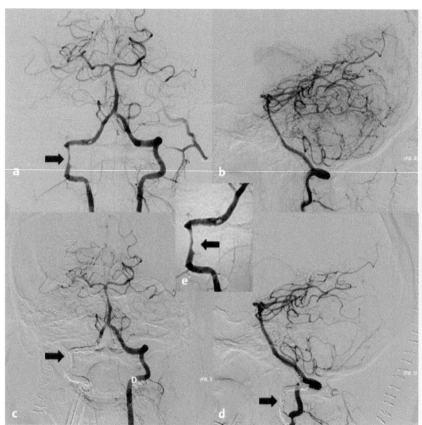

Fig. 21.5 A 31-year-old patient presented to the trauma bay after becoming dizzy and ataxic during a basketball game. Initial imaging demonstrated a right cerebellar infarct and possible right vertebral artery dissection. (a) Digital subtraction angiography (DSA) anteroposterior (AP) view. Injection of the left vertebral artery with reflux into the right vertebral artery and filling of the basilar artery. There is a dissection present in the right vertebral artery (*arrow*), evidenced by the narrowed segment between C1–C2. There is also a focal hypodensity distal to the dissection, representing an intraluminal thrombus. (b) DSA lateral view. Injection of the left vertebral artery. (c) DSA AP view. Injection of the left vertebral artery after coiling of the right vertebral artery (*arrow*). Note how the take-off of the PICA was preserved after coiling and the adequate filling of the distal posterior circulation from the dominant left vertebral artery. (d) DSA lateral view. Injection of the left vertebral artery sowing coil placement in the right vertebral artery (*arrow*). (e) Close-up view of the right vertebral artery dissection (*arrow*) and the intraluminal thrombus.

has been noted (▸ Fig. 21.6).[50,51] In these cases, catheter angiography assists in proper visualization of collateral circulation and provides a better understanding of the patient's vascular anatomy, blood flow, and venous drainage pattern. Coil embolization in combination with stent placement in cases involving the dominant vertebral artery has also been attempted successfully and remains an option in a potentially devastating pathology.[50]

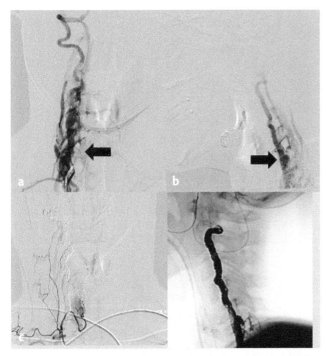

Fig. 21.6 A 44-year-old female presented to the hospital with pulsatile tinnitus on the right side. Due to her history of recent neck trauma, a computed tomography angiography (CTA) was initially done and was suspicious for a vertebrovenous fistula. On digital subtraction angiography (DSA), she was found to have a right vertebral artery focal dissection with pseudoaneurysm formation within the mid right vertebral artery. There was extensive arteriovenous (AV) shunting into the right vertebral vein, paraspinal venous plexus, and the epidural venous plexus. These findings are diagnostic of a vertebrovenous fistula. With this extensive right-sided fistula, the patient was at risk for vertebrobasilar stroke secondary to steal phenomenon and spinal subarachnoid hemorrhage secondary to AV shunting into the epidural venous plexus. Recommendation was made for embolization of the VV fistula. (a) DSA AP view of the VV fistula. Note the extensive amount of contrast in the venous structures (arrow) during the arterial phase of the angiogram. (b) DSA lateral view of the VV fistula and the pseudoaneurysm (arrow). (c) DSA AP view after embolization of the right vertebral artery. First, balloon assisted coiling was performed. Next, Onyx (Medtronic-Minneapolis, MN) was used to embolize the fistula as well as the pseudoaneurysm. (d) DSA lateral view without contrast injection demonstrating the coils and onyx used to embolize the artery and its fistula.

A variety of materials can be utilized for embolization. Control of the hemorrhage can be performed with coils, polyvinyl alcohol (PVA) articles, or with a liquid embolic agent such as n-butyl cyanoacrylate (NBCA) or Onyx.[1] Liquid embolic agents can safely be utilized in cases of traumatic fistulas, as these require precise injection of the embolic agent into smaller caliber vessels.[68]

Detachable coils create a thrombogenic mass which obstructs blood flow and causes a clot to form; these are the embolic agents of choice for performing large vessel occlusion in the context of trauma. Balloon-assisted coiling is performed to avoid distal embolization of the coil mass. One important fact to keep in mind is that it may take longer for a clot to form around the coil mass or for the vessel to thrombose in trauma patients, as they often have depleted reserves of clotting factors.[1]

NBCA (Codman Neuro-DePuy Synthes-Raynham, MA) is a liquid embolic agent which polymerizes upon contact with any ionic solution. It is combined with Ethiodol, a radiopaque iodine-based oil. The viscosity and polymerization time of the agent change in a concentration-dependent manner. Depending upon the dilution, the embolic material forms a cast within a short time (seconds) and occludes the vessel. It is generally used selectively in smaller caliber vessels. Unlike coils, the use of a liquid embolic agent does not preempt the need for clotting factors.

Onyx (Medtronic-Minneapolis, MN), also a liquid embolic agent, is composed of an ethylene vinyl alcohol (EVOH) copolymer mixed in dimethyl sulfoxide (DMSO). Tantalum is added to the solution in order to provide radio-opacity. Onyx is available in a variety of concentrations, allowing for different viscosities, which determine the flow and distance which the embolic material travels. Due to its nonadhesive/cohesive nature and the "lavalike" manner in which it precipitates, Onyx allows for a more controlled injection; greater control is thus afforded during vessel takedowns.[69,70] Liquid embolics, as mentioned earlier are used more often in the takedown of smaller vessels. Detachable coils are usually the agents of choice for larger caliber cervical vessel takedowns.

Stent Placement

The goal of endovascular stent placement is to restore near normal flow to the vessel while avoiding ischemic and hemorrhagic complications. Stenting the affected vessel provides the option of preserving the dominant vessel. One immediate drawback of stent placement in the treatment of trauma patients in the acute setting is the requirement of 6 to 12 months of antiplatelet therapy which may be contraindicated in certain situations where the patient is at an already elevated risk of hemorrhagic complications. While stenting across lower-grade lesions (such as dissections) in the acute period is an attractive option, these lower-grade lesions

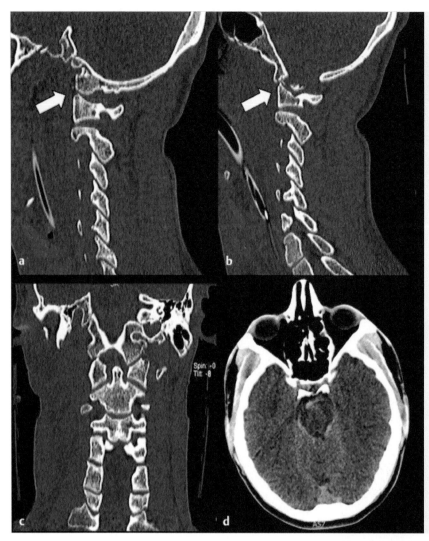

Fig. 21.7 A 20-year-old male presented to the trauma bay as pedestrian struck by a car. He suffered multiple injuries. Notably there was atlanto-occipital dislocation (AOD) on the computed tomography (CT)-Spine. **(a)** CT C-spine sagittal view demonstrating dislocation of the right occipital condyle (*arrow*). **(b)** CT C-spine sagittal view demonstrating a left occipital condyle fracture and dislocation (*arrow*). **(c)** CT C-spine coronal view. **(d)** CT head (axial view) shows subarachnoid hemorrhage raising suspicion for vertebral-basilar injury given his cervical fractures and mechanism of injury.

(grade 1 and 2) have been shown to heal solely with medical management and without any intervention. Stent placement in the treatment of higher-grade injuries, dissections, and pseudoaneurysms has been shown to be safe and efficacious with good outcomes.[29,50,71,72]

There are a variety of stents that have been used off-label in the setting of BCVI. Self-expanding stents (Neuroform, Enterprise, LVIS and Pipeline) are better at tolerating extrinsic compression, but these devices are used as a last resort; this is an off-label indication of these devices. These expanding stents dilate the lumen of the damaged stenotic vessel and incorporate the intimal flap back into the endothelial wall. Balloon-expandable stents are usually not preferred.[73,74] Due to their higher radial force, they are not ideal for the treatment of pseudoaneurysms located in higher cervical regions.[75] Covered stents are generally not used in the intracranial circulation, but can be used to treat extracranial AV fistulas, pseudoaneurysms, and for parent artery reconstruction.[76]

Pseudoaneurysms may be treated by coiling, stenting, or a combination of both. A stent is placed across the aneurysm, a microcatheter is then passed through the stent, and coils are deployed with the stent to prevent the coil mass from herniating out.[76,77,78] Cohen et al recently published a series of nine patients with pseudoaneurysms following BCVI treated with endovascular therapy (flow diversion, stent-assisted coiling, overlapping stents, and balloon-expandable stents) without any periprocedural or delayed complications.[77]

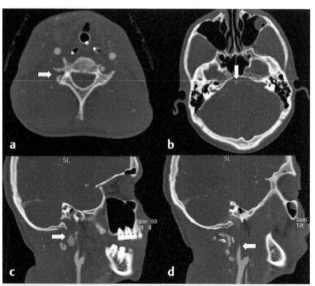

Fig. 21.8 **(a)** Computed tomography angiography (CTA) neck axial view shows no contrast filling the right vertebral artery (*arrow*). **(b)** CTA head axial view. The basilar artery (*arrow*) appears to have a filling defect, likely secondary to a nonocclusive thrombus or dissection. **(c)** CTA neck sagittal view shows a focal dissection of the right cervical ICA with a large 11 × 8 mm pseudoaneurysm (*arrow*). **(d)** CTA neck sagittal view shows dissection and occlusion of the left ICA. Note how the contrast tapers to a point (*arrow*).

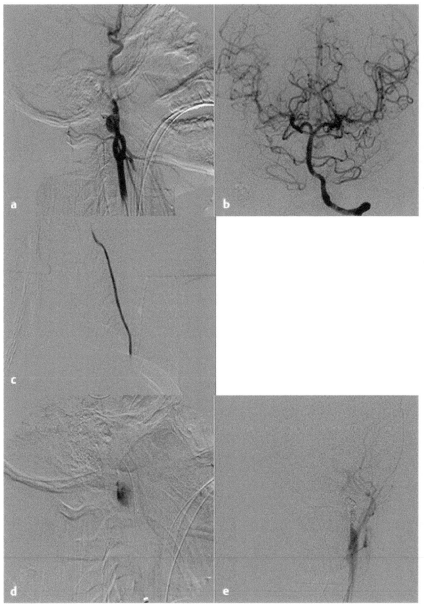

Fig. 21.9 (**a**) Digital subtraction angiography (DSA) lateral view of the right internal carotid artery (ICA). Note the dissection resulting in a posteriorly projecting pseudoaneurysm. (**b**) DSA anteroposterior (AP) view of the left vertebral artery had a fusiform dilatation proximal to the vertebrobasilar junction, concerning for dissection. (**c**) DSA lateral view of the left vertebral artery shows the dissection as the vessel tapers down. (**d**) The right ICA was treated with a self-expanding Acculink (Abbot Vascular, Abbot Park, IL) stent across the pseudoaneurysm. Control angiography performed through the arrow sheath following removal of the stent delivery device demonstrated increased caliber of the artery. There is persistent but sluggish filling of the pseudoaneurysm as seen in the figure. Intracranially, there was improved flow with improved right to left cross filling compared to the prestenting images. Further intervention to occlude the persistent but slow-filling pseudoaneurysm was not performed because it was felt that with the sluggish filling and with the stent across the neck, the pseudoaneurysm was likely to close over a short period of time. (**e**) DSA AP view of the left ICA. The artery was occluded with balloon-assisted coiling.

Flow-diverting stents, mainly the Pipeline Embolization Device (PED, Medtronic, MN), have been shown to effectively treat carotid and vertebral artery pseudoaneurysms.[79,80,81,82,83,84,85] However, this is an off-label indication and should be discussed with the patient or the family member. The use of flow diversion allows for reconstruction of the vessel for traumatic pseudoaneurysms without active bleeding or significant luminal narrowing, or for enlarging chronic pseudoaneurysms.[77,85,86] The PED is self-expandable, maneuverable in narrow segments, and can be used as a stand-alone treatment modality.[75]

Although endovascular treatment approaches reduce the procedural morbidity associated with open surgery, complications related to these techniques do still occur. Immediate complications include iatrogenic dissection, in-stent stenosis or occlusion, and pseudoaneurysm formation at the arterial access site. Stent complications include restenosis due to intimal hyperplasia, acute/subacute thrombus formation, distal stent migration, restenosis of the parent artery, or further injury to the vessel. While the published rates of complications in stent placement vary upon uses in the acute and chronic phase as well as the location of the artery and initial neurological presentation of the patient, the use of stents to treat traumatic vascular pathology remains in high favor.

21.8 Conclusion

As neurointerventional techniques develop, they continue to replace the need for open surgical treatment which carries a higher rate of morbidity. These techniques provide for a faster, safer, and more efficient method of visualizing and treating traumatic arterial injuries following cervical trauma. As advances in screening protocols and imaging modalities have made diagnosing these injuries easier, neurointerventional techniques allow for the prevent of infarctions when medical therapy and open surgery are inadequate; this, in turn, leads to improved clinical outcomes (▶ Fig. 21.7, ▶ Fig. 21.8, ▶ Fig. 21.9, and ▶ Fig. 21.10).

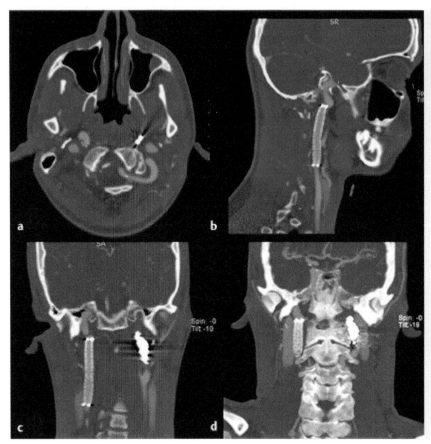

Fig. 21.10 Computed tomography angiography (CTA) images 6-months post procedure. (**a**) CTA of the neck axial view shows the left vertebral artery after Neuroform stent (Stryker Neurovascular, Freemont, CA) placement. (**b**) CTA neck sagittal view showing resolution of the right internal carotid artery (ICA) pseudoaneurysm. (**c, d**) CTA neck coronal view showing stenting of the right ICA and coil embolization of the left ICA. Note the contrast on the left side secondary to adequate filling from both the right ICA and the posterior circulation.

References

[1] Radvany MG, Gailloud P. Endovascular management of neurovascular arterial injuries in the face and neck. Semin Intervent Radiol. 2010; 27(1):44–54

[2] Sperry JL, Moore EE, Coimbra R, et al. Western Trauma Association critical decisions in trauma: penetrating neck trauma. J Trauma Acute Care Surg. 2013; 75(6):936–940

[3] Demetriades D, Asensio JA, Velmahos G, Thal E. Complex problems in penetrating neck trauma. Surg Clin North Am. 1996; 76(4):661–683

[4] Navsaria P, Omoshoro-Jones J, Nicol A. An analysis of 32 surgically managed penetrating carotid artery injuries. Eur J Vasc Endovasc Surg. 2002; 24(4):349–355

[5] Landreneau RJ, Weigelt JA, Megison SM, Meier DE, Fry WJ. Combined carotid-vertebral arterial trauma. Arch Surg. 1992; 127(3):301–304

[6] Lee TS, Ducic Y, Gordin E, Stroman D. Management of carotid artery trauma. Craniomaxillofac Trauma Reconstr. 2014; 7(3):175–189

[7] Anand VK, Raila FA, McAuley JR, Reed JM. Giant pseudoaneurysm of the extracranial vertical artery. Otolaryngol Head Neck Surg. 1993; 109(6): 1057–1060

[8] Tekiner A, Gokcek C, Bayar MA, Erdem Y, Kilic C. Spontaneus resolution of a traumatic vertebral artery pseudoaneurysm. Turk Neurosurg. 2011; 21(1):90–93

[9] Inaraja Pérez GC, Rodríguez Morata A, Reyes Ortega JP, Gómez Medialdea R, Cabezudo García P. Endovascular treatment of a symptomatic vertebral artery pseudoaneurysm. Ann Vasc Surg. 2015; 29(5):1018.e5–1018.e8

[10] Detwiler K, Godersky JC, Gentry L. Pseudoaneurysm of the extracranial vertebral artery. Case report. J Neurosurg. 1987; 67(6):935–939

[11] Roper PR, Guinto FC, Jr, Wolma FJ. Posttraumatic vertebral artery aneurysm and arteriovenous fistula: a case report. Surgery. 1984; 96(3):556–559

[12] Ross DA, Olsen WL, Halbach V, Rosegay H, Pitts LH. Cervical root compression by a traumatic pseudoaneurysm of the vertebral artery: case report. Neurosurgery. 1988; 22(2):414–417

[13] Fusco MR, Harrigan MR. Cerebrovascular dissections: a review. Part II: blunt cerebrovascular injury. Neurosurgery. 2011; 68(2):517–530, discussion 530

[14] Kerwin AJ, Bynoe RP, Murray J, et al. Liberalized screening for blunt carotid and vertebral artery injuries is justified. J Trauma. 2001; 51(2):308–314

[15] Stein DM, Boswell S, Sliker CW, Lui FY, Scalea TM. Blunt cerebrovascular injuries: does treatment always matter? J Trauma. 2009; 66(1):132–143, discussion 143–144

[16] Griessenauer CJ, Fleming JB, Richards BF, et al. Timing and mechanism of ischemic stroke due to extracranial blunt traumatic cerebrovascular injury. J Neurosurg. 2013; 118(2):397–404

[17] Harrigan MR, Falola MI, Shannon CN, Westrick AC, Walters BC. Incidence and trends in the diagnosis of traumatic extracranial cerebrovascular injury in the nationwide inpatient sample database, 2003–2010. J Neurotrauma. 2014; 31(11):1056–1062

[18] Spaniolas K, Velmahos GC, Alam HB, de Moya M, Tabbara M, Sailhamer E. Does improved detection of blunt vertebral artery injuries lead to improved outcomes? Analysis of the National Trauma Data Bank. World J Surg. 2008; 32(10):2190–2194

[19] Miller PR, Fabian TC, Bee TK, et al. Blunt cerebrovascular injuries: diagnosis and treatment. J Trauma. 2001; 51(2):279–285, discussion 285–286

[20] Miller PR, Fabian TC, Croce MA, et al. Prospective screening for blunt cerebrovascular injuries: analysis of diagnostic modalities and outcomes. Ann Surg. 2002; 236(3):386–393, discussion 393–395

[21] Berne JD, Norwood SH, McAuley CE, Vallina VL, Creath RG, McLarty J. The high morbidity of blunt cerebrovascular injury in an unscreened population: more evidence of the need for mandatory screening protocols. J Am Coll Surg. 2001; 192(3):314–321

[22] Berne JD, Norwood SH, McAuley CE, Villareal DH. Helical computed tomographic angiography: an excellent screening test for blunt cerebrovascular injury. J Trauma. 2004; 57(1):11–17, discussion 17–19

[23] Biffl WL, Moore EE, Offner PJ, et al. Optimizing screening for blunt cerebrovascular injuries. Am J Surg. 1999; 178(6):517–522

[24] Burlew CC, Biffl WL, Moore EE, Barnett CC, Johnson JL, Bensard DD. Blunt cerebrovascular injuries: redefining screening criteria in the era of noninvasive diagnosis. J Trauma Acute Care Surg. 2012; 72(2):330–335, discussion 336–337, quiz 539

[25] Biffl WL, Cothren CC, Moore EE, et al. Western Trauma Association critical decisions in trauma: screening for and treatment of blunt cerebrovascular injuries. J Trauma. 2009; 67(6):1150–1153

[26] Crissey MM, Bernstein EF. Delayed presentation of carotid intimal tear following blunt craniocervical trauma. Surgery. 1974; 75(4):543–549

[27] Greenberg MS. Handbook of Neurosurgery. New York, NY: Thieme; 2010

[28] Foreman PM, Griessenauer CJ, Harrigan MR. Blunt cerebrovascular injury. In: Winn HR, ed. Youmans and Winn Neurological Surgery. Vol 4. Philadelphia, PA: Elsevier; 2017:3124–3129

[29] Moon K, Albuquerque FC, Cole T, Gross BA, McDougall CG. Stroke prevention by endovascular treatment of carotid and vertebral artery dissections. J Neurointerv Surg. 2016

[30] Foreman PM, Griessenauer CJ, Falola M, Harrigan MR. Extracranial traumatic aneurysms due to blunt cerebrovascular injury. J Neurosurg. 2014; 120(6):1437–1445

[31] Biffl WL, Ray CE, Jr, Moore EE, et al. Treatment-related outcomes from blunt cerebrovascular injuries: importance of routine follow-up arteriography. Ann Surg. 2002; 235(5):699–706, discussion 706–707

[32] Biffl WL, Moore EE, Offner PJ, Brega KE, Franciose RJ, Burch JM. Blunt carotid arterial injuries: implications of a new grading scale. J Trauma. 1999; 47(5):845–853

[33] Morton RP, Hanak BW, Levitt MR, et al. Blunt traumatic occlusion of the internal carotid and vertebral arteries. J Neurosurg. 2014; 120(6):1446–1450

[34] Redekop GJ. Extracranial carotid and vertebral artery dissection: a review. Can J Neurol Sci. 2008; 35(2):146–152

[35] Biffl WL, Moore EE, Ryu RK, et al. The unrecognized epidemic of blunt carotid arterial injuries: early diagnosis improves neurologic outcome. Ann Surg. 1998; 228(4):462–470

[36] Kraus RR, Bergstein JM, DeBord JR. Diagnosis, treatment, and outcome of blunt carotid arterial injuries. Am J Surg. 1999; 178(3):190–193

[37] Biller J, Hingtgen WL, Adams HP, Jr, Smoker WR, Godersky JC, Toffol GJ. Cervicocephalic arterial dissections. A ten-year experience. Arch Neurol. 1986; 43(12):1234–1238

[38] Zelenock GB, Kazmers A, Whitehouse WM, Jr, et al. Extracranial internal carotid artery dissections: noniatrogenic traumatic lesions. Arch Surg. 1982; 117(4):425–432

[39] Arthurs ZM, Starnes BW. Blunt carotid and vertebral artery injuries. Injury. 2008; 39(11):1232–1241

[40] Biffl WL, Moore EE, Elliott JP, et al. The devastating potential of blunt vertebral arterial injuries. Ann Surg. 2000; 231(5):672–681

[41] Berne JD, Norwood SH. Blunt vertebral artery injuries in the era of computed tomographic angiographic screening: incidence and outcomes from 8,292 patients. J Trauma. 2009; 67(6):1333–1338

[42] Cothren CC, Moore EE. Blunt cerebrovascular injuries. Clinics (São Paulo). 2005; 60(6):489–496

[43] Fassett DR, Dailey AT, Vaccaro AR. Vertebral artery injuries associated with cervical spine injuries: a review of the literature. J Spinal Disord Tech. 2008; 21(4):252–258

[44] Eastman AL, Chason DP, Perez CL, McAnulty AL, Minei JP. Computed tomographic angiography for the diagnosis of blunt cervical vascular injury: is it ready for primetime? J Trauma. 2006; 60(5):925–929, discussion 929

[45] Mas JL, Henin D, Bousser MG, Chain F, Hauw JJ. Dissecting aneurysm of the vertebral artery and cervical manipulation: a case report with autopsy. Neurology. 1989; 39(4):512–515

[46] Caplan LR, Zarins CK, Hemmati M. Spontaneous dissection of the extracranial vertebral arteries. Stroke. 1985; 16(6):1030–1038

[47] Desouza RM, Crocker MJ, Haliasos N, Rennie A, Saxena A. Blunt traumatic vertebral artery injury: a clinical review. Eur Spine J. 2011; 20(9):1405–1416

[48] Cothren CC, Moore EE, Biffl WL, et al. Cervical spine fracture patterns predictive of blunt vertebral artery injury. J Trauma. 2003; 55(5):811–813

[49] Madoz A, Desal H, Auffray-Calvier E, et al. Vertebrovertebral arteriovenous fistula diagnosis and treatment: report of 8 cases and review of the literature. J Neuroradiol. 2006; 33(5):319–327

[50] Herrera DA, Vargas SA, Dublin AB. Endovascular treatment of traumatic injuries of the vertebral artery. AJNR Am J Neuroradiol. 2008; 29(8):1585–1589

[51] Beaujeux RL, Reizine DC, Casasco A, et al. Endovascular treatment of vertebral arteriovenous fistula. Radiology. 1992; 183(2):361–367

[52] Hodge CJ, Jr, Leeson M, Cacayorin E, Petro G, Culebras A, Iliya A. Computed tomographic evaluation of extracranial carotid artery disease. Neurosurgery. 1987; 21(2):167–176

[53] Kitanaka C, Tanaka J, Kuwahara M, et al. Nonsurgical treatment of unruptured intracranial vertebral artery dissection with serial follow-up angiography. J Neurosurg. 1994; 80(4):667–674

[54] Malhotra AK, Camacho M, Ivatury RR, et al. Computed tomographic angiography for the diagnosis of blunt carotid/vertebral artery injury: a note of caution. Ann Surg. 2007; 246(4):632–642, discussion 642–643

[55] Hunter MA, Santosh C, Teasdale E, Forbes KP. High-resolution double inversion recovery black-blood imaging of cervical artery dissection using 3 T MR imaging. AJNR Am J Neuroradiol. 2012; 33(11):E133–E137

[56] Starnes BW, Arthurs ZM. Endovascular management of vascular trauma. Perspect Vasc Surg Endovasc Ther. 2006; 18(2):114–129

[57] Reva VA, Pronchenko AA, Samokhvalov IM. Operative management of penetrating carotid artery injuries. Eur J Vasc Endovasc Surg. 2011; 42(1):16–20

[58] Timberlake GA, Rice JC, Kerstein MD, Rush DS, McSwain NE, Jr. Penetrating injury to the carotid artery. A reappraisal of management. Am Surg. 1989; 55(3):154–157

[59] McKevitt EC, Kirkpatrick AW, Vertesi L, Granger R, Simons RK. Blunt vascular neck injuries: diagnosis and outcomes of extracranial vessel injury. J Trauma. 2002; 53(3):472–476

[60] Sclafani SJ, Panetta T, Goldstein AS, et al. The management of arterial injuries caused by penetration of zone III of the neck. J Trauma. 1985; 25(9):871–881

[61] Colella JJ, Diamond DL. Blunt carotid injury: reassessing the role of anticoagulation. Am Surg. 1996; 62(3):212–217

[62] Martin RF, Eldrup-Jorgensen J, Clark DE, Bredenberg CE. Blunt trauma to the carotid arteries. J Vasc Surg. 1991; 14(6):789–793, discussion 793–795

[63] Fabian TC, Patton JH, Jr, Croce MA, Minard G, Kudsk KA, Pritchard FE. Blunt carotid injury. Importance of early diagnosis and anticoagulant therapy. Ann Surg. 1996; 223(5):513–522, discussion 522–525

[64] Edwards NM, Fabian TC, Claridge JA, Timmons SD, Fischer PE, Croce MA. Antithrombotic therapy and endovascular stents are effective treatment for blunt carotid injuries: results from long term follow up. J Am Coll Surg. 2007; 204(5):1007–1013, discussion 1014–1015

[65] Markus HS, Hayter E, Levi C, Feldman A, Venables G, Norris J, CADISS trial investigators. Antiplatelet treatment compared with anticoagulation treatment for cervical artery dissection (CADISS): a randomised trial. Lancet Neurol. 2015; 14(4):361–367

[66] Engelter ST, Brandt T, Debette S, et al. Cervical Artery Dissection in Ischemic Stroke Patients (CADISP) Study Group. Antiplatelets versus anticoagulation in cervical artery dissection. Stroke. 2007; 38(9):2605–2611

[67] Lyrer P, Engelter S. Antithrombotic drugs for carotid artery dissection. Cochrane Database Syst Rev. 2003(3):CD000255

[68] Alderazi YJ, Cruz GM, Kass-Hout T, Prestigiacomo CJ, Duffis EJ, Gandhi CD. Endovascular therapy for cerebrovascular injuries after head and neck trauma. Trauma. 2015; 17(4):258–269

[69] Medel R, Crowley RW, Hamilton DK, Dumont AS. Endovascular obliteration of an intracranial pseudoaneurysm: the utility of Onyx. J Neurosurg Pediatr. 2009; 4(5):445–448

[70] Weber W, Kis B, Siekmann R, Kuehne D. Endovascular treatment of intracranial arteriovenous malformations with onyx: technical aspects. AJNR Am J Neuroradiol. 2007; 28(2):371–377

[71] Pham MH, Rahme RJ, Arnaout O, et al. Endovascular stenting of extracranial carotid and vertebral artery dissections: a systematic review of the literature. Neurosurgery. 2011; 68(4):856–866, discussion 866

[72] Parkhutik V, Lago A, Tembl JI, Aparici F, Vazquez V, Mainar E. Angioplasty and stenting of symptomatic and asymptomatic vertebral artery stenosis: to treat or not to treat. Eur J Neurol. 2010; 17(2):267–272

[73] Ansari SA, Thompson BG, Gemmete JJ, Gandhi D. Endovascular treatment of distal cervical and intracranial dissections with the neuroform stent. Neurosurgery. 2008; 62(3):636–646, discussion 636–646

[74] Jeon P, Kim BM, Kim DI, et al. Emergent self-expanding stent placement for acute intracranial or extracranial internal carotid artery dissection with significant hemodynamic insufficiency. AJNR Am J Neuroradiol. 2010; 31(8):1529–1532

[75] Wang A, Santarelli J, Stiefel MF. Pipeline embolization device as primary treatment for cervical internal carotid artery pseudoaneurysms. Surg Neurol Int. 2017; 8:3

[76] Yi AC, Palmer E, Luh GY, Jacobson JP, Smith DC. Endovascular treatment of carotid and vertebral pseudoaneurysms with covered stents. AJNR Am J Neuroradiol. 2008; 29(5):983–987

[77] Cohen JE, Gomori JM, Rajz G, et al. Vertebral artery pseudoaneurysms secondary to blunt trauma: endovascular management by means of neurostents and flow diverters. J Clin Neurosci. 2016; 32:77–82

[78] Kansagra AP, Cooke DL, English JD, et al. Current trends in endovascular management of traumatic cerebrovascular injury. J Neurointerv Surg. 2014; 6(1):47–50

[79] Nerva JD, Morton RP, Levitt MR, et al. Pipeline Embolization Device as primary treatment for blister aneurysms and iatrogenic pseudoaneurysms of the internal carotid artery. J Neurointerv Surg. 2015; 7(3):210–216

[80] Amenta PS, Starke RM, Jabbour PM, et al. Successful treatment of a traumatic carotid pseudoaneurysm with the Pipeline stent: case report and review of the literature. Surg Neurol Int. 2012; 3:160

[81] Fischer S, Vajda Z, Aguilar Perez M, et al. Pipeline Embolization Device (PED) for neurovascular reconstruction: initial experience in the treatment of 101 intracranial aneurysms and dissections. Neuroradiology. 2012; 54(4): 369–382

[82] Kerolus M, Tan LA, Chen M. Treatment of a giant vertebral artery pseudoaneurysm secondary to gunshot wound to the neck using pipeline embolization device. Br J Neurosurg. 2016; •••:1–2

[83] Dolati P, Eichberg DG, Thomas A, Ogilvy CS. Application of Pipeline Embolization Device for iatrogenic pseudoaneurysms of the extracranial vertebral artery: a case report and systematic review of the literature. Cureus. 2015; 7(10):e356

[84] Ambekar S, Sharma M, Smith D, Cuellar H. Successful treatment of iatrogenic vertebral pseudoaneurysm using pipeline embolization device. Case Rep Vasc Med. 2014; 2014:341748

[85] Patel PD, Chalouhi N, Atallah E, et al. Off-label uses of the Pipeline Embolization Device: a review of the literature. Neurosurg Focus. 2017; 42(6):E4

[86] Kadkhodayan Y, Shetty VS, Blackburn SL, Reynolds MR, Cross DT, III, Moran CJ. Pipeline embolization device and subsequent vessel sacrifice for treatment of a bleeding carotid pseudoaneurysm at the skull base: a case report. J Neurointerv Surg. 2013; 5(5):e31

22 Bone Graft Options, Substitutes, and Harvest Techniques

Arash J. Sayari, Ankur S. Narain, Fady Y. Hijji, Krishna T. Kudaravalli, Kelly H. Yom, and Kern Singh

Abstract

After trauma to the cervical spine, the first decision in the treatment algorithm is between surgical and conservative management. When surgical therapy is required, cervical fusion procedures are frequently utilized. Consequently, decisions regarding bone grafting options are of significant concern. During graft selection, considerations must be made regarding many factors, such as osteogenic potential, biocompatibility, cost, structural support, site of implantation, immunogenetics, and preservation techniques. While autologous bone graft remains the gold standard in cervical spine fusion procedures, obtaining such grafts is not without disadvantages. To minimize the morbidity of autograft, allograft is the primary alternative utilized in the cervical spine. However, interest in manufactured graft substitutes has been heightened by recent investigations suggesting the efficacy of these alternative grafts with regards to postoperative outcomes. In this chapter, we aim to discuss the various grafting options applied in the cervical spine and delineate the appropriate settings for their use.

Keywords: cervical spine, bone graft, demineralized bone matrix, bone fusion, iliac crest bone graft, allograft, bone graft substitute

22.1 Introduction

Anterior and posterior cervical fusion techniques are commonly utilized in the treatment of traumatic cervical pathologies. The achievement of adequate bony fusion during these procedures is of paramount importance. Adequate fusion not only ensures spinal stability, but is also associated with improvements in postoperative outcomes related to pain, disability, and neurological deficits.[1,2,3,4] Failure of bony fusion or pseudarthrosis following cervical procedures is of significant concern. Symptomatic pseudarthrosis can lead to recurrence of pain and is responsible for a large percentage of revision procedures for cervical pathology.[5,6,7,8]

In order to aid in the fusion, a variety of bone grafts and graft alternatives can be utilized. Bone grafting in humans was first documented as an allograft procedure in the late 1800s when William MacEwen replaced the proximal two-thirds of a humerus in a 4-year-old boy with bone transplanted from his other patients.[9] In the lumbar spine, Albee described the placement of cortical tibial autograft into a split spinous process during the treatment of Pott disease.[10] In cervical spine applications, Smith and Robinson described the technique of anterior cervical discectomy and fusion (ACDF) with a novel method of placing a horseshoe-shaped tricortical graft from the iliac crest.[11] Similarly, Cloward reported a method of obtaining bone graft from the anterosuperior ilium for use in anterior cervical fusion procedures.[12]

Within current practice, autografted bone transplanted from one anatomic site to another remains the gold standard in bone grafting for cervical fusion procedures. However, advances in graft technology have produced viable alternatives to autograft such as allograft, graft enhancers, and graft substitutes. With the plethora of fusion materials available, it is imperative that surgeons understand the relative efficacy of each potential option. As such, the purpose of this chapter is to review the varying types of fusion biologics with a focus on their appropriate use in the setting of cervical trauma (▶ Table 22.1).

22.2 Biology of Bone Grafts and Fusion

The three most commonly cited elements of graft osteointegration are related to its osteoconductive, osteoinductive, and osteogenic potential. Proper understanding of this relationship between the host and graft is crucial as this forms the basis of graft design and choice. Osteoconductive properties relate to the three-dimensional graft–host environment, allowing for further ingrowth of tissue, capillaries, and multipotent stem cells (MSCs). The scaffold by which these MSCs function makes way for the creation of Haversian canals and bone growth.

Table 22.1 Summary of graft options utilized in the cervical spine

Graft type	Osteoconductive	Osteoinductive	Osteogenic	Mechanical support
Autograft				
• Cancellous	+++	+++	+++	+
• Cortical	+	+	+	+++
• Vascularized	++	+	++	+++
• BMA	–	++	+++	–
• PRP	–	+++	–	–
Allograft				
• Cancellous	++	+	–	+
• Cortical	+	+	–	+++
• DBM	++	++	–	–
Ceramics	+	–	–	+++
Growth factors	–	+	+	–

Abbreviations: BMA, bone marrow aspirate; DBM, demineralized bone matrix; PRP, platelet-rich plasma.
-, +, ++, +++ = extent of activity; – = no activity; +++ = maximum activity.
Data from Roberts et al[13] and Khan et al[14]

Osteoinductive properties relate to the graft's availability of growth factors and its ability to stimulate bone growth.[15] Osteoinductive grafts recruit MSCs, which differentiate into chondroblasts and osteoblasts that form novel bone via endosteal ossification.[13] Molecular studies have shown that autograft contains various growth factors that regulate the recruitment and differentiation of the MSCs. The growth factors implicated in bone growth, development, and repair include the transforming growth factor beta (TGF-β), superfamily of proteins (TGF-β1 and bone morphogenetic proteins [BMP] types 2, 4, and 7), fibroblast growth factor alpha (FGF-α), insulin-like growth factor 1 (IGF-I), granulocyte colony-stimulating factors, platelet-derived growth factor-bb (PDGF-bb), and endothelial-derived growth factors.[16] Many of these growth factors also serve as inflammatory cytokines, hence explaining why anti-inflammatory agents are not recommended during the early stages of bone healing and repair.[14]

Finally, the osteogenic potential of a graft is related to its concentration of MSCs and osteoprogenitor cells that can differentiate into osteoblasts and eventually, osteocytes. Only fresh autologous grafts, and autologous and allografted bone marrow transplants possess these properties and contain viable cells capable of directly producing bone.

22.3 Autograft

Autograft is bone graft obtained from a patient's own bone that is transplanted at the recipient site. In cervical procedures for both traumatic and nontraumatic etiologies, autograft is the gold standard graft choice due to its superior osteointegrative potential and lack of immunogenicity. Autograft can be characterized based upon its location with distinctions made between local autograft from the operative site and autograft taken from other anatomic locations. The most commonly utilized location for autograft harvest is the iliac crest. Iliac crest bone grafts (ICBG) have demonstrated successful fusion outcomes in both lumbar and cervical spine applications. In addition, autograft can be classified based on the type of bone graft obtained, such as cancellous, cortical, vascularized, or bone marrow aspirate.

22.3.1 Cancellous Bone Autograft

Cancellous bone, the most commonly used form of autograft, provides a scaffold through which further bone growth can occur. Like cortical bone, graft transplantation involves gradual graft resorption, bony remodeling, and novel bone formation via creeping substitution.[17,18] After transplantation, bleeding and inflammation serve as the foundation for this process. Recruitment of MSCs allows for fibrous granulation in the graft bed in as little as little as 2 days.[13] In addition, macrophages utilize chemotaxis to gather at the site of transplantation in order to begin degradation of necrotic tissue. Revascularization is completed rapidly in an end-to-end or appositional fashion. MSCs from the host and graft cells begin to differentiate into osteoprogenitor cells and eventually osteoblasts that line the graft–host interface to deposit osteoid. However, there is still the presence of necrotic tissue centrally. Inward osteoclastic resorption of this tissue is followed by increased osteoblastic

activity to replace the once vacant lacunae with new bone. The final step is continuous remodeling, which can take up to a year to complete.[18]

The trabecular environment of cancellous bone has a high surface area, thriving with MSCs, osteoblasts, and osteocytes, thus leading to superior osteoconductive, osteoinductive, and osteogenic properties.[14,16,19] This concept is quite apparent in decortication during cervical fusion procedures. When the intramedullary spaces of the posterior elements of the spine are exposed (lamina, pedicles, transverse processes), pluripotent stem cells within the marrow infiltrate the fusion site to provide osteogenic proteins and a rich blood supply to the graft–host interface.

These advantages also support why cancellous graft does not offer the same mechanical strength as cortical graft. In fact, cancellous bone is only one-fourth as dense as cortical bone and should, therefore, be more commonly used for filling small defects rather than being used as supportive strut. However, because of its relatively rapid incorporation, cancellous autograft initially strengthens over the necrotic center. The increased early stability is produced as bone is initially laid down but normalizes over time. Locally available autograft should be used if possible, especially in single-level procedures. It is easily incorporated into the surgical site and has demonstrated fusion rates in the lumbar spine similar to that of ICBG.[20,21]

22.3.2 Cortical Bone Autograft

Autologous cortical bone graft behaves differently, most notably with a rate of revascularization nearly half that of cancellous bone due to its density and highly organized Haversian and Volkmann canals. In both cancellous and cortical autografts, creeping substitution follows in a centripetal pattern to allow for new bone formation. However, osteointegration of cortical autograft is initially dictated by osteoclasts, rather than osteoblasts. The rate of osteoclastic resorption rises from 2 weeks through 6 months post transplantation, after which the rate declines to near-normal levels at 1 year.[14] Along the process of inward resorption, osteoblasts begin laying down bone to eventually replace the transplanted cortical autograft with new, viable bone. As osteoclastic activity dictates cortical autograft remodeling, initial bone loss may result in the graft losing a significant amount of its strength due to removal of its necrotic center, but eventually will fully heal with near-normal mechanical strength. This was demonstrated in a mechanical study performed by Enneking et al on 23 canines in which fibular autografts were examined. The transplants demonstrated increased porosity and weakness at 6 weeks, but 100% of them had achieved normal mechanical strength by 12 months.[22] Given that only 60% of their study subjects had full remodeling of the transplants, this further exemplifies how the mixture of necrotic and viable bone does not influence the overall strength.

As there are fewer osteocytes, osteoblasts, and infiltrating MSCs in cortical bone graft, it consequently exhibits poorer osteogenic, osteoinductive, and osteoconductive potential than cancellous grafts. However, cortical autograft offers increased initial mechanical strength and increased stability when used as a bony fixation construct.

22.3.3 Autologous Vascularized Bone Graft

Vascularized grafts are those transplanted with their arterial and venous vessels anastomosed during grafting, allowing for more rapid graft incorporation. An adequate anastomosis allows for more than 90% survival of osteocytes and other osteoprogenitor cells.[23] In addition, vascular cortical grafts heal quickly because the revascularization component is essentially complete, allowing for a remodeling process similar to that of normal bone by way of primary or secondary bone healing. Thus, there is no sacrifice of early mechanical strength due to creeping substitution as exhibited with nonvascularized autografts. The primary concern with vascularized grafts is difficulty in obtaining and correctly transplanting these grafts. These grafts involve challenging techniques of orthopaedic and microvascular surgery with increased operative times and blood loss during harvest.

The most commonly used vascularized graft is the free fibula strut graft transplanted along with its peroneal artery. Prior to graft harvest, preoperative angiography may be useful to evaluate vascular pedicles.[24] In the case of short peroneal artery pedicles, iliac crest grafts with branches of the deep circumflex iliac artery and distal radius grafts with the intercompartmental supraretinacular artery may be suitable alternatives.

As vascular grafts are most useful in massive spine defects caused by tumors and deformities, their use is not common in the setting of cervical spine trauma. Regardless, consideration for fibular strut grafts continues to be made, as its strength in the axial plane is nearly five times that of ICBG.[25]

22.3.4 Autologous Bone Marrow Aspirate

Although bone marrow aspirate (BMA) is not technically a bone graft and is less commonly used than cortical or cancellous grafts in cervical fusions, it deserves mention because of its osteogenic properties and other key advantages. Using minimally invasive techniques, BMA can be easily obtained from the iliac crest or vertebral body. The biological properties of BMA that make it useful as an autograft stem from the presumed concentration of MSCs that reproduce and differentiate into connective tissue. Specific to bone, this differentiation produces osteoblasts via medullary osteogenesis.

While BMA offers theoretical advantages, the true number of stem cells that can differentiate into osteoblasts are variable in BMA and may be as few as 1 in 50,000 in the young patients and 1 in 1,000,000 in the elderly.[14] Recent investigation regarding the influence of BMA on bone remodeling and repair has been focused on its concentration of endothelial progenitor cells and ability to stimulate revascularization.[26] This relates to the osteoinductive properties of BMA as it contains chemotactic mitogens that induce and attract local growth factors.

Unfortunately, given its semiliquid state and lack of structural support, BMA tends to migrate from initial transplantation site. Thus, BMA may be less favorable in anatomic sites, such as the cervical spine, as BMA fluid migration has been linked to heterotopic ossification.[15] Despite efforts being made to mix BMA with cancellous bone and bone graft substitutes to mitigate some of these disadvantages,[27,28] the clinical use of BMA in the cervical spine has been minimal thus far. As recent attempts have been made to incorporate BMA into substrates and extenders, such as demineralized bone matrix, potential still exists for BMA to gain traction in the future.

22.3.5 Autologous Platelet-Rich Plasma

Platelet-rich plasma (PRP) is prepared from an autologous supply of whole blood which then undergoes specific centrifugation protocols to provide a high concentration of platelets. This suspension is filled with growth factors such as TGF-β, PDGF, and vascular endothelial growth factor (VEGF). The conglomerate platelet solution is mixed with calcium chloride to create a platelet clot applied at the surgical site. Recent investigation has found a link between PRP, callus formation, and cell proliferation.[26] Feiz-Erfan et al randomized 50 patients with degenerative disc disease or disc herniation to receive either cervical allograft or cervical allograft plus platelet concentrate.[29] The authors found an 84% overall fusion rate, and a significantly higher rate of fusion in the PRP group when compared to controls. However, this difference was not maintained at 12 months postoperatively. Further research is still required regarding the application of PRP within cervical spine surgery before it can be utilized in a more widespread fashion.

22.3.6 Limitations of Autologous Grafting

Autologous grafting has various limitations related to the harvesting process. Donor site morbidity is of primary concern as it is the most common complication.[30] ICBG morbidity has been linked to the volume harvested, with morbidity rates increasing when the harvested volume is greater than 17 cm^3.[31] Interestingly, in a recent cohort of 25 patients undergoing lumbar fusion with ICBG harvested through the same skin incision, more than two-thirds could not accurately or confidently determine which side was used for ICBG.[32] In the setting of cervical trauma, especially multisystem trauma, operative time and the need for blood transfusions may be of concern, both of which have been shown to be significantly higher in those receiving autograft.[33] Limited physiologic supply is also a challenge that dictates the need for an alternative graft material, particularly in the pediatric population. While autograft remains the gold standard in cervical spine applications, the drawbacks to its use have led to the search for viable alternatives.

22.4 Allograft

Allografting is the process by which tissue is transplanted between two genetically nonidentical members of the same species. Allografting has gained significant traction in orthopaedic surgery over the past 20 years and has become the second most popular bone graft choice.[34] The popularity of allograft is based on its customizability, load resistance, and structural support.

However, allograft is not without limitations, the most prominent being its ability to undergo bony remodeling. Specifically, the healing and remodeling potential for allograft is inferior to that of autograft. Moreover, while fresh frozen grafts maintain their mechanical strength, biomechanical studies have demonstrated that freeze-dried cortical allografts lose more than half of their strength during processing.[35] Another major concern of allograft is viral disease transmission. Stringent processing lowers this risk, but also weakens the biological and mechanical properties for which the graft was initially chosen. The overall risk of viral transmission is less than 1 in 1,000,000 for human immunodeficiency virus (HIV), 1 in 100,000 for hepatitis C, and 1 in 63,000 for hepatitis B.[36,37] The American Association of Tissue Banks (AATB) has created a high-quality tissue bank that ensures availability of such allogeneic tissue. Currently, there are more than 60 such tissue banks in the United States, and improvement in quality control by the AATB and United States Food and Drug Administration (FDA) helps minimize risks for disease transmission and increases the availability of high-quality allografts that are properly processed and distributed.

Unlike autograft, in which there is no concern for histoincompatibility, allograft osteointegration involves more complex processes of humoral and cell-mediated responses that involve the immune system. Regardless of the graft processing, donor antigens (major histocompatibility complex [MHC] class I and II) still illicit a host T-cell response.[14]

22.4.1 Cancellous Bone Allograft

Unlike its autograft counterpart, cancellous allograft has limited bone healing properties with inferior osteoconductive, osteoinductive, and osteogenic properties. Within 2 weeks of graft implantation, osteointegration is led by inflammation mediated by macrophages and lymphocytes. An aggressive host immune response results in not only destruction of osteoinductive growth factors necessary for osteointegration, but also formation of an encapsulated layer of fibrous tissue. The extent of fibrosis depends on the histoincompatibility between the donor and host, which can delay bone graft incorporation for up to 8 years in cases of poor histocompatibility.[14,26]

With newer graft processing technology, attempts have been made to improve clinical results. Boyce et al, in a 1999 review, suggested that sterility and reduction in antigenicity are the two primary factors in allograft success.[34] The utilization of freeze-dried and frozen cancellous allografts has provided some solution to the problem of host immunogenicity. However, while reducing antigenicity, the graft preservation process of freeze-dried cancellous bone depletes the graft of its osteoinductive growth factors and limits its osteoconductivity. This consequently results in poorer remodeling and angiogenesis when compared to fresh and fresh-frozen variants.

22.4.2 Cortical Bone Allograft

While cancellous allograft is incorporated far more rapidly than cortical allograft due to its increased surface area and ability for revascularization, it is the poorer choice for initial mechanical stabilization. Cortical allografts are notable for their immediate

ability to resist mechanical loads, which is a necessity in spinal surgery. However, poor vascularization may compromise their associated strength for up to a year or until revascularization. Unlike cancellous allograft, which involves osteoneogenesis throughout trabeculae, cortical allograft is incorporated by callus formation. Both cancellous and cortical allograft elicit a host inflammatory response and fibrous tissue formation, but new periosteal formation at the graft–host edges results in a callus that is unique to cortical allograft.

Clinically, cortical allografts are used for interbody fusions of the cervical spine and have exhibited promising results. A review by Butterman et al in 1996 demonstrated that freeze-dried fibular and ilium allografts have similar fusion rates of 92%.[38] Comparisons of iliac autograft and fresh frozen and freeze-dried allografts also revealed similar rates of graft collapse and fusion rates in single-level cervical fusion procedures. Early studies have suggested significantly higher rates of graft subsidence and nonunion in allografted two-level ACDF.[38] A more recent study comparing autograft ICBG and fibular allograft demonstrated similar fusion rates between one- and two-level ACDF procedures, although the time to union was longer with allograft.[39] Yue et al further reported successful allograft fusion rates of 92.6% at an average of more than 7 years after surgery in 71 patients undergoing ACDF,[40] indicating that freeze-dried and fresh frozen allografts are efficacious in ACDF procedures.

22.4.3 Demineralized Bone Matrix

Demineralized bone matrix (DBM) is a form of allograft that has undergone acid and mineral phase extraction or decalcification. Growth factors, noncollagenous proteins, and collagen are left behind in the organic phase, creating a bony lattice in which MSCs are recruited and new bone is deposited. The trabecular environment contributes to the strong osteoconductive potential of DBM, despite the lack of structural strength.

Due to the fact that bone demineralization does not deplete DBM of growth factors, the osteoinductive properties of DBM are superior to cancellous and cortical allograft. In this type of graft, MSC differentiation into osteoblasts is more readily induced, promoting bony healing. Proprietary techniques limit the published details available in regard to the preparation of DBM. The most widely utilized decalcification techniques include a 0.5 molar hydrochloric acid (HCl) wash.[14] Other techniques include acetic, lactic, and nitric acid preparations; however, it has been suggested that these methods yield poorer-quality DBM. In order to maximize DBM–host interaction, Boyce et al recommended demineralization to less than 40% of original levels.[34]

DBM can be supplied in many different forms (gel, putty, flexible strips, paste), both with and without bone chips. The corticocancellous bone chips in this setting allow for an adjunctive load resistance and provide a further osteoconductive and osteoinductive environment. DBM can also be used with locally available autograft obtained during exposure. A systematic review of 12 studies was performed by Zadegan et al in 2016 to examine various outcome measures after the use of DBM, including fusion rates.[41] The authors determined that DBM, alone or in combination with other materials, demonstrated fusion rates of 88.8 to 100%. This rate was lower than autograft at 1 year postoperatively, although this difference was nonsignificant. Due to these results, DBM is most commonly used as a bone graft extender paired with other forms of allograft or a metal cage to offer mechanical strength. However, more high-quality evidence is required to determine the true efficacy of DBM in the setting of cervical spine procedures.

22.5 Bone Graft Substitutes

In the setting of cervical trauma requiring urgent surgical intervention, autograft may not be a viable option if immediate structural stability is desired. Mineralized bone matrices and bone graft substitutes not only lend this property, but also create a biological environment that promotes bone formation.

22.5.1 Ceramic Matrices

Ceramic matrices can be produced as inorganic preparations that include hydroxyapatite (HA) and/or tricalcium phosphate (TCP) to mimic the mineral phase of bone.[42] An advantage of ceramic matrices is the ability to withstand sterilization without losing strength. Ceramics also have extensive osteoconductive properties, with a three-dimensional environment that allows for bony ingrowth. Similar to DBM, ceramics are most often used as graft extenders in combination with local autograft, BMA, and/or interbody cages.

Coralline HA, an alternative HA derived from sea coral, notably marketed as Pro Osteon (Zimmer Biomet, Warsaw, IN), is available in both 50 and 65% porosity. While most investigations cite fusion rates between 70 and 100%, a study by Bruneau et al utilizing HA with plating during ACDF demonstrated fusion in 98% of single-level and 100% of two-level ACDFs.[43] Similarly, a randomized controlled trial (RCT) using Pro Osteon 200 (50% porosity) versus ICBG had promising clinical results, although HA was found to be structurally inferior and associated with collapse or fracture.[44] Surgeons may experience better fusion rates with TCP, as it has the highest compressive strength of the ceramics.[45,46] Biphasic calcium phosphate (BCP) is used as a preparation of 60% HA and 40% TCP. In an RCT, Cho et al compared 60/40 BCP to ICBG in a polyetheretherketone (PEEK) cage and demonstrated 100% fusion in both groups by 6 months.[47]

Primary concerns regarding ceramics involve resorption capacity and mechanical strength. TCP has a calcium-to-phosphate ratio of 1.5 that results in rapid resorption and poor structural support; on the other hand, HA has a calcium-to-phosphate ratio of 1.67 which leads to resorption far too slow for bony remodeling.[48] Thus, pure formations alone are useful for filling voids, although optimal TCP–HA combinations may allow for more versatile use in cervical fusions.

Other ceramics exist without adequate testing in the cervical spine. These include calcium phosphate, currently marketed as OSTEOSET (Wright Medical, Memphis, TN), calcium sulphate, and calcium pyrophosphate.

22.5.2 Growth Factors

As previously mentioned, various mitogenic cytokines lend osteoinductive properties linked to bone growth. BMP is the most widely studied example and its use in cervical fusion is of particular interest. Initially approved for use in the lumbar spine, recombinant human BMP-2 (rhBMP-2) has been used off-label with much success. Baskin et al performed a prospective RCT involving 33 patients comparing rhBMP-2 in an absorbable collagen sponge (ACS) carrier to autologous ICBG. In the study, both grafts were placed in a fibular allograft prior to insertion and both groups had anterior plating.[49] All 33 patients demonstrated fusion by 6 months, but the investigational group had significantly improved arm pain by 24 months. Similar results have also been reported after posterior cervical fusion.[50] Other nonrandomized clinical studies have also reported 100% fusion rates, suggesting the effectiveness of rhBMP-2 in the cervical spine.[51,52,53,54]

Despite these promising results, there are concerns surrounding the use of rhBMP-2 in the cervical spine. A bivariate analysis by Smucker et al suggested a 10-fold increased risk of swelling-related complications when rhBMP-2 was used during ACDF. Although dose-related responses have been attributed to higher complication rates,[49,53] increased dysphagia, incidence of hematomas requiring evacuation, and length of stay in the hospital are complications linked to rhBMP-2.[52,55] Recently, Arnold et al aggregated data from the control arm of two RCTs evaluating cervical disc arthroplasty and compared this to a subanalysis of a third investigational RCT in which patients received rhBMP-2/ACS during ACDF.[56] This investigation clearly delineated that rhBMP-2 successfully induced fusion, but there was also an increased risk of heterotopic ossification when compared to allograft. Additional reports regarding the costs of rhBMP-2 have also been addressed. There have been documented savings in the long term, with the total cost offset by the need for fewer outpatient services and revision procedures.[57,58] However, long-term cost analyses in the setting of cervical procedures have not yet been conducted. Overall, rhBMP-2 has exhibited promising results in the setting of the cervical spine, and its adoption by practitioners must be done with acknowledgment of the potential risk for complications.

Other factors are available to induce bone formation, including PDGF, TGF-β, and BMP-7/osteogenic protein-1 (OP-1). However, data regarding their use in the cervical spine is currently limited.

22.5.3 Other Substitutes

Currently, there are no FDA-approved synthetic bone graft substitutes for use in anterior cervical fusions. However, there is an ongoing FDA trial with an estimated completion date of May 2019 evaluating P-15.[59] This 15 amino acid synthetic polypeptide has been linked to new bone formation by acting as a binding site on a domain of type I collagen. The P-15 bone putty, known as i-FACTOR (Cerapedics Inc., Westminster, CO), is a conglomerate of P-15 and deproteinated HA that has demonstrated 89% fusion rate compared to 85.8% using local autografts.[59] B2A is an additional synthetic polypeptide created to bind host BMP-2 and amplify the response[60]; however, data regarding B2A utilization in the cervical spine is limited.

Polymethylmethacrylate (PMMA) has proven useful throughout the field of orthopaedics and may induce fusion at long-term follow-up. However, limited ossification, graft migration, and poor fusion at short-term follow-up limits its use in cervical fusion procedures.[48,61]

22.6 Harvest Techniques

Under most circumstances, the recipient site should be approached first so that the surgeon is aware of the required graft volume. When preparing the graft site, parallel cavities can be made to accept the graft, but care should be taken with the burr to avoid bony necrosis at the graft site. Graft success depends on graft site preparation and a detailed application of surgical techniques.

Classically, the iliac crest is the most common anatomic site of selection for autograft harvesting. If the patient has a history of pelvic trauma or has been previously subjected to a similar procedure, preoperative imaging is warranted. The iliac crest is palpable and is thickest 5 cm posterior to the anterior superior iliac spine (ASIS). There exists a "safe" zone, roughly 35 mm in length, 10 mm in width, and 30 mm in depth at the iliac tubercle.[62] The ASIS and iliac tubercle should be marked, and a 6 to 8 cm line can be drawn parallel to the crest. Erring 1 to 2 cm medial or lateral to the iliac tubercle allows for avoidance of a scar over the ridge of the crest.

When a full-thickness graft is required, a simple technique involves vertical cuts starting perpendicular to the crest that are then connected.[63] This technique places a major point of weakness at the ilium, risking fracture. This risk can be mitigated by remaining at least 3 cm posterior to the ASIS, as recommended by biomechanical studies.[63,64] Using an oscillating saw, a window can also be created, leaving the edge of the iliac crest intact.[65] Staying at least 2.5 cm posterior to the ASIS also avoids injuring the lateral femoral cutaneous nerve, which usually courses anteriorly along the psoas major.[66]

For cancellous autograft, minimally invasive techniques can be used. Inserting a Meunier trephine between the two tables of the ilium, a fracture can be induced at its base by back-and-forth motion of the hands, releasing the graft into the sleeve of the trephine. A standard graft will include anywhere from 0.6 to 1.2 mL of compact graft. If more is needed, the trephine can be reinserted into the same location and angled 45 degrees anterior or posterior. A second incision will rarely be required. When the graft is retrieved, attention should be paid to the time to graft insertion and graft hydration, and the insertion endplates should come into maximal contact with the graft, avoiding any soft-tissue interposition.[14] Posterior approaches to the iliac crest have also been described and may be more appropriate during posterior lumbar procedures, as the graft may be accessed by the same incision.[32,67]

The Reamer/Irrigator/Aspirator System (RIAS) is another technique that allows the surgeon to accumulate large quantities of cancellous autograft from sites other than the iliac crest. Studies have suggested that femoral canal cancellous autograft may contain higher quantities of growth factors as compared to ICBG.[16] However, this technique is not routinely practiced during cervical spine procedures and is outside the scope of this discussion.

22.7 Conclusions

Osteoconductive, osteoinductive, and osteogenic properties are primarily targeted during graft selection for cervical spine procedures. Autologous bone graft has a long-standing history of success in the cervical spine, and although various donor sites have been suggested, the iliac crest remains the recommended anatomical site. As autologous grafting is not without complications, there has been significant investigation into alternatives that possess similar grafting properties to autograft. Allograft has demonstrated similar osteoconductive and osteoinductive properties, but is nonosteogenic and lends the risk of disease transmission. DBM offers the distinct advantage over other forms of allograft in that it can be provided in various forms and can also be paired with bone graft substitutes. Growth factors, such as rhBMP-2, have also gained significant traction within cervical spine surgery, but concerns still remain regarding its association with complications. Future comparative research, including several pending FDA trials, is necessary to fully elucidate the efficacy of alternative bone grafting materials.

References

[1] Bohlman HH, Emery SE, Goodfellow DB, Jones PK. Robinson anterior cervical discectomy and arthrodesis for cervical radiculopathy. Long-term follow-up of one hundred and twenty-two patients. J Bone Joint Surg Am. 1993; 75(9):1298–1307

[2] Lowery GL, Swank ML, McDonough RF. Surgical revision for failed anterior cervical fusions. Articular pillar plating or anterior revision? Spine. 1995; 20(22):2436–2441

[3] Newman M. The outcome of pseudarthrosis after cervical anterior fusion. Spine. 1993; 18(16):2380–2382

[4] Phillips FM, Carlson G, Emery SE, Bohlman HH. Anterior cervical pseudarthrosis. Natural history and treatment. Spine. 1997; 22(14):1585–1589

[5] Liu X, Min S, Zhang H, Zhou Z, Wang H, Jin A. Anterior corpectomy versus posterior laminoplasty for multilevel cervical myelopathy: a systematic review and meta-analysis. Eur Spine J. 2014; 23(2):362–372

[6] Slizofski WJ, Collier BD, Flatley TJ, Carrera GF, Hellman RS, Isitman AT. Painful pseudarthrosis following lumbar spinal fusion: detection by combined SPECT and planar bone scintigraphy. Skeletal Radiol. 1987; 16(2):136–141

[7] van Eck CF, Regan C, Donaldson WF, Kang JD, Lee JY. The revision rate and occurrence of adjacent segment disease after anterior cervical discectomy and fusion: a study of 672 consecutive patients. Spine. 2014; 39(26): 2143–2147

[8] Whitecloud TS, III. Anterior surgery for cervical spondylotic myelopathy. Smith-Robinson, Cloward, and vertebrectomy. Spine. 1988; 13(7):861–863

[9] MacEwen W. Observation concerning transplantation of bone: illustrated by a case of interhuman osseous transplantation whereby over two thirds of the shaft of a humerus was restored. Proc R Soc Lond. 1881; 32:232–247

[10] Albee FH. Transplantation of portions of the tibia into the spine for Pott's disease: a preliminary report. JAMA. 1911; 57:885

[11] Smith GW, Robinson RA. The treatment of certain cervical-spine disorders by anterior removal of the intervertebral disc and interbody fusion. J Bone Joint Surg Am. 1958; 40-A(3):607–624

[12] Cloward RB. The anterior approach for removal of ruptured cervical disks. J Neurosurg. 1958; 15(6):602–617

[13] Roberts TT, Rosenbaum AJ. Bone grafts, bone substitutes and orthobiologics: the bridge between basic science and clinical advancements in fracture healing. Organogenesis. 2012; 8(4):114–124

[14] Khan SN, Cammisa FP, Jr, Sandhu HS, Diwan AD, Girardi FP, Lane JM. The biology of bone grafting. J Am Acad Orthop Surg. 2005; 13(1):77–86

[15] Pape HC, Evans A, Kobbe P. Autologous bone graft: properties and techniques. J Orthop Trauma. 2010; 24 Suppl 1:S36–S40

[16] Schmidmaier G, Herrmann S, Green J, et al. Quantitative assessment of growth factors in reaming aspirate, iliac crest, and platelet preparation. Bone. 2006; 39(5):1156–1163

[17] Berven S, Tay BK, Kleinstueck FS, Bradford DS. Clinical applications of bone graft substitutes in spine surgery: consideration of mineralized and demineralized preparations and growth factor supplementation. Eur Spine J. 2001; 10 Suppl 2:S169–S177

[18] Burchardt H. The biology of bone graft repair. Clin Orthop Relat Res. 1983 (174):28–42

[19] Giannoudis PV, Dinopoulos H, Tsiridis E. Bone substitutes: an update. Injury. 2005; 36 Suppl 3:S20–S27

[20] Ito Z, Imagama S, Kanemura T, et al. Bone union rate with autologous iliac bone versus local bone graft in posterior lumbar interbody fusion (PLIF): a multicenter study. Eur Spine J. 2013; 22(5):1158–1163

[21] Sengupta DK, Truumees E, Patel CK, et al. Outcome of local bone versus autogenous iliac crest bone graft in the instrumented posterolateral fusion of the lumbar spine. Spine. 2006; 31(9):985–991

[22] Enneking WF, Burchardt H, Puhl JJ, Piotrowski G. Physical and biological aspects of repair in dog cortical-bone transplants. J Bone Joint Surg Am. 1975; 57(2):237–252

[23] Ashton BA, Allen TD, Howlett CR, Eaglesom CC, Hattori A, Owen M. Formation of bone and cartilage by marrow stromal cells in diffusion chambers in vivo. Clin Orthop Relat Res. 1980(151):294–307

[24] Wuisman PI, Jiya TU, Van Dijk M, Sugihara S, Van Royen BJ, Winters HA. Free vascularized bone graft in spinal surgery: indications and outcome in eight cases. Eur Spine J. 1999; 8(4):296–303

[25] Wittenberg RH, Moeller J, Shea M, White AA, III, Hayes WC. Compressive strength of autologous and allogenous bone grafts for thoracolumbar and cervical spine fusion. Spine. 1990; 15(10):1073–1078

[26] Flynn JM. Fracture Repair and Bone Grafting. OKU 10: Orthopaedic Knowledge Update. Rosemont, IL: American Academy of Orthopaedic Surgeons; 2011:11–12

[27] Niu CC, Tsai TT, Fu TS, Lai PL, Chen LH, Chen WJ. A comparison of posterolateral lumbar fusion comparing autograft, autogenous laminectomy bone with bone marrow aspirate, and calcium sulphate with bone marrow aspirate: a prospective randomized study. Spine. 2009; 34(25):2715–2719

[28] Vadalà G, Di Martino A, Tirindelli MC, Denaro L, Denaro V. Use of autologous bone marrow cells concentrate enriched with platelet-rich fibrin on corticocancellous bone allograft for posterolateral multilevel cervical fusion. J Tissue Eng Regen Med. 2008; 2(8):515–520

[29] Feiz-Erfan I, Harrigan M, Sonntag VK, Harrington TR. Effect of autologous platelet gel on early and late graft fusion in anterior cervical spine surgery. J Neurosurg Spine. 2007; 7(5):496–502

[30] Fernyhough JC, Schimandle JJ, Weigel MC, Edwards CC, Levine AM. Chronic donor site pain complicating bone graft harvesting from the posterior iliac crest for spinal fusion. Spine. 1992; 17(12):1474–1480

[31] Betz RR, Lavelle WF, Samdani AF. Bone grafting options in children. Spine. 2010; 35(17):1648–1654

[32] Pirris SM, Nottmeier EW, Kimes S, O'Brien M, Rahmathulla G. A retrospective study of iliac crest bone grafting techniques with allograft reconstruction: do patients even know which iliac crest was harvested? Clinical article. J Neurosurg Spine. 2014; 21(4):595–600

[33] Murphy ME, McCutcheon BA, Grauberger J, et al. Allograft versus autograft in cervical and lumbar spinal fusions: an examination of operative time, length of stay, surgical site infection, and blood transfusions. J Neurosurg Sci. 2016

[34] Boyce T, Edwards J, Scarborough N. Allograft bone. The influence of processing on safety and performance. Orthop Clin North Am. 1999; 30(4):571–581

[35] Hamer AJ, Strachan JR, Black MM, Ibbotson CJ, Stockley I, Elson RA. Biochemical properties of cortical allograft bone using a new method of bone strength measurement. A comparison of fresh, fresh-frozen and irradiated bone. J Bone Joint Surg Br. 1996; 78(3):363–368

[36] Laurencin CT. Musculoskeletal Allograft Tissue Banking and Safety. Bone Graft Substitutes. W. Conshohocken, PA: ASTM International; 2003:30–67

[37] Buck BE, Malinin TI, Brown MD. Bone transplantation and human immunodeficiency virus. An estimate of risk of acquired immunodeficiency syndrome (AIDS). Clin Orthop Relat Res. 1989(240):129–136

[38] Buttermann GR, Glazer PA, Bradford DS. The use of bone allografts in the spine. Clin Orthop Relat Res. 1996(324):75–85

[39] Suchomel P, Barsa P, Buchvald P, Svobodnik A, Vanickova E. Autologous versus allogenic bone grafts in instrumented anterior cervical discectomy and fusion: a prospective study with respect to bone union pattern. Eur Spine J. 2004; 13(6):510–515

[40] Yue WM, Brodner W, Highland TR. Long-term results after anterior cervical discectomy and fusion with allograft and plating: a 5- to 11-year radiologic and clinical follow-up study. Spine. 2005; 30(19):2138–2144

[41] Zadegan SA, Abedi A, Jazayeri SB, Vaccaro AR, Rahimi-Movaghar V. Demineralized bone matrix in anterior cervical discectomy and fusion: a systematic review. Eur Spine J. 2017; 26(4):958–974

[42] Helm GA. Bone graft substitutes for use in spinal fusions. Clin Neurosurg. 2005; 52:250–255

[43] Bruneau M, Nisolle JF, Gilliard C, Gustin T. Anterior cervical interbody fusion with hydroxyapatite graft and plate system. Neurosurg Focus. 2001; 10(4):E8

[44] McConnell JR, Freeman BJ, Debnath UK, Grevitt MP, Prince HG, Webb JK. A prospective randomized comparison of coralline hydroxyapatite with autograft in cervical interbody fusion. Spine. 2003; 28(4):317–323

[45] Sugawara T, Itoh Y, Hirano Y, Higashiyama N, Mizoi K. β-tricalcium phosphate promotes bony fusion after anterior cervical discectomy and fusion using titanium cages. Spine. 2011; 36(23):E1509–E1514

[46] Dai LY, Jiang LS. Anterior cervical fusion with interbody cage containing beta-tricalcium phosphate augmented with plate fixation: a prospective randomized study with 2-year follow-up. Eur Spine J. 2008; 17(5):698–705

[47] Cho DY, Lee WY, Sheu PC, Chen CC. Cage containing a biphasic calcium phosphate ceramic (Triosite) for the treatment of cervical spondylosis. Surg Neurol. 2005; 63(6):497–503, discussion 503–504

[48] Chau AM, Mobbs RJ. Bone graft substitutes in anterior cervical discectomy and fusion. Eur Spine J. 2009; 18(4):449–464

[49] Baskin DS, Ryan P, Sonntag V, Westmark R, Widmayer MA. A prospective, randomized, controlled cervical fusion study using recombinant human bone morphogenetic protein-2 with the CORNERSTONE-SR allograft ring and the ATLANTIS anterior cervical plate. Spine. 2003; 28(12):1219–1224, discussion 1225

[50] Yan L, Chang Z, He B, et al. Efficacy of rhBMP-2 versus iliac crest bone graft for posterior C1-C2 fusion in patients older than 60 years. Orthopedics. 2014; 37(1):e51–e57

[51] Tumialán LM, Pan J, Rodts GE, Mummaneni PV. The safety and efficacy of anterior cervical discectomy and fusion with polyetheretherketone spacer and recombinant human bone morphogenetic protein-2: a review of 200 patients. J Neurosurg Spine. 2008; 8(6):529–535

[52] Vaidya R, Carp J, Sethi A, Bartol S, Craig J, Les CM. Complications of anterior cervical discectomy and fusion using recombinant human bone morphogenetic protein-2. Eur Spine J. 2007; 16(8):1257–1265

[53] Shields LB, Raque GH, Glassman SD, et al. Adverse effects associated with high-dose recombinant human bone morphogenetic protein-2 use in anterior cervical spine fusion. Spine. 2006; 31(5):542–547

[54] Boakye M, Mummaneni PV, Garrett M, Rodts G, Haid R. Anterior cervical discectomy and fusion involving a polyetheretherketone spacer and bone morphogenetic protein. J Neurosurg Spine. 2005; 2(5):521–525

[55] Buttermann GR. Prospective nonrandomized comparison of an allograft with bone morphogenic protein versus an iliac-crest autograft in anterior cervical discectomy and fusion. Spine J. 2008; 8(3):426–435

[56] Arnold PM, Anderson KK, Selim A, Dryer RF, Kenneth Burkus J. Heterotopic ossification following single-level anterior cervical discectomy and fusion: results from the prospective, multicenter, historically controlled trial comparing allograft to an optimized dose of rhBMP-2. J Neurosurg Spine. 2016; 25(3):292–302

[57] Carreon LY, Glassman SD, Djurasovic M, et al. RhBMP-2 versus iliac crest bone graft for lumbar spine fusion in patients over 60 years of age: a cost-utility study. Spine. 2009; 34(3):238–243

[58] Ackerman SJ, Mafilios MS, Polly DW, Jr. Economic evaluation of bone morphogenetic protein versus autogenous iliac crest bone graft in single-level anterior lumbar fusion: an evidence-based modeling approach. Spine. 2002; 27(16) Suppl 1:S94–S99

[59] Arnold PM, Sasso RC, Janssen ME, et al. Efficacy of i-Factor bone graft versus autograft in anterior cervical discectomy and fusion: results of the prospective, randomized, single-blinded Food and Drug Administration Investigational Device Exemption Study. Spine. 2016; 41(13):1075–1083

[60] Sardar Z, Alexander D, Oxner W, et al. Twelve-month results of a multicenter, blinded, pilot study of a novel peptide (B2A) in promoting lumbar spine fusion. J Neurosurg Spine. 2015; 22(4):358–366

[61] Bärlocher CB, Barth A, Krauss JK, Binggeli R, Seiler RW. Comparative evaluation of microdiscectomy only, autograft fusion, polymethylmethacrylate interposition, and threaded titanium cage fusion for treatment of single-level cervical disc disease: a prospective randomized study in 125 patients. Neurosurg Focus. 2002; 12(1):E4

[62] Missiuna PC, Gandhi HS, Farrokhyar F, Harnett BE, Dore EM, Roberts B. Anatomically safe and minimally invasive transcrestal technique for procurement

of autogenous cancellous bone graft from the mid-iliac crest. Can J Surg. 2011; 54(5):327–332

[63] Hu RW, Bohlman HH. Fracture at the iliac bone graft harvest site after fusion of the spine. Clin Orthop Relat Res. 1994(309):208–213

[64] Varga E, Hu R, Hearn TC, Woodside T, Yang JP. Biomechanical analysis of hemipelvic deformation after corticospongious bone graft harvest from the posterior iliac crest. Spine. 1996; 21(13):1494–1499

[65] Behairy YM, Al-Sebai W. A modified technique for harvesting full-thickness iliac crest bone graft. Spine. 2001; 26(6):695–697

[66] Murata Y, Takahashi K, Yamagata M, Shimada Y, Moriya H. The anatomy of the lateral femoral cutaneous nerve, with special reference to the harvesting of iliac bone graft. J Bone Joint Surg Am. 2000; 82(5):746–747

[67] Merritt AL, Spinnicke A, Pettigrew K, Alamin TF. Gluteal-sparing approach for posterior iliac crest bone graft: description of a new technique and assessment of morbidity in ninety-two patients after spinal fusion. Spine. 2010; 35(14):1396–1400

23 Nonoperative Management and Treatment of Cervical Spine Injuries

Jacob Hoffman and Mark L. Prasarn

Abstract

Nonoperative treatment modalities are essential in the management of both bony and ligamentous cervical spine injuries following trauma, and are incorporated into the initial and, oftentimes, definitive treatment regimen for these patients. Adequate evaluation and immobilization of the cervical spine at the scene followed by a thorough physical examination, assessment of spinal stability, and completion of an imaging work-up at the hospital is crucial. It is also important to minimize motion of the cervical spine as well as to prevent further neurological deterioration via restoration of its natural anatomic alignment. This may be accomplished via closed reduction techniques in select patients. Nonoperative modalities can be used for definitive treatment in many cases, thereby achieving excellent functional outcomes.

Keywords: nonoperative treatment, cervical spine, trauma, ligamentous injury, immobilization, spinal stabilization, decompression

23.1 Introduction

Cervical spine trauma encompasses a broad range of injuries ranging from mild ligamentous injury to fracture-dislocations with catastrophic spinal cord injury. Nonoperative modalities have remained essential in the initial and, oftentimes, definitive care for most injuries. The majority of cervical spine fractures and stable ligamentous injuries can be treated with nonoperative means while avoiding the inherent risks of surgical intervention. After appropriate examination, diagnosis, and patient discussion, a good functional outcome without long-term disability can be anticipated with nonoperative management in most cases.

Beginning at the scene of the trauma through the definitive intervention, nonoperative treatment modalities are used in all cases. Patients should be immobilized, quickly evaluated, and treated definitively (if indicated). Strict adherence to proper immobilization techniques are followed to minimize motion of the injured cervical spine and prevent catastrophic neurological injury. All injuries should be assumed to be unstable until proven otherwise.

Definitive treatment goals are the same for nonoperative management as for operative intervention. These include (1) preservation of neurological function, (2) improvement in neurological deficit if already present, (3) reduction of spinal deformity and maintenance of acceptable alignment, (4) minimization of loss of spinal mobility, (5) achievement of a healed and stable spinal column, and (6) prevention of long-term pain and disability.

23.2 At the Scene

In acute trauma cases, Advanced Trauma Life Support (ATLS) protocol mandates life-threatening injuries take priority in treatment. Compromise to airway, respiration, and circulation should be promptly addressed. The greatest risk of spinal cord injury occurs at the time of high-energy impact. However, neurological deficits can develop at any point during the initial treatment period. Up to 25% of spinal cord injuries occur after a patient has been assumed under medical care.[1] It is paramount that first responders work quickly to immobilize the cervical spine to prevent neurological decline.

The care of spine trauma patients at the scene has dramatically improved over the past several decades; extraction, immobilization, and transport of trauma patients in adherence with ATLS protocols for resuscitation have been credited. ATLS protocol instructs medical personnel to assume that spinal injury has occurred in all trauma patients. At the scene, the patient should be placed immediately into a cervical collar, head immobilization device, and spine backboard.

In athletes with suspected cervical spine injuries, health care providers are presented with unique challenges that are not present within the general population. Equipment worn for personal protection is an obstacle for medical personnel to gain access to the airway, neck, and chest. In 2015, the National Athletic Trainers Association updated their executive summary of acute spinal injury treatment.[2] In their recommendations, equipment can be removed by the highest-level trained personnel prior to transfer to the hospital, if this is deemed appropriate. It is also an option to leave everything but the facemask in place until arrival at the emergency room. The injured athlete should then be placed into a rigid cervical stabilization device and placed onto a spinal backboard.

23.3 At the Hospital

The patient should arrive in the emergency department on a backboard with a cervical collar in place. In the face of global instability, motion can still occur in spite of all attempts at rigid collar immobilization. The patient should be moved on and off the backboard as few times as possible until the stability of the spine can be adequately assessed. For most injuries, the collar provides an increased level of stability, although it does not provide complete immobilization.[3] With complete ligamentous disruption, the collar has minimal effect on providing restriction to cervical movement. Manual stabilization of the spine is much more significant in restricting motion.[4]

During the primary and secondary surveys, clinicians must maintain a high index of suspicion for cervical spine injury. Any trauma patient with head or maxillofacial injuries should be presumed to have a cervical spine injury. Common causes of missed cervical spine injuries include the polytrauma patient, altered mental status due to intoxication or traumatic brain injury, or a noncontiguous spinal injury.[5,6] Many patients with cervical spine trauma require rapid sequence intubation due to other significant injuries. Often intubation and placing the patient on mechanical ventilation occurs prior to the secondary survey and imaging. In a study comparing four various intubation techniques, use of the Lightwand (Aaron Medical, St. Petersburgh, FL) showed the least amount of cervical motion while the commonly used Macintosh blade showed the greatest.[7] Using a technique that produces less motion may lessen the risk of secondary neurological injury during airway management.

Distracting injuries in the polytrauma patient can often mask the presence of a significant spine injury. Trauma patients with facial trauma or closed head injuries should raise suspicion for associated cervical trauma. Meticulous examination of the spine must always be performed including inspecting the patient's cervical posture. Any gross malalignment in angulation or rotation might suggest dislocation or subluxation. The physician should palpate the posterior cervical spine noting for step-offs between spinous processes or pain out of proportion in the awake patient. A meticulous neurological examination of the patient is performed during the secondary survey. The exam is carefully documented according to American Spinal Injury Association (ASIA) guidelines. Throughout the hospitalization, the patient should undergo serial examinations. If possible, the examinations should be performed by members of the same team of providers who are familiar with the patient's previous exam. In spinal shock, distal motor function cannot be fully assessed until the bulbocavernosus reflex returns.

Once the patient has been deemed hemodynamically stable to receive a computed tomography (CT) scan, a coordinated effort should be made to move the patient off the backboard. A full trauma scan including imaging of the brain, face, spine, chest, abdomen, and pelvis should be obtained in one trip to the scanner, with one movement off and on the triage bed. The entire axis of the spine should be carefully reviewed for noncontiguous fractures. In blunt trauma and in the presence of a spine fracture, there is a 19% incidence of noncontinuous spine injuries.[5]

The risk of decubitus ulceration is directly proportional to the length of time on a backboard—8 hours on a backboard is associated with a 100% likelihood of a decubitus ulcer.[8] The patient should be moved from the board as soon as possible. Appropriate spine immobilization must be continued while removing the patient from a spinal board.

Contrary to all available evidence suggesting that the log roll is an ineffective and potentially dangerous technique for spine immobilization, it is still universally used. In fact, studies conducted prior to 2004 showed dramatic and unacceptable motion with a log roll.[8] Recently, many studies have reevaluated this controversial practice. Compared with any other method of transfer, the log roll maneuver has been shown to cause more segmental motion at the level of the unstable, injured segment.[3,9,10,11,12,13,14,15,16,17] Lift and slide techniques are superior as they tend to create less motion at the injured segment.[13]

23.4 Imaging Studies

All traumatically injured patients with suspected spinal injuries should have the entire spinal axis imaged and carefully reviewed. In the absence of a facet dislocation and in the presence of significant spine injury, the appropriateness of a magnetic resonance imaging (MRI) scan must be determined. The spinal motion needed to transfer the patient on and off the MRI

table must be kept in mind when deciding on the necessity of this imaging modality. The strongest argument for an MRI is a suspected neurological deficit that is not explained by the injury seen on a CT scan. The other indication for MRI is to evaluate the posterior ligamentous complex which is felt to be critical for stability of the spinal column. If the patient has an unstable injury which requires surgery (and has been identified clinically or by other imaging studies), it is not necessary to obtain an MRI just to assess the dorsal ligamentous complex.

Specific injury mechanisms and fracture patterns should prompt the treating team to search for commonly associated nonspinal injuries. In many instances, the definitive treatment of cervical spine fractures may be delayed due to the life-threatening condition present in these acutely injured patients. In addition, the mechanism of injury is useful for identifying patients at risk for other injuries, and clinicians must not become solely preoccupied with cervical pathology. In a retrospective review of 492 cervical spine CT scans with spinal traumatic pathology, 60% of patients had injury to an additional anatomic region or organ system.[5]

23.5 Closed Reduction of the Cervical Spine

After appropriate imaging and medical stabilization has occurred, patients with cervical facet subluxations or dislocations or burst-type fractures may undergo closed reduction with the use of skeletal skull traction. The reduction achieved by this means allows for realignment and stabilization in the acute phase of treatment. Contraindications to skeletal skull traction include distractive cervical injuries, patients with certain skull fractures, and stable fracture patterns.[18,19]

When a closed reduction of a dislocated segment is needed, it should be performed expediently in the awake and alert patient. Serial neurological examinations should be performed during any reduction maneuvers. If the patient is obtunded or intoxicated and reliable neurological examinations are impossible, then an emergent MRI should be obtained prior to attempting reduction to rule out significant disc herniation.[20] Closed reduction provides a rapid means of reducing cervical spine deformity, indirectly decompressing the neural elements and providing stability. It has been shown to be safe and can dramatically improve neurological status if performed within the first few hours following the injury. In an animal model, it was shown that decompression within 3 hours showed better and quicker neurological recovery.[21] A small series of patients with no cord function who received reduction in an emergent manner immediately began to recover.[22] Therefore, a closed reduction should be performed as early as possible in the stable patient who is able to give a reliable neurological exam. In the medically compromised patient, the priority is to achieve hemodynamic stability prior to performing urgent reduction or obtaining an MRI.

There remains controversy surrounding MRI in patients with acute cervical spine dislocations, prior to reduction. Advocates of a prereduction MRI consider the potential for displacement of an unrecognized disc herniation or other space-occupying lesion an undue risk for the patient. Eismont et al reported on a series of six patients who roentgenographically demonstrated herniation of an intervertebral disc with marked protrusion of disc material into the spinal canal following subluxation or dislocation of a cervical facet. For the first patient in this series, no myelogram or CT scan was performed, and the patient awoke with complete quadriplegia following dorsal open reduction and internal fixation under general anesthesia. Following a myelogram and ventral decompression surgery, the cause was identified as an extruded intervertebral disc. The authors recommended obtaining an MRI in all patients prior to attempting closed reduction and definitive surgery.[23,24,25] Several other cases with neurological deficits after open reduction under general anesthesia have been reported.[23,25] There have also been reports of progression of neurological deficits during traction while the patient was awake, which later resolved.[26] Some surgeons recommend decompression and open reduction should there be a disc herniation on imaging.

A prereduction MRI may result in a large number of patients undergoing surgical decompression, open reduction, and stabilization prior to manipulative reduction in the emergency department. Some have advocated performing immediate closed reduction in the patient who is awake and can reliably participate in serial neurological examinations. In a study of 11 patients who underwent MRI before and after awake closed reduction, Vaccaro et al reported that no patients had neurological decline during reduction despite a prevalence of disc herniation prior (18%) and after (56%) manipulation.[20] Darsaut et al attempted to determine the effect of disc herniation during closed reduction in a series of 17 patients who had a cervical dislocation that was reduced under MRI monitoring. They demonstrated that this technique could be used successfully as a research tool.[27]

A commonly used algorithm is based on the patient's neurological status. If the patient is unable to participate reliably in the physical examination, then an MRI is obtained as expeditiously as possible. The principal disadvantage of obtaining an MRI is the loss of potentially vital time to neural canal decompression. It has been shown that neurological recovery after injury is directly related to the duration of external compression on the spinal cord.[28] If the patient has a significant spinal cord injury, the risk is that the cord will remain compressed for a longer period of time. If the patient has an ASIA A, B, or C injury and is able to cooperate with the reduction and serial neurological examinations, strong consideration should be given to an immediate, rapid reduction. In this situation, the MRI would be obtained after reduction. In the setting of an obtunded patient without an accurate exam, an emergent MRI should be obtained prior to attempting any reduction maneuver. Should there be a herniated disc present, an anterior decompression is recommended prior to reduction and stabilization. ▶ Fig. 23.1 reviews the decision tree regarding patients with acute subaxial cervical subluxations and dislocations.

23.6 Reduction Techniques

As early as the 4th century BC, reduction maneuvers have been attempted to correct spinal deformity.[29] The goal of reduction is to reestablish the anatomic alignment of the cervical spinal axis in a graded, controlled manner. Restoration of alignment indi-

rectly decompresses the canal and if completed rapidly, may prevent progression of neurological injury. Gardner–Wells tongs are applied with the pins placed 1 cm above the pinna of the ear just below the equator of the head. By placing the pins at this site, the distractive force of the Gardner–Wells tongs will parallel the longitudinal axis of the cervical spine. A flexion moment can be obtained with a posterior placement of pins while anterior placement causes an extension moment. Pins are tightened to 3.6 kg of pressure. While tightening, a precalibrated indicator on the pin protrudes a measured amount once the correct torque is obtained.

It is recommended that the initial applied weight be no more than 4.5 kg. Using more weight can be catastrophic if the patient has unrecognized ligamentous instability. After every application of increased weight, a neurological examination and lateral radiograph should be obtained. The radiographs should be scrutinized to ensure that a distraction-type injury is not present that might be worsened by the traction. Additional weight should be added incrementally until reduction is obtained. Once reduction is achieved, the weight should be decreased to the minimum amount needed to maintain the reduction. Routine examinations are continued and definitive stabilization can occur once medically appropriate. Pulmonary and skin issues can be addressed with use of a kinetic treatment bed until surgery. If reduction cannot be obtained, then an MRI should be obtained and the patient should be taken for urgent open reduction in the operating theatre.

If the patient has a sudden decline in neurological status during a closed reduction attempt, it may be due to a variety of causes such as displacement of herniated disc, hemorrhage or edema within the parenchyma of the neural elements, vascular injury to the spinal cord, and/or hemorrhage into the epidural, subdural, or subarachnoid spaces. Caution should be used in patients with ossified posterior longitudinal ligaments (OPLL), as a segment of the OPLL may displace and cause increased stenosis after reduction.[26] If an alert, cooperative patient experiences a decline in neurological status during attempted closed reduction, immediate reversal of the reduction maneuver sequence must be performed. The patient should be reexamined and then an emergent MRI should be performed. The patient can be taken to the operation theatre for decompression, reduction, and stabilization if a space-occupying lesion is identified and is causing cord compression.[6,26]

Gardner–Wells tongs are used due to the high pull-out strength of the construct when steel pins are used.[30] If using weights over 25 kg, MRI-compatible tongs with titanium pins are insufficient. Weights of over 60 kg have been used safely for closed reduction when stainless steel pins are used.[26] The use of a halo may be considered since it provides four titanium pins to distribute the forces over more pins. The major disadvantage of stainless steel pins is their MRI incompatibility. A potential reason stainless steel pins may fail is due to an underlying skull fracture.[30] Potential complications with the use of skeletal skull traction include cranial perforation, dislodgement, pin site infection, propagation of an unrecognized skull fracture, or superficial temporal artery laceration.[19,31,32,33] Complications with prolonged immobilization can also occur including cervical pressure ulcers, pneumonia, and venous thromboembolic events.[19] The patient should be taken expediently for definitive stabilization as physiological status allows to avoid these complications (▶ Fig. 23.2).

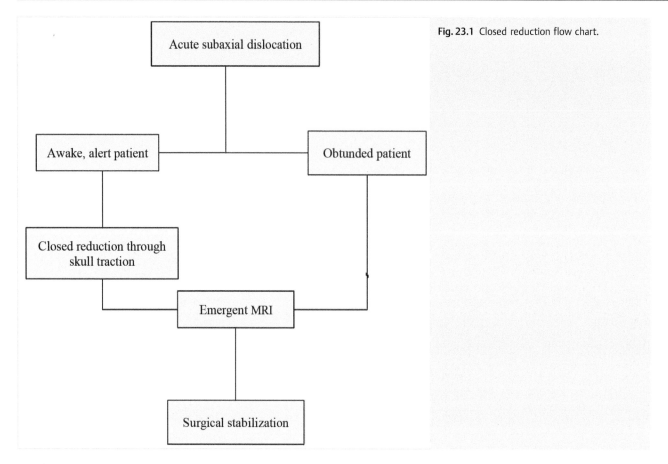

Fig. 23.1 Closed reduction flow chart.

23.7 Definitive Treatment

The majority of cervical spine injuries should be treated nonoperatively. When making the decision for nonoperative management, surgeons must survey the entire clinical picture. Surgical intervention may be indicated in the setting of progressive neurological deficit or any injury deemed to be unstable. As it is thought that the posterior ligamentous complex is the key to stability, ligamentous injuries in those who are skeletally mature require spinal fusion to maintain stability. The presence of a neurological injury is not an absolute indication for surgery.

The remaining spectrum of cervical spinal injuries can initially be treated with nonoperative management. A variety of closed treatment options can be used including bedrest, long-term skeletal traction, halo apparatus, external orthosis, or casting. Many significant fractures can be treated with an initial period of bedrest in a kinetic treatment bed followed by bracing and mobilization once early healing has been achieved. The absence of significant pain should be the clinical indicator of the patient's readiness to be cleared from the kinetic treatment bed and mobilized. Upright films in the external orthosis should be obtained to confirm that the spinal column is stable under physiological loads.

23.8 Timing of Surgical Intervention

Debate continues over the appropriate timing of traction or surgery in cases of acute spinal cord injury. Although early surgical intervention has been shown to prevent complications associated with prolonged bedrest, there has not been great historical

evidence that it will improve neurological function.[34,35,36,37] Complete cord injuries and neurologically intact patients are very likely to remain neurologically unchanged with appropriate surgical or nonoperative care. Incomplete lesions typically improve with either surgical or nonsurgical care. Late surgery with decompression of the cervical spinal canal in incomplete cord injuries has been shown to improve neurological function even several years following the traumatic event.[38] In the acute setting, there has been sparse evidence supporting early surgery, although the Surgical Timing in Acute Spinal Cord Injury Study (STASCIS) demonstrated that those undergoing cervical decompression within 24 hours showed a 2.8 times greater likelihood of a 2 grade AIS improvement as compared to those having late decompression.[39]

23.9 Upper Cervical Injuries

Upper cervical fractures or discoligamentous injuries can be potentially devastating with high mortality rates and poor long-term functional outcomes. With the aging population, there has been an increase in upper cervical fractures and ligamentous injuries. Low-energy falls coupled with poor bone quality due to osteopenia can lead to significant C1 and C2 fractures. Elderly patients with neurological deficits have poor survival rates compared to younger cohorts.[40]

Ligamentous injury to the craniocervical junction can lead to occipitocervical dissociation. Occipitocervical injuries are associated with high-energy trauma and are often found postmortem.[41] Atlanto-occipital dislocations can oftentimes be difficult to diagnose. However, early, routine use of CT scans has

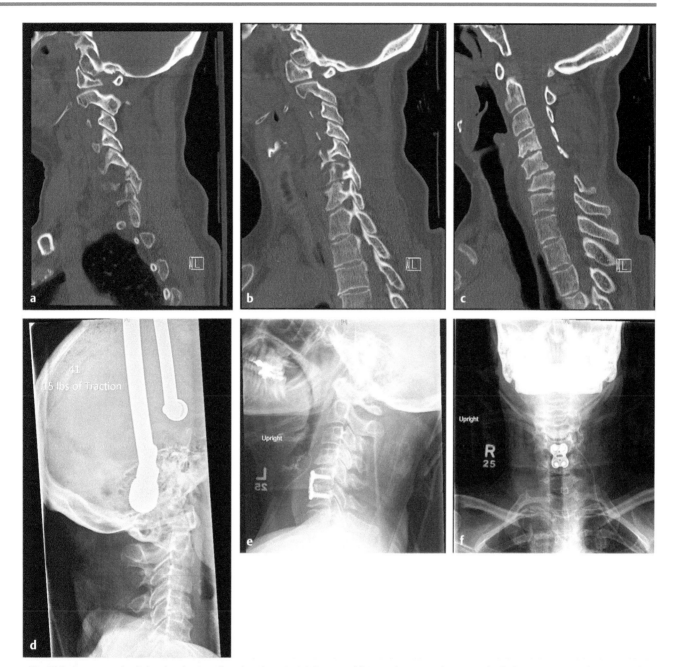

Fig. 23.2 Case example of closed reduction of a subaxial cervical dislocation. (**a**) Sagittal computed tomography (CT) reconstruction showing a right sided C5–C6 facet dislocation and a perched facet on the left (**b**) with significant kyphosis at C5–C6 (**c**). Patient presented awake, alert, and neurologically intact and therefore underwent urgent closed reduction with Gardner–Wells tong skull traction up to 45 lb (**d**). The weight was reduced to 15 lb and then the patient was taken for C5–C6 anterior decompression and fusion without complication (**e**) and (**f**).

improved diagnosis.[42] When encountering this injury, the treating physician must be vigilant about making the diagnosis to ensure the patient's survival and prevent catastrophic neurological deterioration. At the scene, these patients should be carefully immobilized on a backboard with a rigid collar. For additional stabilization, the head is secured with sandbags and tape. At the earliest possible moment after initial work-up, a halo vest is applied until definitive surgical stabilization is performed. Any form of traction for type II injuries (axial distraction) can be catastrophic and is strictly contraindicated. If diagnosis is made early, these injuries can be successfully treated with dorsal occipital cervical fusion with at least

3 months of halo vest immobilization.[42,43,44] However, there still remains a paucity of literature, mostly including case reports, on which dislocations can be treated nonoperatively.[45]

Fractures of the occipital condyle and C1 are often treated nonoperatively. In 1988, Anderson and Montessano proposed the most widely used classification system of occipital condyle fractures based on fracture morphology.[46] Type I fractures are nondisplaced, comminuted variants. Type II fractures involved a basilar skull fracture with extension into the occipital condyle. Type III fractures are produced from a rotational force causing an alar ligament tensional avulsion. Tuli et al[47] proposed an additional classification system based on stability. Isolated type

I fractures are considered stable and can be treated without immobilization. Type IIA fractures are stable fractures without ligamentous disruption and require a rigid collar. Demonstration of significant instability on imaging or ligamentous disruption on MRI (Type IIB) invokes the need for surgical stabilization. Good outcomes have been shown with initial management of occipital condyle fractures treated with nonoperative modalities even in cases of neurological injury.[48,49,50]

An axial force transmitted through the cranium onto the atlas causes a compressive force leading to a burst or Jefferson fracture of C1. Most fractures are considered stable and are treated in a cervical collar.[51] Unstable atlas ring fractures (> 7 mm overhang of the sum total of the lateral masses) indicate ligamentous disruption of the transverse ligament and typically require surgical stabilization.[52]

Odontoid fractures are the most common C2 fractures. They are classified based on the anatomic location and degree of displacement of the fracture. Many can be treated with a rigid orthosis or halo vest. Anderson and D'Alonzo[53] type I avulsion injuries are rare and can be treated with either a soft or rigid collar. Fractures through the body of the atlas (type III) typically heal uneventfully and have a good prognosis without surgery. Transverse type II fractures through the waist of the odontoid have much controversy regarding their treatment due to a high associated nonunion rate. A dorsally displaced odontoid fracture is more likely to be treated with surgery.[54,55,56,57,58] Polin reported on a series of 36 patients with type II odontoid fractures treated with a rigid collar versus a halo. They showed no difference in outcomes when either modality was used.[58] Previous studies have shown nonunion rates ranging from 54 to 75% when treated in either a halo vest or a rigid collar.[59,60,61,62] A posteriorly displaced fracture in patients > 65 years old is at high risk of nonunion.[60,63] Elderly patients treated in a halo vest have a high morbidity and mortality rate.[64] The clinical relevance of nonunion in elderly patient continues to be debated. Some authors report that these can be followed and may not require surgical intervention. In a series of persistent nonunions, no progression of atlantoaxial instability or neurological deterioration, including myelopathic symptoms during the follow-up period, was noted.[59] Contrary to this, Kepler et al showed a 17% incidence of new neurological deficits in a similar cohort.[65] Definitive treatment is individually based and involves shared decision-making by the patient and family.

Transverse ligament ruptures can be managed in an orthosis or halo if a bony avulsion occurs.[66,67] Nonoperative management avoids the significant loss of motion following a C1–C2 arthrodesis. If there is a complete ligamentous disruption, Dickman et al demonstrated a 100% failure to heal. These injuries often result in a significant incidence of neurological injury, and there is frequent association with other upper cervical injuries. Atlantoaxial arthrodesis is indicated in complete ligamentous disruption without bony avulsion in either neurologically compromised or intact patients.[68]

The vast majority of other axis injuries can be stabilized with an orthosis or a halo vest. Most C2 body fractures are considered stable and can be treated with a collar.[69] Traumatic spondylolisthesis of the axis most commonly occurs secondary to a hyperextension and axial load mechanism. Neurological deficit rarely occurs. The exception is for the atypical fracture that occurs ventral to the dorsal vertebral body cortex.[70] These atypical fractures may require surgery to prevent neurological decline. Severe hangman's fractures with instability through the C2–C3 disc space require surgery. Most other axis injuries can be managed successfully nonoperatively.[52,69,70,71,72,73,74] In a retrospective review of 41 patients with hangman's fractures, 11 (27%) patients were treated with a cervical collar, 27 (66%) were treated in a halo, and 3 (7%) were treated with surgical intervention. Of the surgical patients, one had an atypical fracture that failed halo immobilization and the two others had associated cervical fractures. All patients achieved union at 4 to 6 week follow-up (▶ Fig. 23.3).[75]

23.10 Subaxial Injuries

Subaxial cervical spine is a common location of injury due to the substantial amount of motion present in this region. Injuries to the subaxial spine encompass a wide spectrum of conditions varying from isolated spinal process fractures to facet fracture dislocations. If not properly diagnosed, subaxial injuries can lead to devastating outcomes including loss of function, neurological injury, and long-term disability. Isolated, minimally displaced, subaxial lamina, transverse process, and spinous process fractures can be treated with a cervical collar. Compression fractures of a single level can be treated nonoperatively, if intact ligaments are present. In addition, injuries due to a flexion-compression mechanism with intact dorsal ligaments are treated with a cervical orthosis.

Burst fractures result from an axial load leading to a compressive force with disruption of both the anterior and posterior elements of the vertebral body. Oftentimes, there is retropulsion of fracture fragments resulting in neurological injury. One classification system that surgeons may use to help determine whether these fractures can be treated nonoperatively is the Subaxial Injury Classification (SLIC) system.[76] The composite score is determined by summing scores from each category —injury morphology, neurological status, and injury to the posterior ligamentous complex. A score of 3 or less can be treated conservatively versus scores greater than 5 that are treated surgically (▶ Table 23.1). In an evaluation of the SLIC system, scores of 4 were treated nonoperatively in 65% of cases.[77] In the setting of cord compression with neurological injury from retropulsed bone fragments, the patient should undergo urgent ventral decompression and stabilization. Injuries that may be classified as a SLIC 4, or are otherwise indeterminate, require continued investigation to guide treatment.

Flexion-distraction injuries often lead to facet fractures, subluxations, or dislocations. Subaxial facet fracture dislocations result from high-energy trauma. As previously discussed, nonoperative treatment consists of awake closed reduction in the emergency department after appropriate patient selection. If a reduction fails, or in cases involving a displaced disc without a reliable neurological exam, the patient should be taken urgently for decompression and stabilization. After closed reduction, surgical stabilization is usually necessary because up to 40% of cases remain unstable even after 3 months of halo immobilization.[78,79] In addition, there can be significant associated morbidity and even mortality with the use of halos.[64,80]

In elderly patients, after falls without obvious injury on imaging, physicians should closely evaluate for central cord syndrome. A hyperextension moment in the setting of spondylosis and

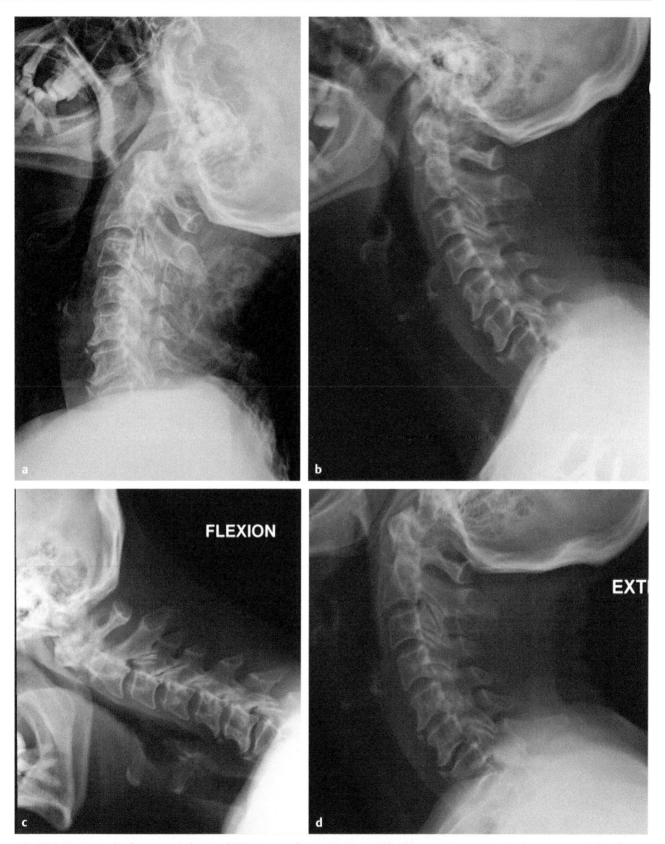

FLEXION

EXT

Fig. 23.3 Case example of nonoperatively treated C2 hangman's fracture. A 67-year-old polytrauma victim was involved in a motor vehicle collision and sustained a C2 hangman's fracture and C6 transverse process fracture. (a) The patient was treated nonoperatively in a cervical collar. At the 3-month follow-up lateral (b), flexion (c), and extension (d) views show complete fracture healing and a stable cervical spine. The patient remained neurologically intact throughout treatment and was asymptomatic at their 3-month follow-up visit.

Table 23.1 Subaxial Cervical Spine Injury Classification (SLIC)

Fracture morphology	Score
None	0
Compression	1
Burst	2
Distraction	3
Rotation/translation	4
Discoligamentous complex	
None	0
Indeterminate	2
Disrupted	3
Neurologic function	
Intact	0
Root injury	1
Complete cord injury	2
Incomplete cord injury	3
Ongoing compression with deficits	+ 1
Total[a]	

[a]Nonoperative management is recommended for a total score of ≤ 3. A score of 4 can be treated with either surgical or nonoperative management as indicated. A score of ≥ 5 indicates surgical intervention.

Table 23.2 Treatment options for cervical injuries

Cervical injuries	Observation	Collar	Halo	Surgery
Atlanto-occipital dissociation				√
Jefferson fracture—stable		√	√	
Jefferson fracture—unstable			√	√
Axis body fracture		√	√	
Type I odontoid fracture	√	√		
Type II odontoid fracture		√	√	√
Type III odontoid fracture		√	√	
Unilateral facet dislocation				√
Bilateral facet dislocation				√
Subaxial compression fracture		√	√	
Unilateral facet fracture		√	√	√
Spinous process fracture	√	√		

stenosis acutely narrows the spinal canal and can cause neural compression at the time of impact. Instability may not be present after injury. In patients with severe spondylosis and stenosis, central cord syndrome may rapidly develop into a high-grade spinal cord injury.[81] These patients should undergo prompt decompression and possibly stabilization. In the acute setting, a collar can be placed for comfort. ▶ Table 23.2 summarizes the current treatment options for cervical fractures.[82]

23.11 Keys to Nonoperative Care

The cervical spine must be accurately assessed at the initial encounter. Continuous reassessment should be performed to ensure the accurate determination of spinal stability. Stability is reevaluated when the patient is mobilized and examined upright. Upright radiographs in the orthosis or definitive method of treatment provide another chance to determine the level of stability and effectiveness of treatment. Mehta et al reported that in 25% of patients with thoracolumbar fractures, the upright radiographs resulted in a change in treatment.[83] Humphry et al reported on four patients with cervical instability which was confirmed on erect radiographs, despite negative CT and MR images.[84]

In cervical injuries, imaging studies must be scrutinized for any subluxation to determine if any ligamentous or facet instability was not previously appreciated. Kyphosis alone does not necessarily mean dorsal ligamentous disruption. It must be determined whether the kyphosis is a result of ventral column collapse or dorsal column distraction. One of the most effective ways to determine the significance of a dorsal ligamentous injury is to simply palpate the spinous processes. MRI is often used to evaluate these structures as well.

The original upright radiograph is then used to measure for progressive kyphosis, listhesis, or further height loss. Keep in mind that increased kyphosis from the original supine film on a backboard may not be meaningful since normal individuals show more kyphosis when standing in the absence of spinal injury.

References

[1] Podolsky S, Baraff LJ, Simon RR, Hoffman JR, Larmon B, Ablon W. Efficacy of cervical spine immobilization methods. J Trauma. 1983; 23(6):461–465

[2] Trainers NA. Appropriate care of the spine injured athlete. Updated from 1998 document. 2015. http://www.nata.org/sites/default/files/Executive-Summary-Spine-Injury.pdf

[3] Prasarn ML, Horodyski M, Dubose D, et al. Total motion generated in the unstable cervical spine during management of the typical trauma patient: a comparison of methods in a cadaver model. Spine. 2012; 37(11):937–942

[4] Del Rossi G, Heffernan TP, Horodyski M, Rechtine GR. The effectiveness of extrication collars tested during the execution of spine-board transfer techniques. Spine J. 2004; 4(6):619–623

[5] Nelson DW, Martin MJ, Martin ND, Beekley A. Evaluation of the risk of noncontiguous fractures of the spine in blunt trauma. J Trauma Acute Care Surg. 2013; 75(1):135–139

[6] Rizzolo SJ, Vaccaro AR, Cotler JM. Cervical spine trauma. Spine. 1994; 19(20):2288–2298

[7] Wendling AL, Tighe PJ, Conrad BP, Baslanti TO, Horodyski M, Rechtine GR. A comparison of 4 airway devices on cervical spine alignment in cadaver models of global ligamentous instability at c1–2. Anesth Analg. 2013; 117(1):126–132

[8] Curry K, Casady L. The relationship between extended periods of immobility and decubitus ulcer formation in the acutely spinal cord-injured individual. J Neurosci Nurs. 1992; 24(4):185–189

[9] McGuire RA, Neville S, Green BA, Watts C. Spinal instability and the log-rolling maneuver. J Trauma. 1987; 27(5):525–531

[10] Bearden BG, Conrad BP, Horodyski M, Rechtine GR. Motion in the unstable cervical spine: comparison of manual turning and use of the Jackson table in prone positioning. J Neurosurg Spine. 2007; 7(2):161–164

[11] Conrad BP, Horodyski M, Wright J, Ruetz P, Rechtine GR, II. Log-rolling technique producing unacceptable motion during body position changes in patients with traumatic spinal cord injury. J Neurosurg Spine. 2007; 6(6):540–543

[12] Del Rossi G, Horodyski M, Conrad BP, Dipaola CP, Dipaola MJ, Rechtine GR. Transferring patients with thoracolumbar spinal instability: are there alternatives to the log roll maneuver? Spine. 2008; 33(14):1611–1615

[13] Del Rossi G, Horodyski M, Heffernan TP, et al. Spine-board transfer techniques and the unstable cervical spine. Spine. 2004; 29(7):E134–E138

[14] Del Rossi G, Horodyski MH, Conrad BP, Di Paola CP, Di Paola MJ, Rechtine GR. The 6-plus-person lift transfer technique compared with other methods of spine boarding. J Athl Train. 2008; 43(1):6–13

[15] DiPaola CP, DiPaola MJ, Conrad BP, et al. Total motion generated in the unstable cervical spine during management of the typical trauma patient- a comparison of methods in a cadaver model.pdfr motion produced by manual and Jackson-. J Bone Jt Surg. 2008; 90(8):1698–1704

[16] DiPaola MJ, DiPaola CP, Conrad BP, et al. Cervical spine motion in manual versus Jackson table turning methods in a cadaveric global instability model. J Spinal Disord Tech. 2008; 21(4):273–280

[17] Rechtine GR, Conrad BP, Bearden BG, Horodyski M. Biomechanical analysis of cervical and thoracolumbar spine motion in intact and partially and completely unstable cadaver spine models with kinetic bed therapy or traditional log roll. J Trauma. 2007; 62(2):383–388, discussion 388

[18] Lauweryns P. Role of conservative treatment of cervical spine injuries. Eur Spine J. 2010; 19 Suppl 1:S23–S26

[19] Uche EO, Nwankwo OE, Okorie E, Muobike A. Skull traction for cervical spinal injury in Enugu: A 5-year retrospective multicenter analysis of the clinical outcomes of patients treated with two common devices. Niger J Clin Pract. 2016; 19(5):580–584

[20] Vaccaro AR, Falatyn SP, Flanders AE, Balderston RA, Northrup BE, Cotler JM. Magnetic resonance evaluation of the intervertebral disc, spinal ligaments, and spinal cord before and after closed traction reduction of cervical spine dislocations. Spine. 1999; 24(12):1210–1217

[21] Lieben MA, Carlson GD, Minato Y, et al. Early time-dependent decompression for injury: evoked potentials. Electroencephalogr Clin Neurophysiol. 1997; 14(12):951–962

[22] Brunette DD, Rockswold GL. Neurologic recovery following rapid spinal realignment for complete cervical spinal cord injury. J Trauma. 1987; 27(4):445–447

[23] Olerud C, Jónsson H, Jr. Compression of the cervical spine cord after reduction of fracture dislocations. Report of 2 cases. Acta Orthop Scand. 1991; 62(6):599–601

[24] Eismont FJ, Arena MJ, Green BA. Extrusion of an intervertebral disc associated with traumatic subluxation or dislocation of cervical facets. Case report. J Bone Joint Surg Am. 1991; 73(10):1555–1560

[25] Jeanneret B, Magerl F, Ward EH, Ward JC. Posterior stabilization of the cervical spine with hook plates. Spine. 1991; 16(3) Suppl:S56–S63

[26] Wimberley DW, Vaccaro AR, Goyal N, et al. Acute quadriplegia following closed traction reduction of a cervical facet dislocation in the setting of ossification of the posterior longitudinal ligament: case report. Spine. 2005; 30(15):E433–E438

[27] Darsaut TE, Ashforth R, Bhargava R, et al. A pilot study of magnetic resonance imaging-guided closed reduction of cervical spine fractures. Spine. 2006; 31(18):2085–2090

[28] Delamarter RB, Sherman J, Carr JB. Pathophysiology of spinal cord injury. Recovery after immediate and delayed decompression. J Bone Joint Surg Am. 1995; 77(7):1042–1049

[29] Sanan A, Rengachary SS. The history of spinal biomechanics. Neurosurgery. 1996; 39(4):657–668, discussion 668–669

[30] Blumberg KD, Catalano JB, Cotler JM, Balderston RA. The pullout strength of titanium alloy MRI-compatible and stainless steel MRI-incompatible Gardner-Wells tongs. Spine. 1993; 18(13):1895–1896

[31] Choo JHN, Liu WY, Kumar VP. Complications from the Gardner-Wells tongs. Injury. 1996; 27(7):512–513

[32] Soyer J, Iborra JP, Fargues P, Pries P, Clarac JP. Abces cerebral secondaire a l'utilisation de traction crainienne par etrier de Gardner-Wells. Chirugie. 1999; 124:432–434

[33] Nimityongskul P, Bose WJ, Hurley DP, Jr, Anderson LD. Superficial temporal artery laceration. A complication of skull tong traction. Orthop Rev. 1992; 21(6):761–, 764–765

[34] McKinley W, Meade MA, Kirshblum S, Barnard B. Outcomes of early surgical management versus late or no surgical intervention after acute spinal cord injury. Arch Phys Med Rehabil. 2004; 85(11):1818–1825

[35] Pollard ME, Apple DF. Factors associated with improved neurologic outcomes in patients with incomplete tetraplegia. Spine. 2003; 28(1):33–39

[36] Rutges JP, Oner FC, Leenen LP. Timing of thoracic and lumbar fracture fixation in spinal injuries: a systematic review of neurological and clinical outcome. Eur Spine J. 2007; 16(5):579–587

[37] Vaccaro AR, Daugherty RJ, Sheehan TP, et al. Neurologic outcome of early versus late surgery for cervical spinal cord injury. Spine. 1997; 22(22):2609–2613

[38] Bohlman HH, Anderson PA. Anterior decompression and arthrodesis of the cervical spine: long-term motor improvement. Part I—improvement in incomplete traumatic quadriparesis. J Bone Joint Surg Am. 1992; 74(5): 671–682

[39] Fehlings MG, Vaccaro A, Wilson JR, et al. Early versus delayed decompression for traumatic cervical spinal cord injury: results of the Surgical Timing in Acute Spinal Cord Injury Study (STASCIS). PLoS One. 2012; 7(2):e32037

[40] Morita T, Takebayashi T, Irifune H, Ohnishi H, Hirayama S, Yamashita T. Factors affecting survival of patients in the acute phase of upper cervical spine injuries. Arch Orthop Trauma Surg. 2017; 137(4):543–548

[41] Alker GJ, Jr, Oh YS, Leslie EV. High cervical spine and craniocervical junction injuries in fatal traffic accidents: a radiological study. Orthop Clin North Am. 1978; 9(4):1003–1010

[42] Reis A, Bransford R, Penoyar T, Chapman JR, Bellabarba C. Diagnosis and treatment of craniocervical dissociation in 48 consecutive survivors. Evid Based Spine Care J. 2010; 1(2):69–70

[43] Govender S, Vlok GJ, Fisher-Jeffes N, Du Preez CP. Traumatic dislocation of the atlanto-occipital joint. J Bone Joint Surg Br. 2003; 85(6):875–878

[44] Cooper Z, Gross JA, Lacey JM, Traven N, Mirza SK, Arbabi S. Identifying survivors with traumatic craniocervical dissociation: a retrospective study. J Surg Res. 2010; 160(1):3–8

[45] Kaplan NB, Molinari C, Molinari RW. Nonoperative management of craniocervical ligamentous distraction injury: literature review. Global Spine J. 2015; 5(6):505–512

[46] Anderson PA, Montesano PX. Morphology and treatment of occipital condyle fractures. Spine. 1988; 13(7):731–736

[47] Tuli S, Tator CH, Fehlings MG, Mackay M. Occipital condyle fractures. Neurosurgery. 1997; 41(2):368–376, discussion 376–377

[48] Maddox JJ, Rodriguez-Feo JA, Maddox GE, Gullung G, McGwin G, Theiss SM. Non-operative treatment of occipital condyle fractures. Spine. 2012; 37(16): E964–E968

[49] Karam YR, Traynelis VC. Occipital condyle fractures. Neurosurgery. 2010; 66(3) Suppl:56–59

[50] Young WF, Rosenwasser RH, Getch C, Jallo J. Diagnosis and management of occipital condyle fractures. Neurosurgery. 1994; 34(2):257–260, discussion 260–261

[51] Vieweg U, Meyer B, Schramm J, U. V. Differential treatment in acute upper cervical spine injuries: a critical review of a single-institution series. Surg Neurol. 2000; 54(3):203–210, discussion 210–211

[52] Hadley MN, Dickman CA, Browner CM, Sonntag VK. Acute traumatic atlas fractures: management and long term outcome. Neurosurgery. 1988; 23(1):31–35

[53] Anderson LD, D'Alonzo RT. Fractures of the odontoid process of the axis. J Bone Joint Surg Am. 1974; 56(8):1663–1674

[54] Hanssen AD, Cabanela ME. Fractures of the dens in adult patients. J Trauma. 1987; 27(8):928–934

[55] Wang G-J, Mabie KN, Whitehill R, Stamp WG. The nonsurgical management of odontoid fractures in adults. Spine. 1984; 9(3):229–230

[56] van Holsbeeck E, Stoffelen D, Fabry G. Fractures of the odontoid process. Conservative and operative treatment. Prognostic factors. Acta Orthop Belg. 1993; 59(1):17–21

[57] Bettini N, Cervellati S, Di Silvestre M, Palmisani M, Bianco T, Savini R. The nonsurgical treatment of fractures of the dens epistrophei. Chir Organi Mov. 1991; 76(1):17–24

[58] Polin RS, Szabo T, Bogaev CA, Replogle RE, Jane JA. Nonoperative management of types II and III odontoid fractures: the Philadelphia collar versus the halo vest. Neurosurgery. 1996; 38(3):450–456, discussion 456–457

[59] Hart R, Saterbak A, Rapp T, Clark C. Nonoperative management of dens fracture nonunion in elderly patients without myelopathy. Spine. 2000; 25(11):1339–1343

[60] Koivikko MP, Kiuru MJ, Koskinen SK, Myllynen P, Santavirta S, Kivisaari L. Factors associated with nonunion in conservatively-treated type-II fractures of the odontoid process. J Bone Joint Surg Br. 2004; 86(8):1146–1151

[61] Ryan MD, Taylor TKF. Odontoid fractures in the elderly. J Spinal Disord. 1993; 6(5):397–401

[62] Clark C, White A. Fracture of the dens. J Bone Joint Surg Am. 1985; 67(9):1340–1348

[63] Stoney J, O'Brien J, Wilde P. Treatment of type-two odontoid fractures in halothoracic vests. J Bone Joint Surg Br. 1998; 80(3):452–455

[64] Tashjian RZ, Majercik S, Biffl WL, Palumbo MA, Cioffi WG. Halo-vest immobilization increases early morbidity and mortality in elderly odontoid fractures. J Trauma. 2006; 60(1):199–203

[65] Kepler CK, Vaccaro AR, Dibra F, et al. Neurologic injury because of trauma after type II odontoid nonunion. Spine J. 2014; 14(6):903–908

[66] Pennington RGC, Gnanalingham KK, Van Dellen JR. Unilateral avulsion fracture of the transverse atlantal ligament: successful treatment in a rigid cervical collar. Br J Neurosurg. 2004; 18(4):382–384

[67] Lo PA, Drake JM, Hedden D, Narotam P, Dirks PB. Avulsion transverse ligament injuries in children: successful treatment with nonoperative management. Report of three cases. J Neurosurg. 2002; 96(3) Suppl:338–342

[68] Dickman CA, Mamourian A, Sonntag VKH, Drayer BP. Magnetic resonance imaging of the transverse atlantal ligament for the evaluation of atlantoaxial instability. J Neurosurg. 1991; 75(2):221–227

[69] Fujimura Y, Nishi Y, Kobayashi K. Classification and treatment of axis body fractures. J Orthop Trauma. 1996; 10(8):536–540

[70] Starr JK, Eismont FJ. Atypical hangman's fractures. Spine. 1993; 18(14):1954–1957

[71] Seljeskog EL, Chou SN, Words KEY. Spectrum of the hangman's fracture. J Neurosurg. 1976; 45(1):3–8

[72] Hadley MN, Dickman CA, Browner CM, Sonntag VKH. Acute axis fractures: a review of 229 cases. J Neurosurg. 1989; 71(5 Pt 1):642–647

[73] German JW, Hart BL, Benzel EC. Nonoperative management of vertical C2 body fractures. Neurosurgery. 2005; 56(3):516–521, discussion 516–521

[74] Greene KA, Dickman CA, Marciano FF, Drabier JB, Hadley MN, Sonntag VK. Acute axis fractures. Analysis of management and outcome in 340 consecutive cases. Spine. 1997; 22(16):1843–1852

[75] Al-Mahfoudh R, Beagrie C, Woolley E, et al. Management of typical and atypical hangman's fractures. Global Spine J. 2016; 6(3):248–256

[76] Vaccaro AR, Hulbert RJ, Patel AA, et al. Spine Trauma Study Group. The subaxial cervical spine injury classification system: a novel approach to recognize the importance of morphology, neurology, and integrity of the disco-ligamentous complex. Spine. 2007; 32(21):2365–2374

[77] Samuel S, Lin J-L, Smith MM, et al. Subaxial injury classification scoring system treatment recommendations: external agreement study based on retrospective review of 185 patients. Spine. 2015; 40(3):137–142

[78] Beyer CA, Cabanela ME. Unilateral facet dislocations and fracture-dislocations of the cervical spine: a review. Orthopedics. 1992; 15(3):311–315

[79] Beyer CA, Cabanela ME, Berquist TH. Unilateral facet dislocations and fracture-dislocations of the cervical spine. J Bone Joint Surg Br. 1991; 73(6):977–981

[80] Bradley JF, III, Jones MA, Farmer EA, Fann SA, Bynoe R. Swallowing dysfunction in trauma patients with cervical spine fractures treated with halo-vest fixation. J Trauma. 2011; 70(1):46–48, discussion 48–50

[81] Harrop JS, Sharan A, Ratliff J. Central cord injury: pathophysiology, management, and outcomes. Spine J. 2006; 6(6) Suppl:198S–206S

[82] Prasarn M, Rechtine GR. Non-operative management of spinal injuries. In: Spine Surgery: Techniques, Complications Avoidance, and Management. Benzel BC.; 2016

[83] Mehta JS, Reed MR, McVie JL, Sanderson PL. Weight-bearing radiographs in thoracolumbar fractures: do they influence management? Spine. 2004; 29(5):564–567

[84] Humphry S, Clarke A, Hutton M, Chan D. Erect radiographs to assess clinical instability in patients with blunt cervical spine trauma. J Bone Joint Surg Am. 2012; 94(23):e1741–e1744

24 Rehabilitation after Spinal Cord Injury: Approaches and Caveats

George M. Ghobrial and Allan D. Levi

Abstract

Given an increase in the prevalence of acute traumatic cervical spinal cord injury (SCI) in the United States, the need for the development of effective rehabilitation strategies is concomitantly rising. Rehabilitation, however, is a multifaceted process which requires a cogent understanding of the pathophysiology of SCI. It is essential to institute this rehabilitation process expeditiously following the initial trauma to maximize recovery, to improve functional outcomes, and to prevent further deconditioning. Numerous technological advances resulting from increased research and clinical trials into effective rehabilitation strategies, such as the use of epidural stimulation, various cellular replacement therapies, and exoskeletons, have provided clinicians with a wider armamentarium of tools with which to approach the rehabilitation process following acute traumatic cervical SCI. Nonetheless, an optimized rehabilitation program can drastically improve quality of life and can significantly enhance recovery in patients with cervical SCI.

Keywords: spinal cord injury, rehabilitation, clinical trials, quality of life, Charcot arthropathy, syringomyelia, epidural stimulation, exoskeleton, cellular replacement therapy

24.1 Introduction

The development of effective rehabilitative strategies for acute traumatic spinal cord injury (SCI) in the past several decades has been an ongoing pursuit as experimental therapies proposed by physicians and scientists have not demonstrated efficacy in altering the natural disease course.[1,2] The post-World War II era saw a paradigm shift in rehabilitation led by Munro and Guttmann, who directed all efforts toward the individual's achievement of independence, obtaining his or her previous standard of living,[3] and integrating sporting activities into rehabilitation.[4] Approximately 30 people sustain an SCI in the United States each day, and the likelihood of recovery of functional independence from a complete cervical motor injury, classified as American Spinal Injury Association (ASIA) Impairment Scale Grade A, is very uncommon.[5] One rough approximation has been that 10% of patients with cervical ASIA Impairment Scale (AIS) Grade A injuries will improve to an incomplete motor injury (AIS C or AIS D).[6] Moreover, because of improvements in the long-term care of patients with SCI and increased long-term survival, the nationwide prevalence of patients with SCI in the United States alone has surpassed 2 million.[6] As such, these numbers are estimated to increase, and the relevance and renewed interest of the public in SCI rehabilitation for those with complete and incomplete SCI has steadily grown. Research advances in epidural stimulation,[7] cellular replacement therapy,[5] and exoskeleton use[8,9,10,11] have encouraged novel rehabilitation measures.[5] As a clinician, understanding the importance of appropriate rehabilitation for a patient with traumatic cervical SCI is paramount. This aspect of care is likely to have a broader impact on maximizing quality of life (QOL) in the long term. The process of developing curative therapies via clinical trials, meanwhile, will be slow and arduous in comparison.

24.1.1 The Importance of the Postoperative Recovery Period of SCI on Long-Term Quality of Life

The impact of the spinal surgeon on patient QOL extends beyond acute decompression and stabilization of traumatic cervical SCI, and the initial inpatient stay.[12,13] These patients tend to score lower on self-reported health-related QOL (HRQOL) surveys. The scores, themselves, are influenced by increasing degrees of disability.[14,15,16,17] Patients with SCI undergo significant negative changes in body composition characterized by muscle atrophy with fat replacement, increasing the risk for comorbid conditions such as neuropathic pain, depression, obesity, osteoporosis, diabetes, heart disease, and life-threatening pneumonia.[18,19,20] Physical activity has been shown to reduce cardiovascular disease risk, obesity, diabetes, and osteoporosis in the general public, and increasingly so in patients with SCI.[21,22] These changes in body composition have been demonstrated in several ways. Castro et al performed serial muscle biopsies in adults with complete SCI and found significant increases in fat composition as early as 6 months postinjury.[23] Less invasively, these results have been similarly confirmed with magnetic resonance imaging (MRI)[23] and bone densitometry[24] studies. Reversibility of these changes has been demonstrated by noninvasive means with targeted rehabilitative measures tailored for the motor-impaired patient.[15,16,17,25,26] Therefore, it behooves the spinal surgeon to understand that spinal surgery is just the beginning of a lifetime of increased health care needs and societal expenses for these patients.

Modern clinical trials and investigational studies have been predominantly pharmacological and have focused on mitigating the damaging effects of inflammation on the spinal cord (i.e., limiting the pervasive effects of secondary injury to the volume of at-risk spinal cord tissue).[27] Pharmacologic treatments and clinical trials targeting novel disease mechanisms to cure SCI will be discussed in subsequent chapters.

In this chapter, the rehabilitative care of the SCI patient with acute, cervical, traumatic SCI will be discussed. The focus of this care begins during the transition from the inpatient setting to long-term rehabilitation. It is possible that advances in the rehabilitation of SCI patients may outpace therapies targeting primary and secondary injury, given the greater technological knowledge gap among other numerous hurdles that hamper progress toward enrollment in clinical studies. In the final section of this chapter, the authors discuss several rehabilitative technologies that surgeons may see with increased frequency in the future, such as electrical stimulation and exoskeleton use.

24.2 Initial Assessment, Defining Goals of Rehabilitation, and Maximizing Quality of Life

The general rehabilitation plan is tailored toward the neurologic status of the individual by a physician with a specialization in rehabilitative medicine, a physical therapy team, and an occupational therapist. The goal of this plan is to aid the patient independently, achieve the patient's activities of daily living (ADLs), achieve reintegration into one's preinjury occupation, and help develop a plan for the patient to define ADLs and those ADLs requiring assistance.[14] It is apparent to the health care provider that tetraplegic patients and those with severe cervical SCI will not have similar goals and requirements as the ambulatory cervical SCI patient. It has been increasingly more common for patients in the United States with SCI to be employed preinjury. Hence, the return to work is a major motivational factor for the patient, and can give him or her personal satisfaction, a sense of purpose in society, and an improved QOL.[28] Ferdiana et al evaluated predictors of return to work at 5 years in wheelchair-dependent SCI individuals.[29] The median return to work time was 13 months and was 51% for patients with work rates ≥ 1 hour/week and 43% in patients paid for ≥ 12 hour/week. Intuitively, the most significant return-to-work predictor identified was the level of physical intensity.[29] Wood-Dauphinee and Küchler's strategy for maximizing well-being is multifaceted.[14] Ultimately, the patient's perspective is the most important facet of well-being and is dependent on physical, social, and psychological well-being. The physical component includes all patient-specific ADLs in addition to recreation, sexual functioning, and sleep quality. Social components include, but are not limited to, patient independence, family contacts, role fulfillments, and intimate relationships. Lastly, psychological components include mood, affect, emotional stability, memory, reasoning, and comprehension.

A full physical and detailed neurologic exam should be performed at standardized interim periods with an SCI-specific graded assessment tool such as the "Graded Redefined Assessment of Strength, Sensibility, and Prehension" (GRASSP)[30,31] and the International Standards for Neurological Classification of SCI (ISNCSCI) assessments.[32] Both these tools are helpful for serial assessments when implemented by a trained assessor. The consistent inclusion of GRASSP, ISNCSCI, and any other instruments for measuring SCI rehabilitation progress and the reliability of these assessments are dependent on the availability of trained staff.[30] It is important to understand the accuracy, reliability, and interrater reliability of each test being utilized, so as not to misinterpret small incremental changes in scoring. Moreover, rehabilitation considerations include an assessment of sensory modalities, prehension, range of motion, balance, ambulation and gait, weight-bearing capacity, occupational and domestic needs for carrying out ADLs, and endurance level for each of these activities. Severe SCI limits aerobic and anaerobic conditioning, and a rehabilitation regimen should include cardiovascular as well as strength training for all patients.[33] Rehabilitation for SCI also requires an understanding of tandem orthopedic injuries in polytrauma that affect ambulation or limb functioning. A training program should take any orthopedic injuries and limitations into account, and they should not be neglected. Traumatic brain injury (TBI) can significantly complicate reintegration of the patient within society and interactions with their care team and family. It is important that this not be overlooked, as concurrent TBI can present in up to 20% of SCI patients and can often be missed.[34] With increases in survival and return to higher standards of living, other issues become more prevalent over time in patients with chronic cervical SCI. These needs must be addressed and given equal importance, and can include musculoskeletal injuries and chronic pain, bowel, bladder, and sexual dysfunction, as well as muscle spasticity requiring surgical intervention.[35]

24.3 Therapy Considerations with High Spinal Cord Injury

In the first year after injury, patients with SCI are deconditioned: quadriplegics have a very limited capacity for physical fitness in the first 6 months after SCI.[36,37] Additionally, patients with high and low cervical injuries have 30 and 60% of their upper body strength relative to paraplegics, respectively.[38] There is a general lack of high-quality, detailed studies on the most efficient or efficacious strength-training or muscle development exercises in the context of SCI. Therefore, the most important step is the early adoption and consistency of a strength-training and aerobic program. Studies by Nilsson et al[39] as well as Davis and Shephard[40] have shown both strength and endurance improvements in as little as 8 to 16 weeks. Impairments in normal physiologic responses to exercise including both autonomic and somatic deinnervation affect respiration and respiratory reflexes. Pulmonary capacity has been shown to be diminished as well, observed experimentally by decreased forced vital capacity, forced expiratory volume, and maximal breathing capacity.[41,42] These measures are also posturally dependent, as demonstrated by Estenne and De Troyer, who found a decrease in vital capacity in tetraplegics when they moved from a seated to supine posture.[43] Work by Noreau and Shephard showed that the maximum oxygen uptake of paraplegics and quadriplegics was 15 and 10 mL/kg/min (VO_{2max}), respectively.[37] This 50% change in reserve can be accounted for by the lack of sympathetic outflow. Paraplegic individuals can bring their heart rates to 90% of their theoretical maximum. In the context of a cervical injury, peak heart rates reaching only 100 to 120 beats per minute can be achieved.[42] Functional electrical stimulation (FES) allows for the transcutaneous stimulation of muscle fibers, promoting muscle fatigue and hypertrophy in patients otherwise unable to voluntarily activate these pathways.[42] This is increasingly being recognized as a tool for rehabilitation. With FES, desired upper heart rate ranges can be more easily achieved and maintained in paraplegics, limiting the stress of chronic high-intensity upper extremity cycling and related joint overuse.[44,45,46] However, conflicting data show that while FES is helpful, it is still unable to overcome the lack of sympathetic modulation in patients with complete injury above the third thoracic vertebrae.[46] The use of FES in pilot studies shows promise, but is early in development. McBain et al demonstrate augmentation of cough muscles during the expiratory phase, raising promise for a future means to prevent aspiration and pneumonia, two major life-threatening conditions affecting patients with chronic cervical SCI.[46,47]

One more commonly utilized FES implementation is by improving respiratory function through timed stimulation of abdominal muscles, resulting in increased contraction of the rectus muscle and secondary muscles of respiration.[48] In one meta-analysis by McCaughey et al, FES was shown to increase respiratory function in a preponderance of the included studies.[48] However, these findings are mired by low study quality, with the majority of studies being cohort studies with small sample sizes.

While there are difficulties with demonstrating efficacy of FES for respiratory functional recovery, FES has demonstrated substantial promise for improving recovery for SCI. Sadowsky et al evaluated FES in chronic SCI patients, comparing two cohorts matched by age, gender, and SCI level and severity, finding a significantly greater recovery in the cohort receiving FES cycling.[49] In fact, while a composite score consisting of ASIA motor and sensory components was shown to decrease by 9 points in the observational period, there was a 20-point increase (improvement) in the FES cohort. A clinical trial of physical therapy in chronic (> 18 months postinjury) ASIA C and D grade SCI patients, with and without FES walking, demonstrated a greater benefit for the FES group.[50] Finally, while the quality of many studies in FES in SCI are limited by low enrollment, clear benefits have been shown for stroke rehabilitation where there is clearly a much higher disease prevalence.[51,52]

24.4 Pain following Traumatic SCI

Numerous sources of chronic pain can limit rehabilitation in patients with SCI.[53] The diagnostic process is often time-consuming and rarely straightforward, due to a multifactorial etiology in the more than 75% of patients with SCI that ultimately seek treatment for chronic pain.[54] The earliest type of pain is the most common and least severe type: musculoskeletal. Pain from mechanical instability most commonly occurs after cervical SCI and least commonly in the thoracic and lumbar spine, often presenting in a delayed fashion due to discoligamentous, facet, or bony injuries not surgically addressed in the acute setting.[54] This is usually due to traumatic injury in the first 6 months, which resolves, and then is followed by pain that peaks at 5 years and is likely due to orthopedic injury from overuse.[55] Orthopedic injuries are common in patients with SCI for several reasons.[56] Musculoskeletal pain often results from the recruitment of joints and preserved muscle groups in a compensatory manner that can often exceed the normal tolerances of these joints and musculature. In severe cervical SCI patients, the prevalence of musculoskeletal shoulder pain is high, approaching more than 50%.[33] In addition to the traumatic injuries inflicted at the onset of SCI, overuse of functioning muscles and joints can result in accelerated arthropathy.[57] Joint arthropathy is further accelerated when stabilized by atrophic muscle groups. This is especially the case with muscles lacking antagonist muscle pairs which could ordinarily counterbalance forces during joint movements. Shortening of ligaments, tendons, and atrophic musculature will further contribute to joint arthropathy and pain following SCI.[56] In a review of the literature evaluating effective treatments for shoulder pain secondary to chronic wheelchair use, three randomized controlled trials found exercise in the form of arm ergometry, resistive strength-

ening either with or without electromyographic biofeedback, and routine shoulder girdle stretch exercises to be efficacious therapeutic interventions.[56]

24.5 Neuropathic Pain, Delayed-Onset Pain, and Cord Lesioning

Aside from early-onset musculoskeletal pain, early "at-level" neuropathic pain is a condition developing within days to weeks of injury and is most frequently described by the patient as severe or excruciating pain.[55] This pain is thought to be due to increased hyperactivity of nociceptive afferent C-fibers. The exact cause of posttraumatic neuropathic pain after SCI can often be difficult to isolate, but nonetheless, up to two-thirds of these patients develop chronic neuropathic pain. Sadly, these painful symptoms will persist, and are refractory to oral analgesics.[58,59,60] Intrathecal administration, however, has proven to be efficacious in double-blinded, randomized controlled trial of morphine and clonidine for the treatment of neuropathic pain. Intrathecal administration allows the concentration of analgesics to greatly exceed the concentration that can safely be given orally.[61] Late, "below-level" neuropathic pain occurs both below the level of injury and at a later time point (2 years) after injury.[55,62] This type of pain is severe and poorly responsive to pain medications, and is hypothesized to be the result of deafferentation of rostral targets originating from spinothalamic tract projections.[63]

Somatic pain refers to pain mediated by the spinothalamic tract. While visceral pain and somatic pain are mediated through discrete spinal cord pathways, visceral pain can be alternatively mediated by the autonomic system. Therefore, given the reliable anatomy of somatic pain mediation, this problem has been amenable to cord lesioning procedures.[64] A full discussion of the types of pain and various cord lesioning techniques is beyond the scope of this chapter.

Visceral pain occurs in a very small percentage of the SCI population, occurring relatively late among the types of pain encountered in the context of SCI, and is thought to occur as a result of bowel, bladder, and kidney dysfunction.[53] Numerous pain drivers exist and an aggressive workup is important, so as not to delay diagnosis of a serious medical condition. A full physical exam, history, and diagnostic imaging workup should be promptly obtained. Three neurosurgical conditions can present with neuropathic pain, and will be subsequently discussed in this chapter due to the potential for operative intervention including posttraumatic syringomyelia (PTS), neuropathic pain secondary to nerve root avulsion, and Charcot spinal arthropathy.[65,66]

24.6 Charcot Spinal Arthropathy

Posttraumatic Charcot spinal arthropathy from cervical SCI typically affects the thoracolumbar and lumbosacral spine due to the loss of the protective feedback mechanisms provided by the innervation of the mobile spine.[66,67,68,69,70,71] Jacobs et al, in a review of 23 patients with a mean age of 43 years, found that the average length of time between SCI and symptomatic presentation of Charcot spinal arthropathy was 20 years.[66]

In another study by Haus et al, the average duration between SCI and onset of Charcot spinal arthropathy diagnosis was 7.6 years.[72] The typical computed tomography (CT) findings are characterized by bony erosion of the vertebral body and posterior elements with reactive bone formation in the facets and adjacent vertebral bodies. Charcot arthropathy of the cervicothoracic spine is exceedingly rare, and limited to small case series.[73] The increased proportion of calcified bone, coupled with microinstability attributed to atrophy and deinnervation of paraspinal muscles, places this population at a high risk for pseudoarthrosis. Commonly, patient complaints may be insidious, and may include an inability to sit up straight with gradually worsening posture. The patient may not complain of pain at all but may describe audible positioning changes, which is the result of bone-on-bone erosion. An inability to sit up and maintain horizontal gaze is distressing to an SCI patient lacking lower extremity compensatory mechanisms, and severely limits ADLs. Ultimately, complete vertebral bodies may be absent on initial diagnostic imaging, with the development of a pannus of cortical bone and scar around the lesion. Radiographic workup may show the complete erosion of one or even two lumbar vertebrae. Moreover, the findings of seroma or paraspinal inflammation at the site of spinal deformity may make osteomyelitis difficult to completely rule out,[74] with the incidence of coinfection of this seroma to be as high as 17%.[66,75,76] Also, due to the pronounced inflammation and pain that can be generated by these shearing forces, patients can present with autonomic dysreflexia, which can be life-threatening due to volatility in heart rate and blood pressure.[69,77,78]

The surgical treatment of this problem is challenging, and even in the hands of experienced spinal surgeons, significant rates of hardware failure and pseudoarthrosis (between 35 and 75%) have been reported.[66,72] Due to the degree of inflammation and lack of anatomical landmarks, patients are at an elevated risk for many other complications including surgical site infection, cerebrospinal fluid (CSF) leak, hardware breakage, persistent deformity, and bleeding.[79] As the QOL and longevity increase for the SCI patient population, an additional level of symptomatic Charcot spinal arthropathy can occur, at an adjacent or distal level, even after the patient overcomes this first onset, as reported by Haus.[72]

The surgical management of Charcot arthropathy historically involved combined anterior and posterior approaches to achieve adequate deformity correction and achieve normal alignment.[71] Due to the high morbidity and increased familiarity with three-column osteotomies, all posterior approaches have seen increased utilization.[68,80] Due to the high degree of shear forces placed on the construct, and the increased time required to achieve fusion, it is not uncommon for surgeons to plan constructs in numerous ways aimed to mitigate these high shearing and rotational forces. Therefore, strategies to increase construct stability and resist forces include but are not limited to long-segment fusions, larger diameter pedicle screws, increased diameter titanium and cobalt-chrome, four-rod constructs, and cross-linking.

24.7 Posttraumatic Syringomyelia

PTS is an uncommon condition of cystic cavitation of the spinal cord, which results from abnormal flow dynamics. This cyst later manifests as a clinical decline with ascending deficits in a stepwise pattern, and takes place years to decades after the traumatic insult.[81] Even though the incidence of traumatic SCI has declined in the two most prevalent age groups, 15 to 25 years and 25 to 44 years, substantial increases in the elderly are still being seen.[82] An increase in SCI incidence has generally correlated with an increase in the incidence of PTS in one study by Jain et al.[82] The duration of onset of syringomyelia after SCI resulting in paraplegia ranges from months to several years and has a slightly higher reported incidence of 1 to 4%. This is manifested by slow progression of neurologic deficits above the neurologic level of SCI.[83,84,85,86,87,88] Bastian is credited with the identification of a posttraumatic syrinx in 1867,[89] followed by the first complete description of syringomyelia as a clinicoradiographic entity almost 100 years later in 1966 by Barnett and colleagues.[87] The clinical concern for syringomyelia in a patient with a complete cervical SCI injury should be raised by any description from the patient with an ascendance of motor and sensory deficits above a prior complete SCI.[87] The incidence of PTS has been historically low, ranging from 0.3 to 3.2%, and most often is seen in the context of severe or complete SCI.[87] However, due to the longevity of the SCI population and the widespread use of diagnostically sensitive tools such as MRI, this number is indeed much higher.[90]

The treatment of syringomyelia is primarily surgical in adults, and is aimed at the restoration of the natural flow of CSF.[91,92,93,94,95] The literature for surgical treatment of PTS is limited to very few prospective nonrandomized studies, in which general guidelines for surgical management are provided.[96,97,98] In the adult population, radiographic identification of underlying structural causes of syringomyelia should be the first step in its management. Treatment of the underlying lesion, if identified, is of paramount importance.[99] Syringomyelia can be seen with intramedullary tumors (particularly hemangioblastomas and ependymomas), and MRI with contrast studies should be obtained as part of the early diagnostic workup.[100] Posttraumatic tethering of the spinal cord with CSF flow obstruction can be diagnosed with a cine MRI. If such pathology is identified, restoration of normal CSF flow is initially performed through microsurgical detethering of the arachnoidopathy and subsequent duraplasty. This will permit the restoration of the natural corridors around the level of the spinal cord that is involved. While some surgeons argue that this is adequate,[86,91,96,97,98,99] many surgeons proceed with CSF flow diversion via numerous strategies such as cystopleural shunting, cystosubarachnoid shunting, ventriculoperitoneal shunting, and lumboperitoneal shunting.[12,97,101,102,103] Regardless, flow diversion has a high failure rate alone, regardless of type, and the natural history of adult-onset syringomyelia in non-Chiari etiologies is recurrence.[96,101]

24.8 High-Intensity, High-Volume Targeted Approach to SCI Rehabilitation and Epidural Stimulation

Recent SCI rehabilitation has concentrated on the delivery of high-intensity, high-volume, repetitive rehabilitative exercises, delivering clinical improvements to both complete and incomplete-SCI patients.[104] Approaches such as activity-based restorative therapy were developed from the understanding that motor activation could be achieved with intensive training following motor injury or complete transection.[105,106,107,108,109,110,111,112] This is based off the theory that locomotion after SCI could be preserved by repetitive training in tandem with the simulation of central pattern generators (CPGs), motor reflex pathways operating without brain input, and hence below the level of SCI.[104,111,112] Studies by Grillner and others have explored the underlying function of CPGs in cats. They have shown that spinalized cats can be conditioned to stand, to achieve full hindlimb weight-bearing strength, and to achieve locomotion at varying speeds on a treadmill with intensive physical training.[110,112,113] Weight-bearing activity has been shown to be essential following SCI rehabilitation as Harkema and coinvestigators have shown increased hip extensor activity following injury upon weight-bearing treadmill activity.[111,113] However, motor complete SCI patients are a more complex entity and have not been shown to receive a clinical benefit from intensive locomotor training.[111,114,115]

More recently, epidural stimulation has received attention as a future measure to enhance neurorehabilitation in motor complete and incomplete patients. Manual facilitation of standing or stepping[111,114,115] and sensory cutaneous and nociceptive stimuli can induce electromyographic (EMG) activity in the lower extremities of patients with complete SCI.[116,117,118,119] Epidural stimulation has been shown to rhythmically activate lower extremity muscle groups.[120,121] Harkema et al evaluated the use of epidural stimulation in a 23-year-old male with an anatomic C7–T1 injury with a motor complete injury classified as AIS B.[116] After 170 locomotor training sessions with manually facilitated stepping, over a period of 26 months postsurgical stabilization, minimal EMG activity in the medial hamstrings was noted. Spinal cord stimulator placement occurred at T11–L1, with stimulation sessions during training occurring over approximately 40 to 120 minutes at an approximate voltage and frequency of 0.5 to 10.0 V and 5 to 40 Hz, respectively. The stimulus was perceived by the patient as light paresthesias and was not painful. Epidural stimulation on first attempt resulted in the patient being able to stand without manual facilitation, at 65% of bodyweight. Epidural stimulation was also helpful in increasing the patient's maximum performance with regard to adjusting from sitting to standing and loading lower extremities without support from physical trainers. Improvements in bowel, bladder, and sexual function were also noted.[116] Additionally, increased lean body mass and self-esteem were observed as well. Nearly 2 years later, the patient can flex his knees and control all individual joints. Improvements in blood pressure and body temperature regulation were observed as well.[122] The authors acknowledge that there are many gradations in complete motor injury, and that this affects the reconnectivity of motor axons and motor recovery. Prognostication and specifically an explanation of the dramatic improvement in this single case study are limited by the clinician's limited knowledge of the extent of destruction of the motor fibers.

24.9 Exoskeleton Use in SCI

Exoskeleton use in acute rehabilitation and long-term ADLs represents a novel approach to the complex biological processes of central nervous system regeneration and repair that have curbed progress in many areas of SCI treatment. Accompanying the rapid process of muscle atrophy following SCI, especially in the context of complete SCI, are several cellular mechanisms which remain poorly understood.[18,23] As such, increased exertional effort, while extremely beneficial in the acute SCI period, stems rehabilitation efforts, expends significant levels of energy with or without an orthosis or wheelchair, and can significantly limit a patient's ADLs.[10] The use of passive or actively powered robotic exoskeletons increases efficiency of work through support of weakened stabilizer muscles, increases workloads that can be sustained, and decreases energy use by the wearer. Actively powered robotic exoskeletons utilize an external battery source, support joints at risk for injury, are ergonomic, and are becoming more efficient in design.[11] More recently, Grasmücke and coinvestigators implemented a "Hybrid Assistive Limb Exoskeleton" (Hal, Cyberdyne Inc., Japan) which utilizes EMG stimuli from a wearer with incomplete SCI, to serve as an impulse for gait and limb assistance with the powered exoskeleton.[123] They report, through their experiences, that motivated patients can be trained effectively to use this device to improve ADLs.[8,124] While the Hal exoskeleton or any exoskeleton is not a permanent substitute for daily ambulation, these incremental advancements in exoskeleton technology and efficiency are improving the lives of SCI patients.

24.10 Experimental Strategies to Enhance Neurologic Recovery: Cellular Replacement Therapy

Through separate novel approaches, numerous experimental strategies have been developed that each aims to repair dysfunctional spinal cord pathologies. Recently, promising translational therapies have entered clinical trials that, for the first time, provide an approach to treat the primary injury. Namely, cellular replacement therapy, which consists of replacement of the lost neural architecture with populations of neurons and astrocytes, aims to restore functional connectivity and to enhance neuroprotection in a proinflammatory, postinjury state.[125,126] Cellular replacement therapies will be discussed in a subsequent chapter of this book.

24.11 Final Remarks

Rehabilitative care by the surgeon and other health care practitioners is a multidisciplinary process and requires an understanding of the pathologic and physiologic disease processes associated with SCI. A rigorous rehabilitation program needs to be instituted without delay to avoid the rapid deconditioning that can occur following injury. An increase in rehabilitation requirements is observed in patients with higher levels of SCI and an increased severity of injury. Additionally, SCI has profound monetary and societal implications which should be kept in mind at all times. An aggressive and modern rehabilitation program, however, can improve patient QOL and well-being, and can enhance recovery.

References

[1] Witiw CD, Fehlings MG. Acute spinal cord injury. J Spinal Disord Tech. 2015; 28(6):202–210

[2] Wyndaele M, Wyndaele JJ. Incidence, prevalence and epidemiology of spinal cord injury: what learns a worldwide literature survey? Spinal Cord. 2006; 44(9):523–529

[3] Munro D. The rehabilitation of patients totally paralyzed below the waist, with special reference to making them ambulatory and capable of earning their own living. V. An end-result study of 445 cases. N Engl J Med. 1954; 250(1):4–14

[4] Schültke E. Ludwig Guttmann: emerging concept of rehabilitation after spinal cord injury. J Hist Neurosci. 2001; 10(3):300–307

[5] Gomes-Osman J, Cortes M, Guest J, Pascual-Leone A. A systematic review of experimental strategies aimed at improving motor function after acute and chronic spinal cord injury. J Neurotrauma. 2016; 33(5):425–438

[6] Fawcett JW, Curt A, Steeves JD, et al. Guidelines for the conduct of clinical trials for spinal cord injury as developed by the ICCP panel: spontaneous recovery after spinal cord injury and statistical power needed for therapeutic clinical trials. Spinal Cord. 2007; 45(3):190–205

[7] Angeli CAEV, Edgerton VR, Gerasimenko YP, Harkema SJ. Altering spinal cord excitability enables voluntary movements after chronic complete paralysis in humans. Brain. 2014; 137(Pt 5):1394–1409

[8] Cruciger O, Tegenthoff M, Schwenkreis P, Schildhauer TA, Aach M. Locomotion training using voluntary driven exoskeleton (HAL) in acute incomplete SCI. Neurology. 2014; 83(5):474

[9] Louie DR, Eng JJ, Lam T, Spinal Cord Injury Research Evidence (SCIRE) Research Team. Gait speed using powered robotic exoskeletons after spinal cord injury: a systematic review and correlational study. J Neuroeng Rehabil. 2015; 12:82

[10] Massucci M, Brunetti G, Piperno R, Betti L, Franceschini M. Walking with the advanced reciprocating gait orthosis (ARGO) in thoracic paraplegic patients: energy expenditure and cardiorespiratory performance. Spinal Cord. 1998; 36(4):223–227

[11] Sale P, Franceschini M, Waldner A, Hesse S. Use of the robot assisted gait therapy in rehabilitation of patients with stroke and spinal cord injury. Eur J Phys Rehabil Med. 2012; 48(1):111–121

[12] Fehlings MG, Vaccaro A, Wilson JR, et al. Early versus delayed decompression for traumatic cervical spinal cord injury: results of the Surgical Timing in Acute Spinal Cord Injury Study (STASCIS). PLoS One. 2012; 7(2):e32037

[13] Ahuja CS, Martin AR, Fehlings M. Recent advances in managing a spinal cord injury secondary to trauma. F1000 Res. 2016; 5:5

[14] Wood-Dauphinee S, K, ü, chler T. Quality of life as a rehabilitation outcome: are we missing the boat? Can J Rehabil. 1992; 6:3–12

[15] DeVivo MJ, Richards JS. Community reintegration and quality of life following spinal cord injury. Paraplegia. 1992; 30(2):108–112

[16] Eisenberg MG, Saltz CC. Quality of life among aging spinal cord injured persons: long term rehabilitation outcomes. Paraplegia. 1991; 29(8):514–520

[17] Gerhart KA. Spinal cord injury outcomes in a population-based sample. J Trauma. 1991; 31(11):1529–1535

[18] Castro MJ, Apple DF, Jr, Hillegass EA, Dudley GA. Influence of complete spinal cord injury on skeletal muscle cross-sectional area within the first 6 months of injury. Eur J Appl Physiol Occup Physiol. 1999; 80(4):373–378

[19] Spungen AMAR, Adkins RH, Stewart CA, et al. Factors influencing body composition in persons with spinal cord injury: a cross-sectional study. J Appl Physiol (1985). 2003; 95(6):2398–2407

[20] Cragg JJNV, Noonan VK, Noreau L, Borisoff JF, Kramer JK. Neuropathic pain, depression, and cardiovascular disease: a national multicenter study. Neuroepidemiology. 2015; 44(3):130–137

[21] Hoffman MD. Cardiorespiratory fitness and training in quadriplegics and paraplegics. Sports Med. 1986; 3(5):312–330

[22] Le CT, Price M. Survival from spinal cord injury. J Chronic Dis. 1982; 35(6):487–492

[23] Castro MJ, Apple DF, Hillegass EA, Dudley GA. Influence of complete spinal cord injury on skeletal muscle cross-sectional area within the first 6 months of injury. J Appl Physiol. 1999; 80(4):373–378

[24] Fisher JA, McNelis MA, Gorgey AS, Dolbow DR, Goetz LL. Does upper extremity training influence body composition after spinal cord injury? Aging Dis. 2015; 6(4):271–281

[25] Gorgey ASMK, Mather KJ, Cupp HR, Gater DR. Effects of resistance training on adiposity and metabolism after spinal cord injury. Med Sci Sports Exerc. 2012; 44(1):165–174

[26] Ruther CL, Golden CL, H, arris RT, Dudley GA. Hypertrophy, resistance training, and the nature of skeletal muscle activation. J Strength Cond Res. 1995; 9(3):155–159

[27] Kim YH, Ha KY, Kim SI. Spinal cord injury and related clinical trials. Clin Orthop Surg. 2017; 9(1):1–9

[28] Hilton G, Unsworth C, Murphy G. The experience of attempting to return to work following spinal cord injury: a systematic review of the qualitative literature. Disabil Rehabil. 2018; 40(15):1745–1753

[29] Ferdiana A, Post MW, de Groot S, Bültmann U, van der Klink JJ. Predictors of return to work 5 years after discharge for wheelchair-dependent individuals with spinal cord injury. J Rehabil Med. 2014; 46(10):984–990

[30] Kalsi-Ryan S, Beaton D, Curt A, et al. The Graded Redefined Assessment of Strength Sensibility and Prehension: reliability and validity. J Neurotrauma. 2012; 29(5):905–914

[31] Kalsi-Ryan S, Curt A, Verrier MC, Fehlings MG. Development of the Graded Redefined Assessment of Strength, Sensibility and Prehension (GRASSP): reviewing measurement specific to the upper limb in tetraplegia. J Neurosurg Spine. 2012; 17(1) Suppl:65–76

[32] Marino RJ, Jones L, Kirshblum S, Tal J, Dasgupta A. Reliability and repeatability of the motor and sensory examination of the international standards for neurological classification of spinal cord injury. J Spinal Cord Med. 2008; 31(2):166–170

[33] Holtz ALR. Rehabilitation. In: Spinal Cord Injury. Vol 1. 1st ed. New York, NY: Oxford University Press; 2010

[34] Macciocchi S, Seel RT, Thompson N, Byams R, Bowman B. Spinal cord injury and co-occurring traumatic brain injury: assessment and incidence. Arch Phys Med Rehabil. 2008; 89(7):1350–1357

[35] Cyr LB. Sequelae of SCI after discharge from the initial rehabilitation program. Rehabil Nurs. 1989; 14(6):326–329, 337

[36] Nas K, Yazmalar L, Şah V, Aydın A, Öneş K. Rehabilitation of spinal cord injuries. World J Orthop. 2015; 6(1):8–16

[37] Noreau L, Shephard RJ. Spinal cord injury, exercise and quality of life. Sports Med. 1995; 20(4):226–250

[38] Noreau L, Shephard RJ, Simard C, Paré G, Pomerleau P. Relationship of impairment and functional ability to habitual activity and fitness following spinal cord injury. Int J Rehabil Res. 1993; 16(4):265–275

[39] Nilsson S, Staff PH, Pruett ED. Physical work capacity and the effect of training on subjects with long-standing paraplegia. Scand J Rehabil Med. 1975; 7(2):51–56

[40] Davis GM, Shephard RJ. Strength training for wheelchair users. Br J Sports Med. 1990; 24(1):25–30

[41] Anke A, Aksnes AK, Stanghelle JK, Hjeltnes N. Lung volumes in tetraplegic patients according to cervical spinal cord injury level. Scand J Rehabil Med. 1993; 25(2):73–77

[42] Van Loan MD, McCluer S, Loftin JM, Boileau RA. Comparison of physiological responses to maximal arm exercise among able-bodied, paraplegics and quadriplegics. Paraplegia. 1987; 25(5):397–405

[43] Estenne M, De Troyer A. Mechanism of the postural dependence of vital capacity in tetraplegic subjects. Am Rev Respir Dis. 1987; 135(2):367–371

[44] Hettinga DM, Andrews BJ. Oxygen consumption during functional electrical stimulation-assisted exercise in persons with spinal cord injury: implications for fitness and health. Sports Med. 2008; 38(10):825–838

[45] Taylor JA, Picard G, Widrick JJ. Aerobic capacity with hybrid FES rowing in spinal cord injury: comparison with arms-only exercise and preliminary findings with regular training. PM R. 2011; 3(9):817–824

[46] Qiu S, Alzhab S, Picard G, Taylor JA. Ventilation limits aerobic capacity after functional electrical stimulation row training in high spinal cord injury. Med Sci Sports Exerc. 2016; 48(6):1111–1118

[47] McBain RA, Boswell-Ruys CL, Lee BB, Gandevia SC, Butler JE. Electrical stimulation of abdominal muscles to produce cough in spinal cord injury: effect of stimulus intensity. Neurorehabil Neural Repair. 2015; 29(4):362–369

[48] McCaughey EJ, Borotkanics RJ, Gollee H, Folz RJ, McLachlan AJ. Abdominal functional electrical stimulation to improve respiratory function after spinal cord injury: a systematic review and meta-analysis. Spinal Cord. 2016; 54(9):628–639

[49] Sadowsky CL, Hammond ER, Strohl AB, et al. Lower extremity functional electrical stimulation cycling promotes physical and functional recovery in chronic spinal cord injury. J Spinal Cord Med. 2013; 36(6):623–631

[50] Kapadia N, Masani K, Catharine Craven B, et al. A randomized trial of functional electrical stimulation for walking in incomplete spinal cord injury: effects on walking competency. J Spinal Cord Med. 2014; 37(5):511–524

[51] Howlett OA, Lannin NA, Ada L, McKinstry C. Functional electrical stimulation improves activity after stroke: a systematic review with meta-analysis. Arch Phys Med Rehabil. 2015; 96(5):934–943

[52] Quandt F, Hummel FC. The influence of functional electrical stimulation on hand motor recovery in stroke patients: a review. Exp Transl Stroke Med. 2014; 6:9

[53] Mariano AJ. Chronic pain and spinal cord injury. Clin J Pain. 1992; 8(2):87–92

[54] Siddall PJ, Loeser JD. Pain following spinal cord injury. Spinal Cord. 2001; 39(2):63–73

[55] Siddall PJ, McClelland JM, Rutkowski SB, Cousins MJ. A longitudinal study of the prevalence and characteristics of pain in the first 5 years following spinal cord injury. Pain. 2003; 103(3):249–257

[56] Cratsenberg KA, Deitrick CE, Harrington TK, et al. Effectiveness of exercise programs for management of shoulder pain in manual wheelchair users with spinal cord injury. J Neurol Phys Ther. 2015; 39(4):197–203

[57] Bachasson D, Singh A, Shah SB, Lane JG, Ward SR. The role of the peripheral and central nervous systems in rotator cuff disease. J Shoulder Elbow Surg. 2015; 24(8):1322–1335

[58] Davidoff G, Roth E, Guarracini M, Sliwa J, Yarkony G. Function-limiting dysesthetic pain syndrome among traumatic spinal cord injury patients: a cross-sectional study. Pain. 1987; 29(1):39–48

[59] Baastrup C, Finnerup NB. Pharmacological management of neuropathic pain following spinal cord injury. CNS Drugs. 2008; 22(6):455–475

[60] Drewes AM, Andreasen A, Poulsen LH. Valproate for treatment of chronic central pain after spinal cord injury. A double-blind cross-over study. Paraplegia. 1994; 32(8):565–569

[61] Siddall PJ, Molloy AR, Walker S, Mather LE, Rutkowski SB, Cousins MJ. The efficacy of intrathecal morphine and clonidine in the treatment of pain after spinal cord injury. Anesth Analg. 2000; 91(6):1493–1498

[62] Davis L, Martin J. Studies upon spinal cord injuries; the nature and treatment of pain. J Neurosurg. 1947; 4(6):483–491

[63] Vierck CJ, Jr, Siddall P, Yezierski RP. Pain following spinal cord injury: animal models and mechanistic studies. Pain. 2000; 89(1):1–5

[64] Konrad P. Dorsal root entry zone lesion, midline myelotomy and anterolateral cordotomy. Neurosurg Clin N Am. 2014; 25(4):699–722

[65] Snoddy MC, Lee DH, Kuhn JE. Charcot shoulder and elbow: a review of the literature and update on treatment. J Shoulder Elbow Surg. 2017; 26(3):544–552

[66] Jacobs WB, Bransford RJ, Bellabarba C, Chapman JR. Surgical management of Charcot spinal arthropathy: a single-center retrospective series highlighting the evolution of management. J Neurosurg Spine. 2012; 17(5):422–431

[67] Aebli N, Pötzel T, Krebs J. Characteristics and surgical management of neuropathic (Charcot) spinal arthropathy after spinal cord injury. Spine J. 2014; 14(6):884–891

[68] David KS, Agarwala AO, Rampersaud YR. Charcot arthropathy of the lumbar spine treated using one-staged posterior three-column shortening and fusion. Spine. 2010; 35(14):E657–E662

[69] Morita M, Iwasaki M, Okuda S, Oda T, Miyauchi A. Autonomic dysreflexia associated with Charcot spine following spinal cord injury: a case report and literature review. Eur Spine J. 2010; 19 Suppl 2:S179–S182

[70] Suda Y, Shioda M, Kohno H, Machida M, Yamagishi M. Surgical treatment of Charcot spine. J Spinal Disord Tech. 2007; 20(1):85–88

[71] Kalen V, Isono SS, Cho CS, Perkash I. Charcot arthropathy of the spine in long-standing paraplegia. Spine. 1987; 12(1):42–47

[72] Haus BM, Hsu AR, Yim ES, Meter JJ, Rinsky LA. Long-term follow-up of the surgical management of neuropathic arthropathy of the spine. Spine J. 2010; 10(6):e6–e16

[73] Aydinli U, Mohan NK, Kara K. Posttraumatic Charcot (neuropathic) spinal arthropathy at the cervicothoracic junction. World Neurosurg. 2016; 94:580.e1–580.e4

[74] Grassner L, Geuther M, Mach O, Bühren V, Vastmans J, Maier D. Charcot spinal arthropathy: an increasing long-term sequel after spinal cord injury with no straightforward management. Spinal Cord Ser Cases. 2015; 1:15022

[75] Suda Y, Saito M, Shioda M, Kato H, Shibasaki K. Infected Charcot spine. Spinal Cord. 2005; 43(4):256–259

[76] Mikawa Y, Watanabe R, Yamano Y, Morii S. Infected Charcot spine following spinal cord injury. Spine. 1989; 14(8):892–895

[77] Selmi F, Frankel HL, Kumaraguru AP, Apostopoulos V. Charcot joint of the spine, a cause of autonomic dysreflexia in spinal cord injured patients. Spinal Cord. 2002; 40(9):481–483

[78] Shan RS, Linassi AG, Dzus AK, Woo A. Hardware failure and spinal pseudoarthrosis causing autonomic dysreflexia: a report of two cases. Spinal Cord. 2009; 47(12):899–900

[79] Goodwin CR, Ahmed AK, Abu-Bonsrah N, De la Garza-Ramos R, Petteys RJ, Sciubba DM. Charcot spinal arthropathy after spinal cord injury. Spine J. 2016; 16(8):e545–e546

[80] Kim TW, Seo EM, Hwang JT, Kwak BC. Charcot spine treated using a single staged posterolateral costotransversectomy approach in a patient with traumatic spinal cord injury. J Korean Neurosurg Soc. 2013; 54(6):532–536

[81] Heiss JD, Snyder K, Peterson MM, et al. Pathophysiology of primary spinal syringomyelia. J Neurosurg Spine. 2012; 17(5):367–380

[82] Jain NB, Ayers GD, Peterson EN, et al. Traumatic spinal cord injury in the United States, 1993–2012. JAMA. 2015; 313(22):2236–2243

[83] Kramer KM, Levine AM. Posttraumatic syringomyelia: a review of 21 cases. Clin Orthop Relat Res. 1997(334):190–199

[84] Klekamp J, Batzdorf U, Samii M, Bothe HW. Treatment of syringomyelia associated with arachnoid scarring caused by arachnoiditis or trauma. J Neurosurg. 1997; 86(2):233–240

[85] Haney A, Stiller J, Zelnik N, Goodwin L. Association of posttraumatic spinal arachnoid cyst and syringomyelia. J Comput Tomogr. 1985; 9(2):137–140

[86] Fehlings MG, Austin JW. Posttraumatic syringomyelia. J Neurosurg Spine. 2011; 14(5):570–572, discussion 572

[87] Barnett HJ, Botterell EH, Jousse AT, Wynn-Jones M. Progressive myelopathy as a sequel to traumatic paraplegia. Brain. 1966; 89(1):159–174

[88] el Masry WS, Biyani A. Incidence, management, and outcome of posttraumatic syringomyelia. In memory of Mr Bernard Williams. J Neurol Neurosurg Psychiatry. 1996; 60(2):141–146

[89] Bastian HC. On a case of concussion-lesion, with extensive secondary degenerations of the spinal cord, followed by general muscular atrophy. Med Chir Trans. 1867; 50:499–542.1

[90] Foster JB. Neurology of syringomyelia. In: Batzdorf U, ed. Syringomyelia: Current Concepts in Diagnosis and Treatment. Baltimore, MD: Williams & Wilkins; 1991:91–115

[91] Bonfield CM, Levi AD, Arnold PM, Okonkwo DO. Surgical management of post-traumatic syringomyelia. Spine. 2010; 35(21) Suppl:S245–S258

[92] Burchiel K. Neurosurgery: diagnosis and surgical management of cervical syringomyelia. West J Med. 1986; 145(1):84–85

[93] Matsumoto T, Symon L. Surgical management of syringomyelia–current results. Surg Neurol. 1989; 32(4):258–265

[94] Ohata K, Gotoh T, Matsusaka Y, et al. Surgical management of syringomyelia associated with spinal adhesive arachnoiditis. J Clin Neurosci. 2001; 8(1):40–42

[95] Pearce JM. Surgical management of syringomyelia. Br Med J (Clin Res Ed). 1981; 283(6301):1204–1205

[96] Ghobrial GM, Dalyai RT, Maltenfort MG, Prasad SK, Harrop JS, Sharan AD. Arachnolysis or cerebrospinal fluid diversion for adult-onset syringomyelia? A systematic review of the literature. World Neurosurg. 2015; 83(5):829–835

[97] Klekamp J. Treatment of posttraumatic syringomyelia. J Neurosurg Spine. 2012; 17(3):199–211

[98] Klekamp J. Treatment of syringomyelia related to nontraumatic arachnoid pathologies of the spinal canal. Neurosurgery. 2013; 72(3):376–389, discussion 389

[99] Than KD, Mummaneni PV. Perspective: surgical options for adult syringomyelia. World Neurosurg. 2015; 83(4):464–465

[100] Samii M, Klekamp J. Surgical results of 100 intramedullary tumors in relation to accompanying syringomyelia. Neurosurgery. 1994; 35(5):865–873, discussion 873

[101] Ghobrial GM, Amenta PS, Maltenfort M, et al. Longitudinal incidence and concurrence rates for traumatic brain injury and spine injury - a twenty year analysis. Clin Neurol Neurosurg. 2014; 123:174–180

[102] Krebs J, Koch HG, Hartmann K, Frotzler A. The characteristics of posttraumatic syringomyelia. Spinal Cord. 2016; 54(6):463–466

[103] Leahy HP, Beckley AA, Formal CS, Fried GW. Post-traumatic syringomyelia refractory to surgical intervention: a series of cases on recurrent syringomyelia. Spinal Cord Ser Cases. 2015; 1:15013

[104] Sadowsky CLMJ, McDonald JW. Activity-based restorative therapies: concepts and applications in spinal cord injury-related neurorehabilitation. Dev Disabil Res Rev. 2009; 15(2):112–116

[105] Barbeau H, Rossignol S. Recovery of locomotion after chronic spinalization in the adult cat. Brain Res. 1987; 412(1):84–95

[106] De Leon RD, Hodgson JA, Roy RR, Edgerton VR. Full weight-bearing hindlimb standing following stand training in the adult spinal cat. J Neurophysiol. 1998; 80(1):83–91

[107] Grillner S. Neurobiological bases of rhythmic motor acts in vertebrates. Science. 1985; 228(4696):143–149

[108] Grillner S, Wallén P. Central pattern generators for locomotion, with special reference to vertebrates. Annu Rev Neurosci. 1985; 8:233–261

[109] Grillner S, Zangger P. On the central generation of locomotion in the low spinal cat. Exp Brain Res. 1979; 34(2):241–261

[110] Grillner S, Rossignol S. On the initiation of the swing phase of locomotion in chronic spinal cats. Brain Res. 1978; 146(2):269–277

[111] Harkema SJHS, Hurley SL, Patel UK, Requejo PS, Dobkin BH, Edgerton VR. Human lumbosacral spinal cord interprets loading during stepping. J Neurophysiol. 1997; 77(2):797–811

[112] Lovely RGGR, Gregor RJ, Roy RR, Edgerton VR. Effects of training on the recovery of full-weight-bearing stepping in the adult spinal cat. Exp Neurol. 1986; 92(2):421–435

[113] Hubli M, Dietz V. The physiological basis of neurorehabilitation–locomotor training after spinal cord injury. J Neuroeng Rehabil. 2013; 10(5):5

[114] Dietz V, Colombo G, Jensen L. Locomotor activity in spinal man. Lancet. 1994; 344(8932):1260–1263

[115] Harkema SJ. Plasticity of interneuronal networks of the functionally isolated human spinal cord. Brain Res Brain Res Rev. 2008; 57(1):255–264

[116] Harkema S, Gerasimenko Y, Hodes J, et al. Effect of epidural stimulation of the lumbosacral spinal cord on voluntary movement, standing, and assisted stepping after motor complete paraplegia: a case study. Lancet. 2011; 377(9781):1938–1947

[117] Jilge B, Minassian K, Rattay F, et al. Initiating extension of the lower limbs in subjects with complete spinal cord injury by epidural lumbar cord stimulation. Exp Brain Res. 2004; 154(3):308–326

[118] Kuhn RA. Functional capacity of the isolated human spinal cord. Brain. 1950; 73(1):1–51

[119] Nadeau S, Jacquemin G, Fournier C, Lamarre Y, Rossignol S. Spontaneous motor rhythms of the back and legs in a patient with a complete spinal cord transection. Neurorehabil Neural Repair. 2010; 24(4):377–383

[120] Dimitrijevic MR, Gerasimenko Y, Pinter MM. Evidence for a spinal central pattern generator in humans. Ann N Y Acad Sci. 1998; 860:360–376

[121] Minassian K, Jilge B, Rattay F, et al. Stepping-like movements in humans with complete spinal cord injury induced by epidural stimulation of the lumbar cord: electromyographic study of compound muscle action potentials. Spinal Cord. 2004; 42(7):401–416

[122] Edgerton VR, Harkema S. Epidural stimulation of the spinal cord in spinal cord injury: current status and future challenges. Expert Rev Neurother. 2011; 11(10):1351–1353

[123] Sczesny-Kaiser M, Kowalewski R, Schildhauer TA, et al. Treadmill training with HAL exoskeleton: a novel approach for symptomatic therapy in patients with limb-girdle muscular dystrophy-preliminary study. Front Neurosci. 2017; 11:449

[124] Aach M, Cruciger O, Sczesny-Kaiser M, et al. Voluntary driven exoskeleton as a new tool for rehabilitation in chronic spinal cord injury: a pilot study. Spine J. 2014; 14(12):2847–2853

[125] Badner A, Siddiqui AM, Fehlings MG. Spinal cord injuries: how could cell therapy help? Expert Opin Biol Ther. 2017; 17(5):529–541

[126] Krucoff MO, Rahimpour S, Slutzky MW, Edgerton VR, Turner DA. Enhancing nervous system recovery through neurobiologics, neural interface training, and neurorehabilitation. Front Neurosci. 2016; 10:584

25 Clinical Trials Update: Where Do We Go from Here?

Jetan H. Badhiwala and Michael G. Fehlings

Abstract

Research in spinal cord injury (SCI) first entered the arena of clinical trials just over 30 years ago, commencing with the National Acute Spinal Cord Injury Study (NASCIS) I trial. Since then, there has been a flurry of trial activity in the field, spurred by the devastating cost of SCI to patients and families, and the economic footprint on society at large. Many of these trials have stirred controversy and have attracted criticism for their methodological shortcomings. This chapter provides a critical review of past and current clinical trials in SCI, in particular the findings of prospective randomized controlled trials, the difficulties encountered, and lessons learned that can be applied to future trials.

Keywords: spinal cord injury, randomized controlled trial, trial design, outcomes, patient selection, neuroprotective agents, quality-of-life indices, surgical decompression

25.1 Randomized Controlled Trials

25.1.1 Neuroprotection

Neuroprotective strategies attempt to counteract one or more of the secondary injury mechanisms in spinal cord injury (SCI).[1,2] To date, nine randomized controlled trials (RCTs) examining neuroprotective agents in SCI have been published (▶ Table 25.1).

Methylprednisolone, Naloxone, and Tirilazad

Three North American and one Japanese trials evaluated the efficacy of methylprednisolone (MP), theorized to block peroxidation of neuronal membrane lipids early in the secondary injury cascade following SCI.[3]

NASCIS I

The results of the National Acute Spinal Cord Injury Study (NASCIS) I trial[4] were published in 1984. It was the first RCT to evaluate the effect of a potential neuroprotective drug in acute SCI, and ushered in the clinical trial era of SCI. This was a multicenter, double-blinded RCT comparing two intravenous (IV) MP treatment protocols: (1) a high-dose protocol consisting of a 1,000-mg bolus at admission and daily thereafter for 10 days (11,000 mg total); or (2) a low-dose protocol consisting of a 100-mg bolus at admission and daily thereafter for 10 days (1,100 mg total). A total of 330 patients with acute SCI were enrolled from 1979 to 1981. No difference was noted in neurological recovery of motor function or pinprick and light touch sensation at 6 weeks or 6 months. There was also no significant difference in mortality. However, wound infections at both trauma and operative sites were greater in the high-dose group (risk ratio [RR] 3.55; 95% confidence interval [CI], 1.20–10.59).

It is important to recognize that NASCIS I was published in an era where corticosteroid use in acute SCI was ubiquitous, despite the lack of hard clinical evidence of benefit. There was a perceived lack of equipoise with regard to the benefit of corticosteroids, and this raised ethical concerns for randomizing patients to a non-MP arm. For this reason, a placebo control was not included. By failing to show a "dose response," and instead finding potential harm with higher-dose MP, the results of NASCIS I raised questions on the practice of routinely using corticosteroids in acute SCI. Nonetheless, the absence of a placebo control meant this study did little to address the absolute safety and efficacy of MP treatment in acute SCI. Moreover, subsequent data from animal studies suggested the peak serum MP concentrations obtained with the high-dose regimen would have been inadequate to produce a neuroprotective effect.[5]

NASCIS II

The shortcomings of NASCIS I prompted the NASCIS II trial,[6] which began in May 1985. The results of NASCIS I overturned prevailing dogma and provided equipoise, allowing use of a placebo control group in NASCIS II. Patients were randomized to MP, the opioid receptor blocker naloxone, or a placebo. NASCIS II used a higher dose of MP consisting of a 30 mg/kg bolus at admission followed by an infusion of 5.4 mg/kg/hour for the subsequent 23 hours. Naloxone was given as a bolus of 5.4 mg/kg and then a 4.0 mg/kg/hour infusion for the next 23 hours. The results of NASCIS II were published in 1990. A total of 487 patients were randomized. The primary analysis of neurological recovery at 6 months revealed improvements in pinprick and light touch sensation among patients receiving MP, but no differences in motor recovery. However, the analysis was stratified to compare those receiving treatment before versus after 8 hours. Those patients who had received MP within 8 hours of injury had significantly better motor and sensory recovery compared to placebo. This applied to both complete and incomplete injuries. Motor scores in the MP group improved by an additional 4.8 points as compared to placebo ($p = 0.03$). Morbidity and mortality were similar across all three treatment groups, but there was a nonsignificant trend toward more frequent wound infections in the MP group (7.1%) compared to placebo (3.6%). This was a landmark paper. The uptake was profound, and the publication and dissemination of these results led to widespread adoption of the "NASCIS II Protocol" for acute SCI, which was almost considered standard of care.[7] However, the trial went on to generate substantial controversy, including alleged nontransparency of analysis and misinterpretation of results.[7,8,9,10] A consistent criticism levied against NASCIS II is that the primary analysis was negative, and a treatment benefit was only seen in a subgroup analysis.[11] Moreover, subsequent studies, as discussed below, have failed to reproduce the results of NASCIS II, although these have suffered from important methodological limitations, as we have published previously.[5]

Table 25.1 Summary of randomized controlled trials in spinal cord injury

Trial	N	Eligibility criteria	Intervention	Control	Outcome	Key findings
NASCIS I[4]	330 (9 centers)	• Acute SCI • Age > 13 y • Admittance within 48 h after injury • No other severe comorbidity or life-threatening condition	• N=165 • MP (high-dose): 1,000-mg IV bolus and daily thereafter for 10 d	• N=165 • MP (low-dose): 100-mg IV bolus and daily thereafter for 10 d	• NASCIS motor and sensory scores	• No difference in motor or sensory scores at 6 wk or 6 mo • More frequent wound infections with high-dose MP: RR, 3.55; 95% CI, 1.20–10.59
NASCIS II[6]	487 (10 centers)	• Acute SCI • Age > 13 y • Randomization within 12 h of injury • No other severe comorbidity or life-threatening condition	• MP: N=162, 30 mg/kg IV bolus, then 5.4 mg/kg/h infusion for 23 h • Naloxone: N=154, 5.4 mg/kg IV bolus, then 4.0 mg/kg/h infusion for 23 h	• Placebo: N=171, bolus, then infusion	• NASCIS motor and sensory scores	• Improvement in motor function (change score: 16.0 vs. 11.2, p = 0.03) and sensation to pinprick (change scores: 11.4 vs. 6.6, p = 0.02) and touch (change score: 8.9 vs. 4.3, p = 0.03) at 6 mo in patients treated with MP within 8 h of injury, as compared to placebo • No difference in motor or sensory recovery in patients treated with naloxone or MP more than 8 h after injury
NASCIS III[12]	499 (16 centers)	• Acute SCI • Age > 13 y • Randomization within 6 h of injury • Able to receive study drug within 8 h • No other severe comorbidity or life-threatening condition • Weight < 109 kg	• MP: 5.4 mg/kg/h IV infusion for 48 h • Tirilazad: 2.5 mg/kg IV bolus over 15–20 min every 6 h for 48 h • All patients received an IV bolus of MP (30 mg/kg) before randomization	• MP: 5.4 mg/kg/h IV infusion for 24 h	• ASIA grade • ASIA motor scores • FIM	• Nonsignificant trend toward improved motor recovery at 6 wk (p = 0.09) and 6 mo (p = 0.07) after injury with MP for 48 vs. 24 h • Significant improvement in motor recovery at 6 wk (change score: 12.5 vs. 7.6, p = 0.04) and 6 mo (change score: 17.6 vs. 11.2, p = 0.01) in patients treated with MP for 48 vs. 24 h for patients who started treatment at 3–8 h after injury • Patients in the 48-h regimen were more likely to improve 1 full neurologic grade (p = 0.03) at 6 mo, show more improvement in 6-mo FIM (p = 0.08), and to have more severe sepsis and severe pneumonia than patients in the 24-h MP group and tirilazad group • No difference in motor recovery rates between patients treated with tirilazad vs. 24-h MP
Otani et al[13]	158 (42 centers)	• Acute SCI • Able to initiate treatment within 8 h of injury	• MP: 30 mg/kg IV bolus, then 5.4 mg/kg/h infusion for 23 h	• Placebo	• NASCIS motor and sensory scores	• Nonsignificant improvement in motor recovery with MP vs. placebo (3.9 points)

Table 25.1 continued

Trial	N	Eligibility criteria	Intervention	Control	Outcome	Key findings
Matsumoto et al[14]	46 (1 center)	• Acute cervical SCI • Treated without surgery • Randomization within 8 h of injury • No gunshot wound or life-threatening morbidity	• MP: $N = 23$, 30 mg/kg IV bolus, then 5.4 mg/kg/h infusion for 23 h	• Placebo: $N=23$	• Complication rates	• Significantly greater rate of pulmonary complication with MP (34.8%) vs. placebo (4.34%) ($p = 0.009$) within 2 mo • Significantly greater rate of gastrointestinal complication with MP (17.4%) vs. placebo (0) ($p = 0.036$) within 2 mo • Greater prevalence of pulmonary complications in patients over 60 years old ($p = 0.029$) within 2 mo
Geisler et al[15] (GM1 ganglioside 1)	34 (1 center)	• Acute SCI • Age ≥18 y • Able to receive study drug within 72 h of injury	• GM1: 100 mg IV daily for 18 to 32 doses	• Placebo	• Frankel grade • ASIA motor score	• Better distribution of improvement in Frankel grade from baseline to 1-y follow-up with GM1 vs. placebo ($p = 0.034$) • Significantly greater improvement in ASIA motor score from baseline to 1-y follow-up with GM1 (369 points) vs. placebo (21.6 points) ($p = 0.047$)
Geisler et al[16] (GM1 ganglioside 2 [multicenter])	760 (28 centers)	• Acute SCI • Age ≥18 y • Able to receive study drug within 72 h of injury • Substantial motor deficit in at least one of the lower extremities	• GM1 (low-dose): $N = 331$, 300 mg loading dose, then 100 mg daily for 56 d • GM1 (high-dose): $N = 99$, 600 mg loading dose, then 200 mg daily for 56 d • All patients were to receive the NASCIS II dose regimen of MP starting within 8 h of injury	• Placebo: $N = 330$, loading dose, then 56 d	• ASIA grade • ASIA motor and sensory scores • Benzel grade	• No difference in fraction of patients exhibiting marked recovery (at least a two-grade improvement in the modified Benzel classification from baseline) at 26 wk with high-dose (2.0%) vs. low-dose (3.6%) vs. placebo (7.3%) • Greater proportion of patients achieving marked recovery in the GM1 group (11.9%) at 8 wk (end of treatment period) vs. placebo (8.2%)
Pitts et al[18] (TRH)	20 (1 center)	• Acute SCI • Randomization within 12 h of injury	• TRH: 0.2 mg/kg IV bolus followed by 0.2 mg/kg/h infusion over 6 h	• Placebo: equal volume of IV physiological saline	• Sunnybrook score • NASCIS motor and sensory scores	• No treatment effect in patients with complete injuries • For incomplete injuries, significantly higher motor, sensory, and Sunnybrook scores with TRH than placebo treatment at 4 mo
Pointillart et al[21] (nimodipine)	106 (1 center)	• Acute SCI • Age: 15–65 y • Hospitalization within 8 h of injury • No multiple trauma or head injury with GCS<13	• Nimodipine: $N = 27$, 0.015 mg/kg/h for 2 h followed by 0.03 mg/kg/h for 7 d • MP: $N = 27$, 30 mg/kg over 1 h, then 5.4 mg/kg/h infusion for 23 h • nimodipine + MP: $N = 27$	• No medication: $N = 25$	• ASIA grade • ASIA motor and sensory scores	• No significant difference among four groups in any of the ASIA scores • More frequent infectious complications in patients treated with MP • No influence on neurological outcome with early surgery (<8 h)

Table 25.1 continued

Trial	N	Eligibility criteria	Intervention	Control	Outcome	Key findings
Tadie et al[25] (gacyclidine)	280 (31 centers)	• Acute SCI • Age: 16–65 y • Weight < 110 kg • Maximum ASIA motor score 15 points for most severely injured lower limb • Normal consciousness (documented GCS) • Able to receive first injection of gacyclidine within 2 h of injury • Able to undergo surgical decompression within 8 h of injury • Controlled BP before injection of drug (SBP no lower than 90 mm Hg for more than 15 min)	• Gacyclidine: 0.005 mg/kg (N = 70), 0.010 mg/kg (N = 71), or 0.020 mg/kg (N = 70) IV twice at an interval of 4 h, the first injection as early as possible within 2 h of injury, the second one 4 h after the first injection	• Placebo: N = 69	• ASIA grade • ASIA motor and sensory scores • FIM	• No significant difference between groups in ASIA score at 1 y
Vaccaro et al[30] (surgery)	62 (1 center)	• Acute cervical SCI (C3–T1) • ASIA grade A–D • Age: 15–75 y	• Early surgery (<72 h): N = 34	• Late surgery (> 5 d): N = 28	• ASIA grade • Frankel grade • ASIA motor score	• No difference in length of acute post-operative ICU stay, length of inpatient rehabilitation, or improvement in ASIA grade or motor score between early (mean 1.8 d) vs. late (mean 16.8 d)
Casha et al[29] (minocycline)	52 (1 center)	• Age ≥16 y • Acute SCI • ASIA level C0–T11 • Randomization and administration of study drug within 12 h	• Minocycline: N = 27, 200 mg or 400 mg IV twice daily × 7 d	• Placebo: N = 25, equal volume normal saline × 7 d	• ASIA motor score	• 6 points greater motor recovery with minocycline vs. placebo (95% CI, 3–14, $p = 0.20$) • No difference in recovery for thoracic SCI • Difference in motor recovery of 14 points that approached significance for patients with cervical SCI with minocycline vs. placebo (95% CI, 0–28, $p = 0.05$)

Abbreviations: ASIA, American Spinal Cord Injury Association; BP, blood pressure; CI, confidence interval; FIM, functional independence measurement; GCS, Glasgow Coma Scale; ICU, intensive care unit; IV, intravenous; MP, methylprednisolone; NASCIS, National Acute Spinal Cord Injury Study; RR, risk ratio; SBP, systolic blood pressure; SCI, spinal cord injury; TRH, thyrotropin-releasing hormone.

NASCIS III

NASCIS III[12] was borne out of the unresolved question about the optimal duration of MP treatment and parallel preclinical data advancing our understanding of the duration of secondary injury mechanisms post-SCI. The question was whether a longer duration of MP treatment (48 hours) would afford greater neuroprotection and better neurological outcomes than the standard 24-hour regimen, while remaining safe. NASCIS III did not have a placebo arm given the positive results of NASCIS II. A total of 499 patients were randomized to either (1) a 48-hour MP protocol (30 mg/kg bolus followed by 5.4 mg/kg/hour); (2) a 24-hour MP protocol (30 mg/kg bolus followed by 5.4 mg/kg/hour); or (3) a 2.5 mg/kg bolus infusion of tirilazad (a 24-amino steroid shown in animal studies to have neuroprotective potential) every 6 hours for 48 hours. In the overall analysis, the 48-hour MP group showed improved motor recovery at 6 months, though this did not reach statistical significance ($p = 0.07$). Mortality was comparable; however, the 48-hour group had an increased risk of severe pneumonia ($p = 0.02$) and severe sepsis ($p = 0.07$). In the timing-related secondary analysis, for patients receiving treatment initiated 3 to 8 hours after injury, the 48-hour MP group had an additional 6 points in motor recovery at 6 months, as compared to the 24-hour MP group ($p = 0.01$). The authors concluded that patients who receive MP within 3 hours should be maintained on MP for 24 hours, whereas those initiated on therapy 3 to 8 hours after injury should receive the 48-hour protocol, accepting a potentially greater risk of infectious complications.

Other MP Trials

In a Japanese study, Otani et al[13] randomly assigned 158 patients either to the NASCIS II MP protocol, started within 8 hours of injury, or to standard medical care. Patients treated with MP experienced an additional 3.9 points in motor recovery compared to the control group on average, although this did not reach statistical significance. However, concerns regarding losses to follow-up and inadequate blinding threaten the validity of these findings.[5] Matsumoto et al[14] evaluated complication occurrence in 46 patients with cervical SCI randomized to either the NASCIS II MP regimen or a placebo. The MP group had a higher rate of pulmonary ($p = 0.009$) and gastrointestinal ($p = 0.036$) complications. A criticism with this trial is that the treatment groups were substantially unbalanced, with a disproportionately high proportion of less severe injuries (Frankel D) in the placebo group.

GM1 Ganglioside

The initial trial of GM1 (monosialotetrahexosylganglioside)[15] ganglioside was published in 1991. This was a single-center, randomized, double-blinded, placebo-controlled pilot study that evaluated the safety and efficacy of GM1 ganglioside as a neuroprotective agent in acute SCI. A total of 37 patients were enrolled between 1986 and 1987. Patients received 100 mg of either GM1 ganglioside or placebo intravenously per day for 18 to 32 doses, with the first dose given within 72 hours of injury. The authors found improved Frankel grades ($p = 0.034$) and American Spinal Cord Injury Association (ASIA) motor scores ($p = 0.047$) at 1-year follow-up in the GM1 ganglioside group

compared to the placebo group, with no difference in adverse events. This single-center pilot study set the stage for the later multicenter trial of GM1 ganglioside.[16] This study enrolled 760 patients with ASIA A, B, C, and D injuries from 1992 to 1997. Patients were randomized to either 100 mg GM1 ganglioside, 200 mg GM1 ganglioside, or placebo initiated within 72 hours of injury and given daily for 56 days. The primary efficacy outcome was "marked recovery," defined as two grades of improvement on the modified Benzel scale, at 26 weeks. The primary analysis was negative, although there was a nonsignificant trend favoring treatment in a subgroup analysis of patients with ASIA B injuries. Interestingly, the GM1 ganglioside group recovered function earlier, so that at 8 weeks (at the conclusion of therapy), the primary outcome favored the treatment groups. However, the control group "caught up" over the course of follow-up.

TRH

On the basis of preclinical data demonstrating improved long-term behavioral recovery with thyrotropin-releasing hormone (TRH) administered post-SCI,[17] Pitts et al[18] randomized 20 patients with SCI within 12 hours of injury to TRH or placebo. The trial was double-blinded. Patients were stratified by complete or incomplete injury. The treatment group received a 0.2 mg/kg IV bolus of TRH followed by a 0.2 mg/kg/hour infusion over 6 hours; the placebo group received an equal volume of saline. The authors found no treatment effect in the complete injury group. In patients with incomplete SCI, the TRH-treated group had significantly higher motor, sensory, and Sunnybrook scores than the placebo group. Unfortunately, the results of this trial have not been replicated.

Nimodipine

One of the common final pathophysiological mechanisms in SCI is ischemia and associated vascular changes. Nimodipine is a calcium channel blocker with vasodilatory effects. Experimental models of SCI found nimodipine reduced the decrease in spinal cord blood flow in the proximity of the traumatic lesion.[19,20] This provided the impetus for a randomized trial of nimodipine in human SCI. In France, 106 patients with SCI were randomized to one of four groups: nimodipine (0.015 mg/kg/hour for 2 hours followed by 0.03 mg/kg/hour for 7 days), MP (NASCIS II dose), nimodipine plus MP, or neither agents.[21] An effort was made to treat patients requiring surgical decompression as early as possible. The results of this trial were published in 2000. No treatment benefit was observed, and all treatment groups had similar neurological recovery, as measured by ASIA scores, to placebo. Similar to the NASCIS studies, this trial found evidence of greater infectious complications in the MP group. Early surgery (< 8 hours) did not influence neurological outcome relative to surgery at the 8- to 24-hour mark, although patients were not randomized according to early surgery.

Gacyclidine

Another French study evaluated gacyclidine. An important secondary injury mechanism in SCI is neuronal release of excitotoxic glutamate, which results in abnormal levels of Ca^{2+}

influx and eventually local cell death.[22,23] Gacyclidine is an N-methyl-D-aspartate (glutamate receptor) antagonist with the ability to prevent glutamate-induced neuronal death.[24] A clinical trial of gacyclidine for SCI was undertaken and the results published in 2003.[25] There were strict inclusion and exclusion criteria which included: male or nonpregnant female, age 18 to 65 years, weight < 110 kg, maximum ASIA motor score 15 points for most severely injured lower limb, normal consciousness, documented Glasgow Coma Scale (GCS) score, able to receive first injection of gacyclidine within 2 hours of injury, able to undergo decompression surgery within 8 hours, and controlled blood pressure (systolic blood pressure no lower than 90 mm Hg for more than 15 minutes) prior to injection of drug. Patients were randomized to one of four groups: placebo or one of three doses of gacyclidine (0.005, 0.010, or 0.020 mg/kg). The drug was administered as early as possible within 2 hours of injury and again at 4 hours after the first injection. A total of 272 patients were evaluated. No significant difference was observed in ASIA or functional independence measurement (FIM) scores between any of the treatment or placebo groups at 1 year.

Minocycline

The antibiotic minocycline has been found to have neuroprotective properties in preclinical studies.[26] In the context of SCI, it has been found to improve neurological recovery owing to reduced apoptosis of oligodendrocytes and microglia.[27,28] Casha et al[29] conducted a phase II double-blinded, randomized, placebo-controlled trial of minocycline for acute SCI. Twenty-seven patients were randomized to IV minocycline and 25 to placebo. At 1-year follow-up, patients treated with minocycline experienced 6 points greater motor recovery as compared to placebo, though this did not reach statistical significance. No difference was observed for thoracic SCI. However, a trend toward improved recovery with minocycline, a difference of 14 points, was observed for cases of cervical SCI. Plans are being developed to further investigate the possible efficacy of minocycline in a phase III investigation.

25.1.2 Surgery

There has been one surgical RCT on the topic of SCI to date, relating to the timing of surgical decompression.

Timing of Surgical Decompression

A key area of contention in SCI treatment has been the value of early surgical decompression. Vaccaro et al[30] evaluated early (< 72 hours) versus delayed (> 5 days) surgical decompression for cervical SCI in a randomized trial format. Eligible patients were 15 to 75 years old, had an ASIA grade A to D injury with a neurological level of C3–T1, were admitted within 48 hours of injury to allow for possible surgery within 72 hours of injury, and had radiographically documented spinal cord compression from an acute traumatic event. There were 34 patients in the early surgery group, with a mean time to surgery of 1.8 days. There were 28 patients in the delayed surgery group, with a mean time to surgery of 16.8 days. Follow-up was approximately 1 year. No differences were found in ICU length of stay, length of inpatient

rehabilitation, or improvement in ASIA grade or motor score. This study was limited by its small size. Moreover, a time window of 72 hours may have been too wide, as many authors would consider "early" surgery to be within 24 hours.

Although not a randomized trial, we feel the Surgical Timing in Acute Spinal Cord Injury Study (STASCIS)[31] deserves special mention. This was a multicenter, international, prospective cohort study, the largest of its kind, to address the question of timing of surgical decompression for acute SCI. Adults aged 16 to 80 years with cervical SCI were enrolled from 2002 to 2009 at six North American centers. A total of 313 patients were included. Of these, 182 underwent early surgery (< 24 hours) at a mean of 14.2 hours from injury. The other 131 patients underwent delayed surgery (> 24 hours) at a mean of 28.3 hours. Follow-up data were available for 22 patients at 6 months post-injury. A greater proportion of patients who underwent early surgery achieved an improvement of 2 or more ASIA grades (19.8%) compared to delayed surgery (8.8%). Recognizing that there is heterogeneity in the potential for recovery depending on the severity of the initial injury, the authors conducted a multivariate analysis adjusting for preoperative neurological status and also for steroid administration. Still, the odds of a 2 or greater ASIA grade improvement was 2.8-fold greater among patients who underwent early rather than delayed surgery. This was a pivotal study, and has certainly altered practice, providing robust evidence for early surgical intervention in SCI.

25.2 Lessons Learned

25.2.1 Trial Design

The RCT is the "gold standard" study design. Here, we have given little attention to phase I and phase II trials. Phase I trials are designed to test safety and toxicity, and these generally enroll a dozen or so patients in a nonrandomized fashion. Phase II trials assess the feasibility of a therapeutic strategy and the potential for efficacy. These usually enroll up to 50 patients, without placebo.[8] Phase III trials are poised to evaluate the effectiveness of a therapy, and these follow a randomized format. The goal with a carefully designed and conducted RCT is to eliminate, or at least mitigate, any sources of potential bias. Especially for therapies with unproven benefit, it is important that a placebo group be included, as exemplified by this shortcoming of the NASCIS I trial. The randomization process should ensure concealment of treatment allocation. Patients and study personnel (i.e., outcome assessors) should be blinded to treatment allocation. Some authors have advocated for use of adaptive randomization strategies in SCI RCTs.[8] This format uses bayesian statistical methods with frequent reassessment of accumulated data to update allocation of patients to treatment groups. It has the advantage of potentially enhancing the efficiency of trials by allowing for smaller sample sizes. This is especially relevant to SCI, where there are only 11,000 new cases annually in North America, and accrual of large patient numbers poses a real challenge.[32]

25.2.2 Heterogeneity of SCI

The heterogeneity of human SCI makes it a difficult topic to study. Cases vary with regard to patient population and mechanism, level, and severity of injury; this has important implications for potential responses to therapy. For example, patients with ASIA A (i.e., complete) injuries may be too severely injured to respond to any therapy that does not regenerate the cavitated, necrotic segment. Alternatively, some have argued that these patients actually represent a more homogeneous group than those with incomplete injuries insofar as potential for recovery goes.[33] Several prior clinical trials have disregarded this heterogeneity, perhaps because they were trying to find a "one size fits all" therapy. However, failing to address this heterogeneity may threaten not only the external validity of a study, but also its internal validity. For example, in the trial of MP published by Matsumoto and colleagues,[14] the treatment and placebo groups were unbalanced with regard to severity of injury, with more patients with less severe injuries being allocated to placebo. The bias introduced makes it difficult to trust the findings of this study.

There are two options to address this heterogeneity within the design of an RCT. The first is to decide to focus on a relatively homogeneous population—for example, adult patients with an ASIA A SCI with a neurological level between C4 and C8. The advantage of this approach is that it allows a targeted therapeutic approach, reducing "noise" created from having a heterogeneous population. The drawbacks are that the study findings will only be applicable to a smaller segment of the total SCI population (i.e., limited in external validity), and patient accrual will be slower owing to the more limited eligibility criteria. The second option is to stratify randomization by important variables (e.g., ASIA grade, level of injury), employing a block design. This ensures an equal distribution of important confounders between the two treatment groups. This approach retains a broader generalizability of the findings, but still, there is the possibility of "losing" an important signal in all the noise generated by having such a heterogeneous study population.

25.2.3 Patient Selection

Related to the above discussion on heterogeneity of SCI, precisely defining inclusion and exclusion criteria is of paramount importance. A clinical trial should begin with a clearly defined research question. The PICOT format is useful: P, population; I, intervention; C, control group; O, outcome; and T, timing.

With respect to patient selection, beyond age cutoffs, important issues to consider are level and severity of injury. Thoracic injuries are rare, accounting for only 10 to 15% of SCI.[32] Nonetheless, phase I trials concerned with safety tend to be limited to (usually complete) thoracic injuries, given that any complication in a thoracic ASIA A injury is likely to have a minimal impact on function. Of course, recruitment is likely to be slow owing to numbers. On the other hand, cervical injuries are more common, but a treatment-related adverse event could have devastating consequences regardless of ASIA grade, owing to potential ascending injury. Likewise, C4 or C5 is often the highest level of injury at which patients should be eligible for enrollment in a trial, because of concern of possible respiratory compromise for any potential mishap. It is important to consider that studies examining ASIA A patients would need either an extremely effective therapy or large patient numbers to detect any neurological recovery. Many patients with ASIA B through D injuries will improve naturally, as discussed further

below, meaning large patient numbers would be required to discern any treatment benefit over the natural history of these injuries.[34]

The timing of intervention in relation to the disease course depends on the nature of the intervention and the question being asked. In general, neuroprotective strategies should enroll patients in the acute stages of SCI (< 72 hours), as this is the period where secondary injury mechanisms are involved. Trials of regenerative therapies should target patients in the subacute stages (72 hours to 2 weeks), and rehabilitative trials in the chronic phase (12 + months).[8]

25.2.4 Assessment of Neurological Recovery

Accurate, reliable, and clinically relevant neurological assessment is critical to any trial in SCI. Many systems have been developed and used over the years. The first of these is the Frankel system, which was developed in 1967 and includes five grades of severity: A, complete neurological injury; B, preserved sensation only; C, preserved motor, nonfunctional; D, preserved motor, functional; and E, normal motor function.[35] The primary advantage of this system is its simplicity and ease of use. Analyzing change in Frankel grade permits researchers to plot the neurological recovery of a large series of patients in an intuitive and easy-to-understand way. The real drawback of the Frankel system was the imprecise definition of grade A, C, and D injuries, later to be improved by the ASIA system. The Sunnybrook system,[36] used in the TRH trial,[18] was the next to be developed. This system improved on the clinical grading of acute SCI and quantification of recovery in patients, as compared to the Frankel grade, by defining 10 severity grades and 17 ways in which neurological function could improve or deteriorate. The NASCIS system, used in the NASCIS I trial,[4] incorporated a numerical scoring system of motor and sensory function that evolved from the motor scoring system devised by Lucas and Ducker.[37] However, as discussed further below, this system proved difficult to understand. The ASIA standards, first devised in 1982 and revised several times thereafter (eventually becoming the International Standards of Neurological Classification of Spinal Cord Injury [ISNCSCI]), brought several improvements due to more robust motor and sensory scoring methods.[38] By extension, this system more accurately defined "complete injuries" (based on sacral sparing) and grade C and D injuries (based on motor scores below the injured level). However, grade C and D injuries do have a "ceiling effect," whereby patients rarely improve sufficiently to advance to the next grade. The modified Benzel system, used in the GM1 ganglioside trials,[15,16] defines seven grades of severity and incorporates sphincter control and ambulation. However, because walking cannot usually be assessed in the acute stages of SCI, its use in monitoring patients' recovery in a longitudinal manner is limited.

The NASCIS trials used a complex and difficult to understand scheme consisting of expanded motor (70-point) and sensory (58-point) scores, with only data from the right limbs used in the analysis. The scheme contained five motor and five sensory categorizations, three broad categorizations of completeness, and five completeness-by-level categorizations. Yet, there was no categorization by discrete segmental level.[39] Difficulty in understanding the measurement method has been an important point of contention in acceptance of the NASCIS trials' conclusions. Other critics claimed selective reporting in the NASCIS trial, given the myriad of possible combinations within the measurement scheme.[39] The authors did not precisely define how the scores would be analyzed a priori. They presented some measurement possibilities, but not all of the data were presented. In reality, the findings of the NASCIS trials should stand on their own. However, this point highlights the need to use consistent and standardized measurement schemes in SCI trials—in other words, we need to speak the same language. This not only can increase global uptake of a trial's findings, but also can permit some comparison of the magnitude of treatment effects of different therapies from different trials. To this end, the development, refinement, and international acceptance of the ISNCSCI/ASIA standards has been an important step forward.

25.2.5 Assessment of Functional Outcomes

In the early stages, SCI trials, including NASCIS I, NASCIS II, and the first GM1 ganglioside trial, assessed only neurological outcome or impairment, without assessing functional outcomes. The limitations of this became readily apparent. The authors of NASCIS II, for example, had great difficulty explaining the functional impact on the patient of a 5- or 6-point improvement on the expanded motor score. The third NASCIS trial was the first to incorporate a measurement of activity beyond a measurement of impairment. This was the FIM, which evaluates the overall level of independence of a disabled person, including eating, grooming, and ambulation. The FIM was originally developed for assessing many non-SCI conditions.[40] Other functional outcome measures have since been developed, including the Spinal Cord Injury Measure[41,42] and the Walking Index in Spinal Cord Injury.[43,44]

25.2.6 Assessment of Quality of Life Outcomes

Patient-reported outcomes are being increasingly used in clinical trials in all areas of medicine, and spine surgery is no exception.[45] Hence, in addition to outcomes measuring neurological function and functional independence, there is a need for SCI trials to employ quality of life outcome measures using validated instruments, such as the Short-Form 36 (SF-36),[46] Euro-QoL five dimensions (EQ-5D),[47] or Short-Form six dimensions (SF-6D).[48] These provide a global assessment of patients' self-perceived health. The domains of the SF-36, for example, include physical functioning, bodily pain, mental health, physical role functioning, emotional role functioning, social role functioning, vitality, and general health perceptions. Much of the focus of SCI research to date, rightfully so, has centered on finding therapies that result in objective improvements in motor and/or sensory function. Without this, one would assume the impact on quality of life would be irrelevant. Although somewhat true, the efficacy of therapy aside, studying the impact of SCI on patients' self-perceived quality of life is an extremely important endeavor, because it informs clinicians, families, and, most importantly, patients about what they can expect for their quality of life after this life-altering event, as reported by other patients.

25.2.7 Assessment of Imaging Outcomes

In recent years, there have been substantial advances in our ability to image the injured spinal cord at high resolution, especially with MRI. Work in our own group has led to the development of clinically feasible microstructural MRI protocols to quantify cervical spinal cord tissue injury using diffusion tensor imaging (DTI), magnetization transfer (MT), and T2*-weighted imaging.[49] We have found the signal intensity ratio of white matter to gray matter on T2*-weighted imaging to be a useful biomarker of white matter injury, showing stronger correlation with focal motor and sensory deficits than cross-sectional area, fractional anisotropy, and the MT ratio.[50] It is indeed more a probability than a possibility that SCI trials in the future will employ these or similar techniques, both at baseline for their prognostic utility and as an outcome measure.

25.2.8 Definition of Primary and Secondary Outcomes

The outcomes of any clinical trial should be carefully and precisely defined a priori, as this has a profound impact on how the results are interpreted. The time-related treatment effect in the NASCIS II trial,[6] for example, was only seen in a subgroup analysis, which the trial would not have been powered to detect. The primary analysis showed no benefit, and NASCIS II is considered a "negative" trial.[11] Another example is the multicenter GM1 ganglioside study.[16] This was a "negative" trial, with no significant difference found in the achievement of "marked recovery" according to the modified Benzel scale at 26 weeks. However, had the outcome been defined a priori as being measured at the conclusion of treatment, the authors could have claimed benefit, and this would have been considered a "positive" trial. Of course, we are more interested in long-term outcome than any short-term benefit, but this example speaks to how the definition of outcomes in a clinical trial can have a bearing on the interpretation and uptake of its results.

One issue with assessing neurological outcomes in SCI trials is that owing to the heterogeneity of SCI, as discussed above, patients differ with regard to potential for recovery. In the NASCIS III trial,[12] baseline scores were included as covariates in the analysis of variance (ANOVA), so as to adjust for the effect of baseline measures on neurological change. Likewise, some authors have advocated for using percent changes in ASIA motor or sensory scores, rather than absolute changes.[8]

25.2.9 Method of Outcomes Assessment

The validity of any RCT's findings hinges upon the assumption that the outcomes were assessed in a reliable way, and can be trusted. However, neurological examination of the SCI patient poses several challenges, particularly in the acute setting (i.e., the initial examination). For example, the exam may be difficult to perform, and the data unreliable, in the context of intoxication, altered level of consciousness from a concomitant head injury, or the presence of neurogenic and/or systemic shock. Often, the polytrauma patient may be intubated and/or sedated. Outcome assessors need to be rigorously trained and re-evaluated, and there should be high interrater reliability. In this regard, the multicenter GM1 ganglioside study was the first of its kind to provide training in the performance of ISNCS-CI exams and to perform reliability assessments of the trained examiners.[39,51]

The optimal interval after injury to obtain an accurate and reliable examination has been questioned by many groups.[52] Burns et al[34] found that 24 to 48 hours after injury, ASIA A patients can be predicted with approximately 97.4% accuracy. The real issue pertains to the "instability" of the baseline neurological exam in patients with incomplete injuries, as many of these patients experience an early grade change. In fact, it is estimated that approximately 60% of patients with ASIA grades B through D injuries improve to a higher grade.[34] This is thought to be due to the spinal cord's inherent ability for recovery, driven by resolution of acute injury events or secondary mechanisms of injury, or regrowth or regeneration. Ultimately, Burns et al[34] proposed that ASIA B or higher grade injuries should be excluded from some early trials. Other authors have suggested that, if possible, acute studies should begin 24 to 48 hours after injury; accurate scoring of neurological function is imperative in studies that need to start before the 24-hour mark.[8]

25.3 Future and Ongoing Clinical Trials

25.3.1 RISCIS (Riluzole)

Riluzole is a benzothiazole anticonvulsant drug that is approved by the United States FDA for the treatment of amyotrophic lateral sclerosis (ALS), where it has been shown to improve survival by modulation of excitatory neurotransmission and neuroprotective mechanisms.[53] During the secondary injury cascade of SCI, there is constitutive activation of voltage-gated Na^+ channels, resulting in an increase in intracellular Na^+ concentrations.[54] This results in cellular swelling through reversal of the osmotic gradient, and also intracellular acidosis.[54,55] Furthermore, the influx of Na^+ promotes influx of Ca^{2+} through the Na^+–Ca^{2+} exchanger, leading to extracellular release of the excitatory neurotransmitter glutamate.[55] The ensuing events lead to local cell death from cytotoxic edema, intracellular acidosis, and glutaminergic excitotoxicity. Riluzole exerts its neuroprotective properties through sodium channel blockade and mitigation of glutamatergic toxicity. In animal models of SCI, the Fehlings group has found riluzole prevents aberrant sodium release and glutamate imbalance, leading to functional recovery.[56,57] A phase I clinical trial evaluating the safety and pharmacokinetics of riluzole in the setting of acute SCI was completed in 2011 (ClinicalTrials.gov NCT00876889).[58] This trial showed improved ASIA motor scores and a similar complication profile compared to matched patients in the North American Clinical Trials Network (NACTN) SCI Registry. The results of this trial provided the impetus for a phase IIB/III RCT, Riluzole in Acute Spinal Cord Injury Study (RISCIS), which commenced in

January 2014 and is currently ongoing (ClinicalTrials.gov NCT01597518).[59] The findings of this trial will provide level 1 evidence regarding the efficacy of riluzole for acute SCI. Many of the points discussed in this chapter were considered in the design of RISCIS. We use this as a platform to summarize and further discuss some of the key issues and considerations in SCI trial design.

RISCIS follows a double-blinded, placebo-controlled, RCT design. There are 28 participating centers, 19 in the United States, 4 in Canada, 3 in Australia, and 2 in New Zealand. Patients are randomized in a 1:1 ratio to riluzole or placebo. Randomization sequence is stratified by site and uses randomly permuted block sizes of 2 and 4. Allocation is concealed by use of an opaque envelope that contains a unique number corresponding to the number on a prestocked medication container containing either riluzole or placebo. Subjects, treating physicians, and data collectors are blinded to treatment allocation.

Investigation of the neuroprotective potential of riluzole in acute SCI is backed by good science, with several preclinical models demonstrating benefit in traumatic and nontraumatic (i.e., degenerative cervical myelopathy) forms of SCI.[60,61,62,63] Moreover, the drug has an established safety profile from its use in humans with ALS.[64] RISCIS has a clear research question: Does riluzole improve neurological recovery in adults suffering an acute SCI compared to placebo, as measured by change in ASIA motor score from baseline to 180 days post-SCI? It is useful to consider the PICOT format.

Eligible patients are adults age 18 to 75 years (inclusive). The trial focuses on a somewhat more homogeneous population of cervical SCI. Included patients have suffered an acute SCI, with an ASIA grade of A, B, or C and a neurological level of C4–C8 based on initial evaluation. Patients must be able to receive the investigational drug within 12 hours of injury. Patients must also be able to cooperate with completion of a standard neurological examination by ASIA (ISNCSCI) standards. As discussed previously, several factors can influence the accuracy of the neurological examination of an SCI patient (e.g., intoxication, sedation, head injury). For this reason, patients with a significant concomitant head injury (GCS < 14) or a preexisting neurological or mental disorder, which could preclude accurate evaluation and follow-up, are excluded.

With regard to the intervention and control, patients in the experimental arm receive 100 mg of riluzole every 12 hours for two doses in the first 24 hours after injury, and 50 mg twice daily for the following 13 days. Medication is administered orally or via nasogastric tube. The control group receives a placebo capsule identical in shape, size, and color to the riluzole capsule at the same schedule.

In terms of outcomes, a variety of validated measures evaluating neurological function, disability, functional outcome, and quality of life have been defined a priori as outcomes of interest. The primary outcome measure is a change in ASIA motor score from baseline to 180 days. This was used to perform a sample size calculation. A sample size of 316 patients was calculated to have 90% power to detect a 9-point difference in change in ASIA motor score with a one-tailed $\alpha = 0.025$. RISCIS aims to enroll 351 patients accounting for losses to follow-up (estimated to be 10%). Secondary efficacy outcomes include change in ASIA grade from baseline to 180 days and score on the Spinal Cord Independence Measure (SCIM) III at 180 days.[65]

The SCIM is a comprehensive rating scale that measures the ability of SCI patients to perform everyday tasks, and provides a measure of functional outcome. Another functional outcome includes sensorimotor upper limb function, as evaluated by the Graded Redefined Assessment of Strength Sensibility and Prehension (GRASSP).[66] Disabling pain is assessed by the Pain Numeric Rating Scale. Quality of life is assessed by the SF-36[46] and EQ-5D.[47] All adverse events are recorded throughout the trial on an ongoing basis. Outcomes were assessed at 180 days based on prior evidence that major functional recovery after SCI occurs by this point in time.[58] Given the heterogeneity in potential for neurological recovery, a preplanned subgroup analysis will compare outcomes among patients separated by ASIA grade.

With respect to timing, riluzole (or placebo) is to be administered within 12 hours of injury. This is based on preclinical data. In rodents with severe cervical SCI, the Fehlings group found administration of riluzole at 1 and 3 hours postinjury contributed to sensorimotor function improvement, improved axonal condition, and reduced apoptosis and inflammation.[57] Because pathological changes in SCI peak approximately fourfold more rapidly in rats than in humans, the optimal timing of riluzole administration in humans was estimated to be within 12 hours.

25.3.2 Spring (Vx-210/Cethrin)

It is well known that axonal growth and regeneration is blocked following central nervous system injury. Several growth inhibitory pathways converge in signaling to Rho, an intracellular GTPase.[67] Activation of Rho and downstream activation of Rho-associated kinase leads to an imbalance in the phosphorylation state of myosin light chain and, as a result, a collapse of the growth cone scaffold and axon growth arrest.[68] C3 transferase, an enzyme derived from *Clostridium botulinum*, inhibits Rho signaling by locking RhoA in the inactive state. Prior studies have found that C3 transferase can promote axonal outgrowth on inhibitory substrates in vitro and in vivo.[67,69] Unfortunately, the wild-type C3 transferase has poor cellular penetration. BA-210, tradename Cethrin, is a recombination engineered variant of C3 transferase that is readily able to cross the dura of the spinal cord and permeate across the cell membrane in a receptor-independent mechanism.[69] Local delivery of BA-210 to the injury site in rats with thoracic spinal cord contusion has been shown to inactivate RhoA, reduce the extent of the lesion, and improve locomotor function.[69] In a phase I/IIa clinical trial, 48 patients with an ASIA A cervical or thoracic SCI received 0.3 to 9 mg of Cethrin applied locally onto the anterior or posterior dural surface overlying the injured spinal cord at surgery.[68] Changes in ASIA motor scores were low in all thoracic patients (1.8 ± 5.1) and larger in cervical patients (18.6 ± 19.3). Pharmacokinetic analysis from this study found low levels of systemic exposure to the drug. Cervical SCI patients treated with 3 mg of Cethrin experienced the greatest improvement in ASIA motor score at 1 year (27.3 ± 13.3). Thirty-one percent of cervical patients converted from ASIA A to C or D and 66% for the cervical cohort. Based on these results, a phase IIb/III double-blind, randomized, placebo-controlled, multicenter trial of Cethrin is now underway (ClinicalTrials.gov NCT02669849). Eligible patients are between 14 and 75 years of age with ASIA A or B acute traumatic cervical SCIs, who are scheduled to undergo surgery within 72 hours of injury.

25.3.3 Inspire (Neuro-Spinal Scaffold)

The Neuro-Spinal Scaffold is a porous bioresorbable polymer scaffold that promotes appositional healing, spares white matter, decreases posttraumatic cyst formation, and normalizes intraparenchymal tissue pressure.[70] The polymer is composed of poly (lactic-co-glycolic acid) covalently conjugated to poly (L-lysine). In animal hemisection models of SCI, a polymer scaffold seeded with neural stem cells has improved functional recovery.[71,72] A pilot study to evaluate the safety and feasibility of implantation of the Neuro-Spinal Scaffold is currently underway (ClinicalTrials.gov NCT02138110). Eligibility criteria include age 16 to 70 years, ASIA A traumatic SCI with a neurological level of T2 to T12/L1, ability to receive the scaffold within 96 hours of injury, and nonpenetrating contusion injury no less than approximately 4 mm diameter by MRI. A report of the first patient to undergo implantation of the scaffold as part of this trial has been published.[70] The patient was a 25-year-old male with a T11–T12 fracture-dislocation sustained in a motocross accident resulting in a T11 ASIA A SCI. A 2 × 10 mm scaffold was implanted directly into the traumatic cavity within the spinal cord parenchyma at T12 through a dorsal root entry zone myelotomy. At 3 months, neurological function had improved to an L1 ASIA C incomplete injury. No procedural complication or safety concern from implantation of the scaffold was seen at 6-month follow-up.

25.3.4 SCiStar (Human Embryonic Stem Cells)

Moving away from neuroprotection toward regenerative strategies, there has been tremendous interest, from both scientists and the general public, in using human embryonic stem cells (hESC) in traumatic SCI. A few small studies have been conducted in the past.[73,74,75] The first phase I human clinical trial of hESC, referred to as the Geron trial, was conducted in 2009. Although the first cohort contained five patients who met the primary safety endpoint, the trial had to be discontinued due to financial constraints.[76,77] However, Asterias Biotechnology received U.S. FDA approval for use of hESC in SCI, and this company bought the rights of Geron to conduct a clinical trial with hESC in humans. Geron's original product, GRNOPC1, was rebranded as AST-OPC-1, composed primarily of oligodendrocyte progenitor cells. A phase I/IIa trial is currently underway, designed to evaluate the safety and activity of escalating doses of AST-OPC-1 in patients 18 to 69 years old with complete cervical SCI (ClinicalTrials.gov NCT02302157).

StemCells, Inc. has developed and tested a product, HuCNS-SC, composed of expanded human fetal forebrain neural stem cells isolated by enriching for stem cells through flow cytometry.[78] Transplantation of these cells was tested in a phase I/II study of patients with thoracic ASIA A to C injuries (ClinicalTrials.gov NCT01321333) and a phase I/II trial of patients with cervical (C5 to C7) ASIA B or C SCI (ClinicalTrials.gov NCT02163876). Results from these trials revealed no safety concerns related to the cells or manual intramedullary injection.[79,80]

A few studies have examined the safety and efficacy of autologous human bone marrow (BMC) transplantation and the administration of granulocyte macrophage colony-stimulating factor (GM-CSF).[73,81] Yoon et al[81] conducted a phase I/II open-label, nonrandomized study in patients with complete SCI. Thirty-five patients underwent BMC transplantation by injection into the SCI site and administration of GM-CSF. BMC transplantation and GM-CSF administration was not found to be associated with any serious adverse events. ASIA grade improved in 30.4% of patients treated in the acute or subacute period, but no significant improvement was observed in the chronic treatment group.

25.3.5 Hypothermia

Systematic hypothermia has been evaluated as a neuroprotective strategy in acute traumatic SCI.[82,83,84] Dididze et al[84] reported on 35 acute cervical SCI patients who received moderate intravascular hypothermia (33 °C) for 48 hours. All patients were complete on admission, but four improved to ASIA B within 24 hours postinjury. Fifteen patients (43%) improved at least one ASIA grade at latest follow-up (10.07 ± 1.03 months). The risk of thromboembolic complications was 14.2%. A multicenter randomized trial in patients 18 to 70 years old with ASIA A, B, or C acute traumatic SCI is currently underway (ClinicalTrials.gov NCT02991690). The experimental group will receive hypothermia via an intravascular catheter inserted through the femoral vein. Patients will be cooled at a maximum rate of 2 to 2.5 °C until a target temperature of 33 °C is reached, which will be maintained for 48 hours. Patients will then be rewarmed at 0.1 °C/hour until normothermia (37 °C) is reached. The control group will receive standard of care medical treatment. The primary outcome measure will be neurological improvement in ASIA grade and motor score. The trial has a target enrollment of 120 patients.

25.4 Conclusion

There has been a tremendous evolution in clinical trials in SCI. The development, validation, and widespread adoption of standardized neurological grading systems, functional outcome measures, and quality of life indices now permit robust trial designs. This, together with advances in imaging techniques, our understanding of the pathophysiology of secondary injury mechanisms in SCI, and streamlined translation of therapeutics from bench to bedside, brings promise to the future of SCI research. Important considerations in SCI trial design include development of a clear research question, use of techniques that mitigate selection bias (i.e., randomization, allocation concealment, blinding), application of methods to address the heterogeneity of SCI with regard to severity and/or level (i.e., definition of a homogeneous population or stratification of randomization by severity/level), use of validated outcome measures (including neurological grading systems and functional and quality of life outcome measures), and an a priori, clear definition of primary and secondary outcomes. Other trial designs may need to be considered, such as the use of adaptive randomization, or propensity-matched analyses of data from large cohort studies or RCTs. Collaborative efforts are needed, and consortia of investigators, such as NACTN and the AO Study Group, will have an important role in leading the way.

References

[1] Tator CH. Biology of neurological recovery and functional restoration after spinal cord injury. Neurosurgery. 1998; 42(4):696–707, discussion 707–708

[2] Sekhon LH, Fehlings MG. Epidemiology, demographics, and pathophysiology of acute spinal cord injury. Spine. 2001; 26(24) Suppl:S2–S12

[3] Hall ED, Braughler JM. Effects of intravenous methylprednisolone on spinal cord lipid peroxidation and Na++K+)-ATPase activity. Dose-response analysis during 1st hour after contusion injury in the cat. J Neurosurg. 1982; 57(2):247–253

[4] Bracken MB, Collins WF, Freeman DF, et al. Efficacy of methylprednisolone in acute spinal cord injury. JAMA. 1984; 251(1):45–52

[5] Fehlings MG, Wilson JR, Cho N. Methylprednisolone for the treatment of acute spinal cord injury: counterpoint. Neurosurgery. 2014; 61 Suppl 1: 36–42

[6] Bracken MB, Shepard MJ, Collins WF, et al. A randomized, controlled trial of methylprednisolone or naloxone in the treatment of acute spinal-cord injury. Results of the Second National Acute Spinal Cord Injury Study. N Engl J Med. 1990; 322(20):1405–1411

[7] Hugenholtz H. Methylprednisolone for acute spinal cord injury: not a standard of care. CMAJ. 2003; 168(9):1145–1146

[8] Tator CH. Review of treatment trials in human spinal cord injury: issues, difficulties, and recommendations. Neurosurgery. 2006; 59(5):957–982, discussion 982–987

[9] Coleman WP, Benzel D, Cahill DW, et al. A critical appraisal of the reporting of the National Acute Spinal Cord Injury Studies (II and III) of methylprednisolone in acute spinal cord injury. J Spinal Disord. 2000; 13(3):185–199

[10] Nesathurai S. Steroids and spinal cord injury: revisiting the NASCIS 2 and NASCIS 3 trials. J Trauma. 1998; 45(6):1088–1093

[11] Hugenholtz H, Cass DE, Dvorak MF, et al. High-dose methylprednisolone for acute closed spinal cord injury–only a treatment option. Can J Neurol Sci. 2002; 29(3):227–235

[12] Bracken MB, Shepard MJ, Holford TR, et al. Administration of methylprednisolone for 24 or 48 hours or tirilazad mesylate for 48 hours in the treatment of acute spinal cord injury. Results of the Third National Acute Spinal Cord Injury Randomized Controlled Trial. National Acute Spinal Cord Injury Study. JAMA. 1997; 277(20):1597–1604

[13] Otani K, Abe H, Kadoya S. Beneficial effect of methylprednisolone sodium succinate in the treatment of acute spinal cord injury. Sekitsui Sekizui J. 1994; 7:633–647

[14] Matsumoto T, Tamaki T, Kawakami M, Yoshida M, Ando M, Yamada H. Early complications of high-dose methylprednisolone sodium succinate treatment in the follow-up of acute cervical spinal cord injury. Spine. 2001; 26(4): 426–430

[15] Geisler FH, Dorsey FC, Coleman WP. Recovery of motor function after spinal-cord injury–a randomized, placebo-controlled trial with GM-1 ganglioside. N Engl J Med. 1991; 324(26):1829–1838

[16] Geisler FH, Coleman WP, Grieco G, Poonian D, Sygen Study Group. The Sygen multicenter acute spinal cord injury study. Spine. 2001; 26(24) Suppl:S87–S98

[17] Faden AI, Jacobs TP, Smith MT. Thyrotropin-releasing hormone in experimental spinal injury: dose response and late treatment. Neurology. 1984; 34(10):1280–1284

[18] Pitts LH, Ross A, Chase GA, Faden AI. Treatment with thyrotropin-releasing hormone (TRH) in patients with traumatic spinal cord injuries. J Neurotrauma. 1995; 12(3):235–243

[19] Fehlings MG, Tator CH, Linden RD. The effect of nimodipine and dextran on axonal function and blood flow following experimental spinal cord injury. J Neurosurg. 1989; 71(3):403–416

[20] Guha A, Tator CH, Smith CR, Piper I. Improvement in post-traumatic spinal cord blood flow with a combination of a calcium channel blocker and a vasopressor. J Trauma. 1989; 29(10):1440–1447

[21] Pointillart V, Petitjean ME, Wiart L, et al. Pharmacological therapy of spinal cord injury during the acute phase. Spinal Cord. 2000; 38(2):71–76

[22] Li S, Mealing GA, Morley P, Stys PK. Novel injury mechanism in anoxia and trauma of spinal cord white matter: glutamate release via reverse Na+-dependent glutamate transport. J Neurosci. 1999; 19(14):RC16

[23] Taylor CP, Geer JJ, Burke SP. Endogenous extracellular glutamate accumulation in rat neocortical cultures by reversal of the transmembrane sodium gradient. Neurosci Lett. 1992; 145(2):197–200

[24] Hirbec H, Gaviria M, Vignon J. Gacyclidine: a new neuroprotective agent acting at the N-methyl-D-aspartate receptor. CNS Drug Rev. 2001; 7(2):172–198

[25] Tadie M, Gaviria M, Mathe J-F, et al. Early care and treatment with a neuro-protective drug, gacyclidine, in patients with acute spinal cord injury. Rachis. 2003; 15:363–376

[26] Yrjänheikki J, Keinänen R, Pellikka M, Hökfelt T, Koistinaho J. Tetracyclines inhibit microglial activation and are neuroprotective in global brain ischemia. Proc Natl Acad Sci U S A. 1998; 95(26):15769–15774

[27] Lee SM, Yune TY, Kim SJ, et al. Minocycline reduces cell death and improves functional recovery after traumatic spinal cord injury in the rat. J Neurotrauma. 2003; 20(10):1017–1027

[28] Wells JE, Hurlbert RJ, Fehlings MG, Yong VW. Neuroprotection by minocycline facilitates significant recovery from spinal cord injury in mice. Brain. 2003; 126(Pt 7):1628–1637

[29] Casha S, Zygun D, McGowan MD, Bains I, Yong VW, Hurlbert RJ. Results of a phase II placebo-controlled randomized trial of minocycline in acute spinal cord injury. Brain. 2012; 135(Pt 4):1224–1236

[30] Vaccaro AR, Daugherty RJ, Sheehan TP, et al. Neurologic outcome of early versus late surgery for cervical spinal cord injury. Spine. 1997; 22(22): 2609–2613

[31] Fehlings MG, Vaccaro A, Wilson JR, et al. Early versus delayed decompression for traumatic cervical spinal cord injury: results of the Surgical Timing in Acute Spinal Cord Injury Study (STASCIS). PLoS One. 2012; 7(2):e32037

[32] Tator CH. Epidemiology and general characteristics of the spinal cord injured patient. In: Tator CH, Benzel E, eds. Contemporary Management of Spinal Cord Injury: From Impact to Rehabilitation. Park Ridge, IL: American Association of Neurological Surgeons; 2000:15–19

[33] Ragnarsson KT, Wuermser LA, Cardenas DD, Marino RJ. Spinal cord injury clinical trials for neurologic restoration: improving care through clinical research. Am J Phys Med Rehabil. 2005; 84(11) Suppl:S77–S97, quiz S98–S100

[34] Burns AS, Lee BS, Ditunno JF, Jr, Tessler A. Patient selection for clinical trials: the reliability of the early spinal cord injury examination. J Neurotrauma. 2003; 20(5):477–482

[35] Frankel HL, Hancock DO, Hyslop G, et al. The value of postural reduction in the initial management of closed injuries of the spine with paraplegia and tetraplegia. I. Paraplegia. 1969; 7(3):179–192

[36] Tator CH, Rowed DW, Schwartz ML. Sunnybrook cord injury scales for assessing neurological injury and recovery. In: Tator CH, ed. Early Management of Acute Spinal Cord Injury. New York, NY: Raven Press; 1982:7–24

[37] Lucas JT, Ducker TB. Motor classification of spinal cord injuries with mobility, morbidity and recovery indices. Am Surg. 1979; 45(3):151–158

[38] Kirshblum SC, Burns SP, Biering-Sorensen F, et al. International standards for neurological classification of spinal cord injury (revised 2011). J Spinal Cord Med. 2011; 34(6):535–546

[39] Lammertse DP. Clinical trials in spinal cord injury: lessons learned on the path to translation. The 2011 International Spinal Cord Society Sir Ludwig Guttmann Lecture. Spinal Cord. 2013; 51(1):2–9

[40] Keith RA, Granger CV, Hamilton BB, Sherwin FS. The functional independence measure: a new tool for rehabilitation. Adv Clin Rehabil. 1987; 1:6–18

[41] Catz A, Itzkovich M, Agranov E, Ring H, Tamir A. The spinal cord independence measure (SCIM): sensitivity to functional changes in subgroups of spinal cord lesion patients. Spinal Cord. 2001; 39(2):97–100

[42] Catz A, Itzkovich M, Steinberg F, et al. The Catz-Itzkovich SCIM: a revised version of the Spinal Cord Independence Measure. Disabil Rehabil. 2001; 23(6):263–268

[43] Ditunno JF, Jr, Ditunno PL, Scivoletto G, et al. The Walking Index for Spinal Cord Injury (WISCI/WISCI II): nature, metric properties, use and misuse. Spinal Cord. 2013; 51(5):346–355

[44] Ditunno JF, Jr, Ditunno PL, Graziani V, et al. Walking index for spinal cord injury (WISCI): an international multicenter validity and reliability study. Spinal Cord. 2000; 38(4):234–243

[45] Witiw CD, Mansouri A, Mathieu F, Nassiri F, Badhiwala JH, Fessler RG. Exploring the expectation-actuality discrepancy: a systematic review of the impact of preoperative expectations on satisfaction and patient reported outcomes in spinal surgery. Neurosurg Rev. 2018; 41(1):19–30

[46] McHorney CA, Ware JE, Jr, Raczek AE. The MOS 36-Item Short-Form Health Survey (SF-36): II. Psychometric and clinical tests of validity in measuring physical and mental health constructs. Med Care. 1993; 31(3):247–263

[47] Rabin R, de Charro F. EQ-5D: a measure of health status from the EuroQol Group. Ann Med. 2001; 33(5):337–343

[48] Brazier J, Roberts J, Deverill M. The estimation of a preference-based measure of health from the SF-36. J Health Econ. 2002; 21(2):271–292

[49] Martin AR, De Leener B, Cohen-Adad J, et al. Clinically feasible microstructural MRI to quantify cervical spinal cord tissue injury using DTI, MT, and T2*-weighted imaging: assessment of normative data and reliability. AJNR Am J Neuroradiol. 2017; 38(6):1257–1265

[50] Martin AR, De Leener B, Cohen-Adad J, et al. A novel MRI biomarker of spinal cord white matter injury: T2*-weighted white matter to gray matter signal intensity ratio. AJNR Am J Neuroradiol. 2017; 38(6):1266–1273

[51] Harrop JS, Maltenfort MG, Geisler FH, et al. Traumatic thoracic ASIA A examinations and potential for clinical trials. Spine. 2009; 34(23):2525–2529

[52] Marino RJ, Ditunno JF, Jr, Donovan WH, Maynard F, Jr. Neurologic recovery after traumatic spinal cord injury: data from the Model Spinal Cord Injury Systems. Arch Phys Med Rehabil. 1999; 80(11):1391–1396

[53] Miller RG, Mitchell JD, Moore DH. Riluzole for amyotrophic lateral sclerosis (ALS)/motor neuron disease (MND). Cochrane Database Syst Rev. 2012(3): CD001447

[54] Agrawal SK, Fehlings MG. Mechanisms of secondary injury to spinal cord axons in vitro: role of Na+, Na(+)-K(+)-ATPase, the Na(+)-H+ exchanger, and the Na(+)-Ca2+ exchanger. J Neurosci. 1996; 16(2):545–552

[55] Stys PK, Sontheimer H, Ransom BR, Waxman SG. Noninactivating, tetrodotoxin-in-sensitive Na+ conductance in rat optic nerve axons. Proc Natl Acad Sci U S A. 1993; 90(15):6976–6980

[56] Schwartz G, Fehlings MG. Evaluation of the neuroprotective effects of sodium channel blockers after spinal cord injury: improved behavioral and neuroanatomical recovery with riluzole. J Neurosurg. 2001; 94(2) Suppl:245–256

[57] Wu Y, Satkunendrarajah K, Teng Y, Chow DS, Buttigieg J, Fehlings MG. Delayed post-injury administration of riluzole is neuroprotective in a preclinical rodent model of cervical spinal cord injury. J Neurotrauma. 2013; 30(6):441–452

[58] Grossman RG, Fehlings MG, Frankowski RF, et al. A prospective, multicenter, phase I matched-comparison group trial of safety, pharmacokinetics, and preliminary efficacy of riluzole in patients with traumatic spinal cord injury. J Neurotrauma. 2014; 31(3):239–255

[59] Fehlings MG, Nakashima H, Nagoshi N, Chow DS, Grossman RG, Kopjar B. Rationale, design and critical end points for the Riluzole in Acute Spinal Cord Injury Study (RISCIS): a randomized, double-blinded, placebo-controlled parallel multi-center trial. Spinal Cord. 2016; 54(1):8–15

[60] Vasconcelos NL, Gomes ED, Oliveira EP, et al. Combining neuroprotective agents: effect of riluzole and magnesium in a rat model of thoracic spinal cord injury. Spine J. 2016; 16(8):1015–1024

[61] Satkunendrarajah K, Nassiri F, Karadimas SK, Lip A, Yao G, Fehlings MG. Riluzole promotes motor and respiratory recovery associated with enhanced neuronal survival and function following high cervical spinal hemisection. Exp Neurol. 2016; 276:59–71

[62] Karadimas SK, Laliberte AM, Tetreault L, et al. Riluzole blocks perioperative ischemia-reperfusion injury and enhances postdecompression outcomes in cervical spondylotic myelopathy. Sci Transl Med. 2015; 7(316):316ra194

[63] Nagoshi N, Nakashima H, Fehlings MG. Riluzole as a neuroprotective drug for spinal cord injury: from bench to bedside. Molecules. 2015; 20(5):7775–7789

[64] Lacomblez L, Bensimon G, Leigh PN, et al. ALS Study Groups I and II. Long-term safety of riluzole in amyotrophic lateral sclerosis. Amyotroph Lateral Scler Other Motor Neuron Disord. 2002; 3(1):23–29

[65] Catz A. Spinal cord independence measure. In: Kreutzer JS, DeLuca J, Caplan B, eds. Encyclopedia of Clinical Neuropsychology. New York, NY: Springer; 2011:2351–2353

[66] Kalsi-Ryan S, Curt A, Verrier MC, Fehlings MG. Development of the Graded Redefined Assessment of Strength, Sensibility and Prehension (GRASSP): reviewing measurement specific to the upper limb in tetraplegia. J Neurosurg Spine. 2012; 17(1) Suppl:65–76

[67] Dubreuil CI, Winton MJ, McKerracher L. Rho activation patterns after spinal cord injury and the role of activated Rho in apoptosis in the central nervous system. J Cell Biol. 2003; 162(2):233–243

[68] Fehlings MG, Theodore N, Harrop J, et al. A phase I/IIa clinical trial of a recombinant Rho protein antagonist in acute spinal cord injury. J Neurotrauma. 2011; 28(5):787–796

[69] Lord-Fontaine S, Yang F, Diep Q, et al. Local inhibition of Rho signaling by cell-permeable recombinant protein BA-210 prevents secondary damage and promotes functional recovery following acute spinal cord injury. J Neurotrauma. 2008; 25(11):1309–1322

[70] Theodore N, Hlubek R, Danielson J, et al. First human implantation of a bioresorbable polymer scaffold for acute traumatic spinal cord injury: a clinical pilot study for safety and feasibility. Neurosurgery. 2016; 79(2):E305–E312

[71] Teng YD, Lavik EB, Qu X, et al. Functional recovery following traumatic spinal cord injury mediated by a unique polymer scaffold seeded with neural stem cells. Proc Natl Acad Sci U S A. 2002; 99(5):3024–3029

[72] Pritchard CD, Slotkin JR, Yu D, et al. Establishing a model spinal cord injury in the African green monkey for the preclinical evaluation of biodegradable polymer scaffolds seeded with human neural stem cells. J Neurosci Methods. 2010; 188(2):258–269

[73] Park HC, Shim YS, Ha Y, et al. Treatment of complete spinal cord injury patients by autologous bone marrow cell transplantation and administration of granulocyte-macrophage colony stimulating factor. Tissue Eng. 2005; 11(5–6):913–922

[74] Lima C, Escada P, Pratas-Vital J, et al. Olfactory mucosal autografts and rehabilitation for chronic traumatic spinal cord injury. Neurorehabil Neural Repair. 2010; 24(1):10–22

[75] Kang KS, Kim SW, Oh YH, et al. A 37-year-old spinal cord-injured female patient, transplanted of multipotent stem cells from human UC blood, with improved sensory perception and mobility, both functionally and morphologically: a case study. Cytotherapy. 2005; 7(4):368–373

[76] Lukovic D, Stojkovic M, Moreno-Manzano V, Bhattacharya SS, Erceg S. Perspectives and future directions of human pluripotent stem cell-based therapies: lessons from Geron's clinical trial for spinal cord injury. Stem Cells Dev. 2014; 23(1):1–4

[77] Geron Completes Divestiture of Stem Cell Assets. Geron Corporation. 2013. Available at: http://ir.geron.com/phoenix.zhtml?c=67323&p=irol-newsArticle&ID=1860364

[78] Irion S, Zabierowski SE, Tomishima MJ. Bringing neural cell therapies to the clinic: past and future strategies. Mol Ther Methods Clin Dev. 2016; 4:72–82

[79] Levi AD, Okonkwo DO, Park P, et al. Emerging safety of intramedullary transplantation of human neural stem cells in chronic cervical and thoracic spinal cord injury. Neurosurgery. 2018; 82(4):562–575

[80] Phase I/II clinical trial of HuCNS-SC cells in chronic thoracic spinal cord injury—interim analysis. 2014. Available at: http://www.stemcellsinc.com/Presentations/ASIA_FINAL.pdf

[81] Yoon SH, Shim YS, Park YH, et al. Complete spinal cord injury treatment using autologous bone marrow cell transplantation and bone marrow stimulation with granulocyte macrophage-colony stimulating factor: phase I/II clinical trial. Stem Cells. 2007; 25(8):2066–2073

[82] Levi AD, Casella G, Green BA, et al. Clinical outcomes using modest intravascular hypothermia after acute cervical spinal cord injury. Neurosurgery. 2010; 66(4):670–677

[83] Levi AD, Green BA, Wang MY, et al. Clinical application of modest hypothermia after spinal cord injury. J Neurotrauma. 2009; 26(3):407–415

[84] Dididze M, Green BA, Dietrich WD, Vanni S, Wang MY, Levi AD. Systemic hypothermia in acute cervical spinal cord injury: a case-controlled study. Spinal Cord. 2013; 51(5):395–400

26 Pharmacologic Treatment of Spinal Cord Injury

Swetha J. Sundar and Michael P. Steinmetz

Abstract

Spinal cord injury (SCI) causes irreversible damage to neuronal pathways and structures, both through the initial insult itself (termed primary injury) and through a complex set of biochemical processes that act to worsen the damage (termed secondary injury). The various mechanisms through which this secondary injury occurs, including ischemic damage, lipid peroxidation, endogenous opioid release, inflammation, and free radical changes, all present potential targets for medical therapy for the body to attempt neurorestoration. In this chapter, we will discuss the use of pharmacologic agents such as corticosteroids, riluzole, lithium, glyburide, gangliosides, naloxone, signaling proteins, and tetracycline that work to mitigate secondary injury after SCI. We will also discuss the roles of blood pressure control and therapeutic hypothermia in minimizing injury following SCI.

Keywords: spinal cord injury, secondary injury, corticosteroids, neurorestoration

26.1 Introduction

Traumatic spinal cord injury (SCI) causes irreversible damage to neuronal pathways through numerous pathophysiologic mechanisms, prompting a multifaceted management schema. In the United States, it is estimated that about 250,000 individuals suffer acute SCI annually, with a 6.3% 1-year mortality rate, significant morbidity and disability to affected individuals, and nearly 10 million dollars in annual costs to the health care system.[1,2,3] Irreversible changes to neuronal components can occur as soon as within 1 hour of initial injury and continue for several days. Presenting factors such as neurologic deficits, age, respiratory status, and level of consciousness can be predictors of survival and better outcomes. Death of SCI patients is usually due to complications secondary to extent of neurologic damage and length of hospital stays, including respiratory failure, cardiac arrest, septicemia, pulmonary embolism, or suicide.[4,5,6] About half of these complications manifest within 1 week of presentation and 75% within 2 weeks, highlighting the importance of optimizing early management protocols of SCI patients.

26.2 Pathophysiology

Both physical and biochemical processes in the spinal cord following acute trauma contribute to the loss of neurologic function. Primary injury is caused directly by mechanical forces at initial impact.[7] Compression of the spinal cord can be transient, such as in hyperextension injuries in patients with advanced cervical degenerative disease (which momentarily reduce the AP diameter of the canal), or persistent, in instances of burst fractures with bony retropulsion or fracture-dislocations. Patients with constant compression are most likely to benefit from urgent surgical intervention to decompress neural elements.[8,9] Primary injury can also occur through direct lacera-

tion or transection of the cord when there are severe distraction injuries, penetrating traumas, or sharp bony fragments in the canal. The transmission of energy to the cord associated with penetrating trauma can cause ischemia by interrupting vascular supply.[10,11] Mechanical forces preferentially damage the gray matter, which sustains irreversible damage within 1 hour of acute injury.[7] Surgery can halt the primary injurious process by decompressing the spinal cord, but otherwise, minimizing effects of the traumatic insult can only come by avoiding the injury itself.

Minutes to hours after the primary injury occurs, a complicated, diverse cascade of biochemical pathways become activated, which entail the secondary injury.[12,13] This process will expand the initial impact through a variety of mechanisms including ischemia, free radical damage, lipid peroxidation, neuronal apoptosis, electrolyte imbalances, inflammatory processes, and neurogenic shock. Secondary injury is a time-sensitive process that worsens the extent of injury and limits the body's attempts at neurorestoration. Damage to microvasculature results in ischemia and hemorrhage, leading to regions of infarcts, increases in lactic acid, and edema. Release of endogenous opioids in response to the initial trauma leads to hypotension and worsening cord ischemia. The autoregulation of the microcirculation becomes disrupted and can cause reperfusion damage to areas of initial infarct.[14,15] Neurologic function can be compromised due to increases in intracellular K^+, causing membrane depolarization and decreased adenosine triphosphate (ATP) production. Ischemic damage generates oxidized free radicals in nonphysiologic quantities, causing a self-propagating cascade of oxidative damage to cell membranes via lipid peroxidation. Intracellular Ca^{2+} rises and calcium-dependent enzymes become activated as well. Mitochondria are damaged due to oxidative stress, and ultimately, the combined result of these biochemical processes is cellular necrosis and apoptosis.[16] Knowledge of these pathways allows for medical therapies that specifically target mechanisms to limit neuronal damage and loss of function after initial injury.

26.3 Medical Management in ICU Setting

Minimizing the secondary injury is an important focus of treating SCI. These patients are best served in an intensive care unit (ICU), which allows for strict blood pressure control and close monitoring of respiratory function.

26.4 Maintaining Perfusion

SCI patients can often be hypotensive, not only from acute volume loss due to trauma, but also because of loss of sympathetic tone, microvascular damage, inflammation, and impaired autoregulatory processes. Patients who initially present with hypotension are noted to have poor long-term outcomes compared to those presenting in a normotensive state.[10,17,18,19,20]

Optimizing oxygenation and perfusion to the cord is the immediate goal of resuscitating SCI patients. Research demonstrates improved outcomes when mean arterial pressure (MAP) is kept greater than 85 mm Hg.[17,21,22,23,24] If fluid resuscitation with crystalloids and/or colloids is not successful in maintaining MAPs, patients should have blood pressure augmentation with pressors. The Guidelines for the Management of Acute Cervical Spine and Spinal Cord Injuries recommend keeping MAPs greater than 85 mm Hg for 1 week, when the cord is most susceptible to autoregulation dysfunction.[25] The desire to increase perfusion must be balanced with the risk of hemorrhage and worsening edema. Additionally, patients with high cervical injury can be hypoxic from impaired respiratory function, secondary to diaphragmatic paralysis, loss of accessory muscle function, or direct neck/tracheal trauma; in these cases, early intubation may be considered.[26]

26.5 Hypothermia

Therapeutic hypothermia has demonstrated neuroprotective properties for pathologies where edema and oxidative stress mediate neuronal damage, such as cardiac arrest, stroke, and traumatic brain injury.[27,28,29,30,31] In traumatic SCI, animal evidence supports that hypothermia is efficacious in improving outcomes in mild to moderate cases.[32] Cooling (32–34 °C) can decrease oxidative stress, limit apoptosis, minimize neuronal swelling, and inhibit the inflammatory process in instances of SCI. However, all the patient's injuries and management goals need to be considered because systemic hypothermia can increase infectious complications and/or impair respiratory status.[33]

26.6 Pharmacologic Agents

26.6.1 Methylprednisolone

The use of corticosteroids for patients with SCI has been repeatedly studied in animal and human models and remains a controversial topic. Methylprednisolone (MP) is a glucocorticoid that is thought to minimize secondary injury by protecting lipid membranes, increasing Na^+/K^+ ATPase activity, reducing inflammation, and scavenging free radicals to minimize lipid peroxidation. When excess Ca^{2+} influx is halted, it is believed that lysosomes and protease release is prevented.[34,35,36,37,38]

The debate regarding MP use for post-SCI stems in part from inconsistent conclusions between multiple animal and human studies. Many studies utilizing MP have demonstrated reductions in lipid peroxidation at various time points. However, animal studies have concluded no functional benefits.[39,40,41,42,43,44,45,46,47] The administration of MP is not risk-free, with side effects of hyperglycemia, gastrointestinal hemorrhage, increased infection risk, and myopathy; the extent of traumatic injury and patient comorbidities must be taken into account when considering its use.[48]

There have been three major clinical trials examining the use of MP for acute SCI, known as the National Acute Spinal Cord Injury Studies (NASCIS). The NASCIS I was a randomized control trial where MP was administered within 48 hours of injury and patients were randomized to receiving either 100 or 1,000 mg over 10 days total.[49,50] Patient outcomes were analyzed at 6 weeks and 6 months, and there were no significant differences demonstrated between the two groups. The patients in the 1,000-mg group did have more wound infections.

The main criticism of the NASCIS I is that dosages of MP were inappropriately low to demonstrate efficacy. This was adjusted for the NASCIS II, a prospective randomized control trial where patients were given either MP, naloxone, or a placebo. The MP group received an initial bolus of 30 mg/kg followed by 5.4 mg/kg/hour infusion for 23 hours. Although overall analyses did not demonstrate significant benefits, subgroup analyses of patients receiving MP within 8 hours of nonpenetrating injuries showed significant improvements in motor and sensory functions when compared to the placebo group. The NASCIS II is largely responsible for the widespread practice of giving patients MP after acute SCI in the 1990s.[51,52]

The NASCIS III was the subsequent trial where patients were randomized to receiving MP for 24 or 48 hours or tirilazad mesylate for 48 hours. The patients receiving 48 hours of MP post-SCI demonstrated improved motor recovery at 6 weeks and 6 months, especially when treatment was initiated within 8 hours of injury, as similarly demonstrated in the NASCIS II trial. However, there was also an increased incidence of infections in the 48-hour MP group compared to the 24-hour MP group. In the subset of patients with penetrating injury, there were no benefits shown with MP use.[53]

Both the NASCIS II and III have been extensively reevaluated since their initial publication, with significant criticisms—the NASCIS II for flawed study design and subgroup analysis, and NASCIS III due to clinically insignificant differences in motor outcomes. These trials have failed to demonstrate relevant benefits for the treatment groups and, moreover, have repeatedly shown increased risk of infectious complications. The use of MP for acute SCI patients remains a treatment option with careful consideration of traumatic injury type and comorbidities, but is not considered a standard of care. Current level I recommendations state that MP administration for acute SCI is not recommended and is not approved by the Food and Drug Administration (FDA).[54,55,56]

26.6.2 Riluzole

More commonly known as an FDA-approved medication for amyotrophic lateral sclerosis (ALS), riluzole is thought to reduce motor neuron degeneration by blocking pathologic sodium influx and inhibiting abnormal glutamatergic transmission. In a phase I clinical trial of 36 acute SCI patients who received 50-mg riluzole within 12 hours of injury, followed by dosing every 12 hours for 28 doses total, there was a significant improvement in ASIA motor scores in cervical SCI patients when compared to a matched cohort.[57] The most significant improvements were seen in ASIA B patients. Currently underway is the Riluzole in Spinal Cord Injury Study (RISCIS), a multicenter double-blinded placebo-controlled RCT that includes cervical SCI patients who receive riluzole within the first 12 hours of injury.[58,59]

26.6.3 Cethrin

The protein Rho is a small guanosine triphosphatase (GTPase) that acts as a molecular modulator by downregulating many actin-mediated pathways, including endocytosis, phagocytosis, motility, and morphogenesis. These processes are critical for axonal growth and neuronal regeneration. Research has shown that Rho-mediated pathways are more active following SCI, meaning that the spinal cord's intrinsic efforts to protect itself from furthering secondary injury are inhibited due to Rho.[60,61, 62,63] Cethrin is a commercial recombinant inhibitor of Rho which is delivered during surgery, directly to the dura over the site of primary injury, as a fibrin sealant. A recent study where patients with acute cervical and thoracic SCI are randomized to receive different doses of Cethrin within 7 days of injury shows improvements in motor scores for cervical patients.[64] The data are encouraging; however, further studies of efficacy and safety are needed before recommendations can be made regarding the use of Cethrin for SCI patients.

26.6.4 Minocycline

Minocycline is a derivative of tetracycline, commonly used as treatment for acne vulgaris, which has shown neuroprotective effects in animal studies of Parkinson disease, multiple sclerosis, stroke, and ALS.[37,65] Animal models of SCI have also demonstrated that minocycline can mitigate the secondary injury by neutralizing free radicals, stabilization of mitochondrial membranes, inhibiting microglial proliferation, and reducing apoptosis.[66] In a randomized controlled trial of patients presenting within 12 hours of initial injury, patients were given a week of intravenous minocycline versus a placebo. Improvements in motor scores were shown for cervical SCI patients, but no such difference was demonstrated for thoracic SCI patients. However, these improvements were not statistically significant and only trends were demonstrated.[66] It is not possible to yet draw conclusions or make recommendations regarding minocycline use for SCI patients, and further studies will be necessary.

26.6.5 Lithium

Lithium is known to have regenerative properties and can stimulate stem cell proliferation.[67] Its role in pain management of chronic SCI has been studied. In a double-blinded, randomized, placebo-controlled clinical trial of 40 chronic SCI patients (ASIA A–C injuries that remained unchanged for at least 6 months postinjury) who received either lithium titrated to 0.6 to 1.2 mmol/L for 6 weeks versus a placebo, although no changes in neurological function were demonstrated, patients who received lithium had significantly improved visual analogue scale (VAS) pain scores.[67] Further studies are planned to investigate lithium's role in acute and chronic SCI patients, especially for pain control.

26.6.6 Glyburide

Glyburide is an oral medication most often used to treat type II diabetes mellitus by inhibiting the sulfonylurea receptor (SUR1)-regulated ATP channels to increase insulin release from pancreatic B cells. Animal studies have shown that hyperglycemia at time of SCI (particularly involving contusions to the spinal cord) causes increased tissue damage and poor functional outcomes.[68] The use of glyburide in SCI patients is thought to mitigate effects of secondary hemorrhage and progressive hemorrhagic necrosis after SCI. A phase I/II trial is currently underway, where enrolled patients with acute SCI (ASIA A–C) will start oral glyburide within 8 hours of injury and continue 72 hours of oral therapy. Future results will help guide therapies.

26.6.7 GM-1 Ganglioside

The outer surfaces of neuronal cell membranes contain complex glycosphingolipids called gangliosides. Experimental research has suggested that administration of gangliosides can aid in neuronal survival and reduction in apoptosis following traumatic injury.[69,70,71] The Maryland GM-1 study was a prospective, double-blinded randomized control trial where acute cervical and thoracic SCI patients received 100 mg of GM-1 as intramuscular injections within the first 72 hours following injury, continuing for 30 days. Follow-up at 1 year showed significant improvements in motor scores for the treatment group when compared to placebo.[72] The Sygen GM-1 study followed, looking at almost 800 patients who were randomized to either a placebo, low-dose GM-1, or high-dose GM-1. All patients involved also received MP. This multicenter study did not show any significant differences but there was a trend toward improved bowel and bladder function.[73] The use of MP for all the patients in this study makes results more challenging to interpret. GM-1 is not currently recommended for use in patients with acute SCI.

26.6.8 Naloxone

With the biochemical cascade (part of the secondary injury phase) that occurs after acute SCI, there is release of endogenous opioids.[74] The use of naloxone, a medication designed for rapid opioid overdose reversal, has been studied in the setting of SCI. Experiments have demonstrated mixed results from giving naloxone. It was provided to patients in one study group for the NASCIS II trial.[75] However, human trials have not shown improvements in outcomes.[51] It remains unclear whether the hypothesis of giving naloxone to counteract the deleterious effects of endogenous opioids is incorrect or whether the opioid reversal agent is unable to reach its target location to provide benefits. Nonetheless, naloxone is not currently recommended for minimizing secondary injury in acute SCI.

26.6.9 Thyrotropin-Releasing Hormone

The effects of thyrotropin-releasing hormone (TRH) have been studied for SCI patients. In a blinded, placebo-controlled study of 20 patients where the experimental group received 6 hours of TRH infusion, no significant differences were seen. For SCI with incomplete injuries, some benefits were demonstrated early in the follow-up period. However, due to the limited sample size and loss of patients to follow-up, further research is needed to make meaningful conclusions about TRH in the setting of SCI.[76]

26.7 Conclusion

There are a number of pathophysiologic mechanisms through which traumatic SCI results in irreversible damage to neuronal structures and significant morbidity to the individual. It is necessary to approach management of SCI through a multifaceted and time-sensitive approach that takes into account these complex biochemical processes so that damage in the acute period can be minimized. Patients must be optimized medically in the ICU setting with close blood pressure monitoring to ensure ideal cord perfusion and avoiding hypothermia. The NASCIS trials evaluating the use of steroids in SCI patients have been criticized for poor study design and, ultimately, have not demonstrated differences in outcomes but have shown an increased risk of infectious complications. As a result, current level I recommendations are against steroid use for acute SCI. Other treatments with initial promise due to the mechanisms they target, such as GM-1 ganglioside or naloxone, are not currently recommended due to flaws in study design, confounding factors, and insufficient evidence to demonstrate improved outcomes. There are currently several pharmacologic treatments being studied that have demonstrated outcome improvements in initial trials, including riluzole, Cethrin, minocycline, glyburide, and lithium. Ultimately, further studies will be necessary to demonstrate consistent safety and efficacy before strong recommendations can be made for SCI patients on a large scale. Given the significant morbidity and mortality SCI patients face and the increasing costs to the health care system, such clinical trials will need to be followed closely in the coming years. The pharmacologic management of SCI offers an arena where significant neurorestoration may be possible and can greatly improve quality of life for a large number of patients.

References

[1] DeVivo MJ, Rutt RD, Black KJ, Go BK, Stover SL. Trends in spinal cord injury demographics and treatment outcomes between 1973 and 1986. Arch Phys Med Rehabil. 1992; 73(5):424–430

[2] Berkowitz M, O'Leary P, Kruse D, et al. Spinal Cord Injury: An Analysis of Medical and Social Costs. New York, NY: Demos Medical; 1998

[3] Wyndaele M, Wyndaele JJ. Incidence, prevalence and epidemiology of spinal cord injury: what learns a worldwide literature survey? Spinal Cord. 2006; 44(9):523–529

[4] DeVivo MJ, Stover SL, Black KJ. Prognostic factors for 12-year survival after spinal cord injury. Arch Phys Med Rehabil. 1992; 73(2):156–162

[5] Daverat P, Gagnon M, Dartigues JF, Mazaux JM, Barat M. Initial factors predicting survival in patients with a spinal cord injury. J Neurol Neurosurg Psychiatry. 1989; 52(3):403–406

[6] Krause JS, Kjorsvig JM. Mortality after spinal cord injury: a four-year prospective study. Arch Phys Med Rehabil. 1992; 73(6):558–563

[7] Dumont RJ, Okonkwo DO, Verma S, et al. Acute spinal cord injury, part I: pathophysiologic mechanisms. Clin Neuropharmacol. 2001; 24(5):254–264

[8] Tator CH. Pathophysiology and Pathology of Spinal Cord Injury. Baltimore, MD: Williams & Wilkins; 1996

[9] Tator CH. Spinal Cord Syndromes with Physiological and Anatomic Correlations. New York, NY: McGraw-Hill; 1996

[10] Amar AP, Levy ML. Pathogenesis and pharmacological strategies for mitigating secondary damage in acute spinal cord injury. Neurosurgery. 1999; 44(5):1027–1039, discussion 1039–1040

[11] Anderson DK, Hall ED. Pathophysiology of spinal cord trauma. Ann Emerg Med. 1993; 22(6):987–992

[12] Juurlink BH, Paterson PG. Review of oxidative stress in brain and spinal cord injury: suggestions for pharmacological and nutritional management strategies. J Spinal Cord Med. 1998; 21(4):309–334

[13] Carlson SL, Parrish ME, Springer JE, Doty K, Dossett L. Acute inflammatory response in spinal cord following impact injury. Exp Neurol. 1998; 151(1):77–88

[14] Kwon BK, Tetzlaff W, Grauer JN, Beiner J, Vaccaro AR. Pathophysiology and pharmacologic treatment of acute spinal cord injury. Spine J. 2004; 4(4):451–464

[15] Faden AI, Simon RP. A potential role for excitotoxins in the pathophysiology of spinal cord injury. Ann Neurol. 1988; 23(6):623–626

[16] Cuzzocrea S, Riley DP, Caputi AP, Salvemini D. Antioxidant therapy: a new pharmacological approach in shock, inflammation, and ischemia/reperfusion injury. Pharmacol Rev. 2001; 53(1):135–159

[17] Sandler AN, Tator CH. Effect of acute spinal cord compression injury on regional spinal cord blood flow in primates. J Neurosurg. 1976; 45(6):660–676

[18] McMichan JC, Michel L, Westbrook PR. Pulmonary dysfunction following traumatic quadriplegia. Recognition, prevention, and treatment. JAMA. 1980; 243(6):528–531

[19] Dolan EJ, Tator CH. The effect of blood transfusion, dopamine, and gamma hydroxybutyrate on posttraumatic ischemia of the spinal cord. J Neurosurg. 1982; 56(3):350–358

[20] Levi L, Wolf A, Belzberg H. Hemodynamic parameters in patients with acute cervical cord trauma: description, intervention, and prediction of outcome. Neurosurgery. 1993; 33(6):1007–1016, discussion 1016–1017

[21] Hickey R, Albin MS, Bunegin L, Gelineau J. Autoregulation of spinal cord blood flow: is the cord a microcosm of the brain? Stroke. 1986; 17(6):1183–1189

[22] Griffiths IR. Spinal cord blood flow in dogs. 2. The effect of the blood gases. J Neurol Neurosurg Psychiatry. 1973; 36(1):42–49

[23] Griffiths IR. Spinal cord blood flow after acute impact injury. In: Harper AM, ed. Blood Flow and Metabolism in the Brain: Proceedings of the 7th International Symposium on Cerebral Blood Flow and Metabolism; Aviemore, Scotland; June 17–20. New York, NY: Churchill-Livingstone; 1975:427–429

[24] Guha A, Tator CH, Rochon J. Spinal cord blood flow and systemic blood pressure after experimental spinal cord injury in rats. Stroke. 1989; 20(3):372–377

[25] Walters BC, Hadley MN, Hurlbert RJ, et al. American Association of Neurological Surgeons, Congress of Neurological Surgeons. Guidelines for the management of acute cervical spine and spinal cord injuries: 2013 update. Neurosurgery. 2013; 60 Suppl 1:82–91

[26] Como JJ, Sutton ER, McCunn M, et al. Characterizing the need for mechanical ventilation following cervical spinal cord injury with neurologic deficit. J Trauma. 2005; 59(4):912–916, discussion 916

[27] Bernard SA, Gray TW, Buist MD, et al. Treatment of comatose survivors of out-of-hospital cardiac arrest with induced hypothermia. N Engl J Med. 2002; 346(8):557–563

[28] Steinberg GK, Ogilvy CS, Shuer LM, et al. Comparison of endovascular and surface cooling during unruptured cerebral aneurysm repair. Neurosurgery. 2004; 55(2):307–314, discussion 314–315

[29] Conrad MF, Crawford RS, Davison JK, Cambria RP. Thoracoabdominal aneurysm repair: a 20-year perspective. Ann Thorac Surg. 2007; 83(2):S856–S861, discussion S890–S892

[30] Fehrenbacher JW, Hart DW, Huddleston E, Siderys H, Rice C. Optimal end-organ protection for thoracic and thoracoabdominal aortic aneurysm repair using deep hypothermic circulatory arrest. Ann Thorac Surg. 2007; 83(3):1041–1046

[31] Marion D, Bullock MR. Current and future role of therapeutic hypothermia. J Neurotrauma. 2009; 26(3):455–467

[32] Parsa AT, Miller JI. Neurosurgical diseases of the spine and spinal cord: Surgical considerations. In: Cottrell JE, Smith DS, eds. Anesthesia and Neurosurgery. 4th ed. St. Louis, MO: Mosby; 2001:531–555

[33] Levi AD, Casella G, Green BA, et al. Clinical outcomes using modest intravascular hypothermia after acute cervical spinal cord injury. Neurosurgery. 2010; 66(4):670–677

[34] Hall ED. The neuroprotective pharmacology of methylprednisolone. J Neurosurg. 1992; 76(1):13–22

[35] Oudega M, Vargas CG, Weber AB, Kleitman N, Bunge MB. Long-term effects of methylprednisolone following transection of adult rat spinal cord. Eur J Neurosci. 1999; 11(7):2453–2464

[36] Young W. Molecular and Cellular Mechanisms of Spinal Cord Injury Therapies. Totowa, NJ: Humana Press; 2000

[37] Hawryluk GW, Rowland J, Kwon BK, Fehlings MG. Protection and repair of the injured spinal cord: a review of completed, ongoing, and planned clinical trials for acute spinal cord injury. Neurosurg Focus. 2008; 25(5):E14

[38] Bracken MB, Shepard MJ, Holford TR, et al. Administration of methylprednisolone for 24 or 48 hours or tirilazad mesylate for 48 hours in the treatment of acute spinal cord injury. Results of the Third National Acute Spinal Cord Injury Randomized Controlled Trial. National Acute Spinal Cord Injury Study. JAMA. 1997; 277(20):1597–1604

[39] Kaptanoglu E, Tuncel M, Palaoglu S, Konan A, Demirpençe E, Kilinç K. Comparison of the effects of melatonin and methylprednisolone in experimental spinal cord injury. J Neurosurg. 2000; 93(1) Suppl:77–84

[40] Taoka Y, Okajima K, Uchiba M, Johno M. Methylprednisolone reduces spinal cord injury in rats without affecting tumor necrosis factor-alpha production. J Neurotrauma. 2001; 18(5):533–543

[41] Braughler JM, Hall ED. Correlation of methylprednisolone levels in cat spinal cord with its effects on (Na++K+)-ATPase, lipid peroxidation, and alpha motor neuron function. J Neurosurg. 1982; 56(6):838–844

[42] Kaptanoglu E, Caner HH, Sürücü HS, Akbiyik F. Effect of mexiletine on lipid peroxidation and early ultrastructural findings in experimental spinal cord injury. J Neurosurg. 1999; 91(2) Suppl:200–204

[43] Koc RK, Akdemir H, Karakücük EI, Oktem IS, Menkü A. Effect of methylprednisolone, tirilazad mesylate and vitamin E on lipid peroxidation after experimental spinal cord injury. Spinal Cord. 1999; 37(1):29–32

[44] Diaz-Ruiz A, Rios C, Duarte I, et al. Lipid peroxidation inhibition in spinal cord injury: cyclosporin-A vs methylprednisolone. Neuroreport. 2000; 11(8):1765–1767

[45] Mu X, Azbill RD, Springer JE. Riluzole improves measures of oxidative stress following traumatic spinal cord injury. Brain Res. 2000; 870(1–2):66–72

[46] Rabchevsky AG, Fugaccia I, Sullivan PG, Blades DA, Scheff SW. Efficacy of methylprednisolone therapy for the injured rat spinal cord. J Neurosci Res. 2002; 68(1):7–18

[47] Haghighi SS, Agrawal SK, Surdell D, Jr, et al. Effects of methylprednisolone and MK-801 on functional recovery after experimental chronic spinal cord injury. Spinal Cord. 2000; 38(12):733–740

[48] Qian T, Campagnolo D, Kirshblum S. High-dose methylprednisolone may do more harm for spinal cord injury. Med Hypotheses. 2000; 55(5):452–453

[49] Bracken MB, Collins WF, Freeman DF, et al. Efficacy of methylprednisolone in acute spinal cord injury. JAMA. 1984; 251(1):45–52

[50] Bracken MB, Shepard MJ, Hellenbrand KG, et al. Methylprednisolone and neurological function 1 year after spinal cord injury. Results of the National Acute Spinal Cord Injury Study. J Neurosurg. 1985; 63(5):704–713

[51] Bracken MB, Shepard MJ, Collins WF, et al. A randomized, controlled trial of methylprednisolone or naloxone in the treatment of acute spinal-cord injury. Results of the Second National Acute Spinal Cord Injury Study. N Engl J Med. 1990; 322(20):1405–1411

[52] Bracken MB, Shepard MJ, Collins WF, Jr, et al. Methylprednisolone or naloxone treatment after acute spinal cord injury: 1-year follow-up data. Results of the second National Acute Spinal Cord Injury Study. J Neurosurg. 1992; 76(1):23–31

[53] Levy ML, Gans W, Wijesinghe HS, SooHoo WE, Adkins RH, Stillerman CB. Use of methylprednisolone as an adjunct in the management of patients with penetrating spinal cord injury: outcome analysis. Neurosurgery. 1996; 39(6):1141–1148, discussion 1148–1149

[54] Hurlbert RJ. Methylprednisolone for acute spinal cord injury: an inappropriate standard of care. J Neurosurg. 2000; 93(1) Suppl:1–7

[55] Hadley MN, Walters BC, Grabb PA, et al. Management of acute central cervical spinal cord injuries. Neurosurgery. 2002; 50(3) Suppl:S166–S172

[56] Early Acute Management in Adults with Spinal Cord Injury. A Clinical Practice Guideline for Health-Care Providers. Washington, DC: Paralyzed Veterans of America; 2007

[57] Fehlings MG, Wilson JR, Frankowski RF, et al. Riluzole for the treatment of acute traumatic spinal cord injury: rationale for and design of the NACTN Phase I clinical trial. J Neurosurg Spine. 2012; 17(1) Suppl:151–156

[58] Fehlings M, Kopjar B. A multi-center, randomized, placebo controlled, double-blinded, trial of efficacy and safety of riluzole in acute spinal cord injury. Available at: https://clinicaltrials.gov/ct2/show/NCT01597518

[59] Fehlings MG, Nakashima H, Nagoshi N, Chow DS, Grossman RG, Kopjar B. Rationale, design and critical end points for the Riluzole in Acute Spinal Cord Injury Study (RISCIS): a randomized, double-blinded, placebo-controlled parallel multi-center trial. Spinal Cord. 2016; 54(1):8–15

[60] Hall A. Rho family GTPases. Biochem Soc Trans. 2012; 40(6):1378–1382

[61] Forgione N, Fehlings MG. Rho-ROCK inhibition in the treatment of spinal cord injury. World Neurosurg. 2014; 82(3–4):e535–e539

[62] Dubreuil CI, Winton MJ, McKerracher L. Rho activation patterns after spinal cord injury and the role of activated Rho in apoptosis in the central nervous system. J Cell Biol. 2003; 162(2):233–243

[63] Madura T, Yamashita T, Kubo T, Fujitani M, Hosokawa K, Tohyama M. Activation of Rho in the injured axons following spinal cord injury. EMBO Rep. 2004; 5(4):412–417

[64] Fehlings MG, Theodore N, Harrop J, et al. A phase I/IIa clinical trial of a recombinant Rho protein antagonist in acute spinal cord injury. J Neurotrauma. 2011; 28(5):787–796

[65] Yong VW, Wells J, Giuliani F, Casha S, Power C, Metz LM. The promise of minocycline in neurology. Lancet Neurol. 2004; 3(12):744–751

[66] Casha S, Zygun D, McGowan MD, Bains I, Yong VW, Hurlbert RJ. Results of a phase II placebo-controlled randomized trial of minocycline in acute spinal cord injury. Brain. 2012; 135(Pt 4):1224–1236

[67] Yang ML, Li JJ, So KF, et al. Efficacy and safety of lithium carbonate treatment of chronic spinal cord injuries: a double-blind, randomized, placebo-controlled clinical trial. Spinal Cord. 2012; 50(2):141–146

[68] Kobayakawa K, Kumamaru H, Saiwai H, et al. Acute hyperglycemia impairs functional improvement after spinal cord injury in mice and humans. Sci Transl Med. 2014; 6(256):256ra137

[69] Skaper SD, Leon A. Monosialogangliosides, neuroprotection, and neuronal repair processes. J Neurotrauma. 1992; 9 Suppl 2:S507–S516

[70] Imanaka T, Hukuda S, Maeda T. The role of GM1-ganglioside in the injured spinal cord of rats: an immunohistochemical study using GM1-antisera. J Neurotrauma. 1996; 13(3):163–170

[71] Ferrari G, Greene LA. Promotion of neuronal survival by GM1 ganglioside. Phenomenology and mechanism of action. Ann N Y Acad Sci. 1998; 845: 263–273

[72] Geisler FH, Dorsey FC, Coleman WP. Correction: recovery of motor function after spinal-cord injury–a randomized, placebo-controlled trial with GM-1 ganglioside. N Engl J Med. 1991; 325(23):1659–1660

[73] Geisler FH, Coleman WP, Grieco G, Poonian D, Sygen Study Group. The Sygen multicenter acute spinal cord injury study. Spine. 2001; 26(24) Suppl: S87–S98

[74] Faden AI, Molineaux CJ, Rosenberger JG, Jacobs TP, Cox BM. Endogenous opioid immunoreactivity in rat spinal cord following traumatic injury. Ann Neurol. 1985; 17(4):386–390

[75] Bracken MB, Holford TR. Effects of timing of methylprednisolone or naloxone administration on recovery of segmental and long-tract neurological function in NASCIS 2. J Neurosurg. 1993; 79(4):500–507

[76] Pitts LH, Ross A, Chase GA, Faden AI. Treatment with thyrotropin-releasing hormone (TRH) in patients with traumatic spinal cord injuries. J Neurotrauma. 1995; 12(3):235–243

Index